UT M. D. Anderson Clinical Conference on Cancer
Volume 27

Hodgkin's Disease and Non-Hodgkin's Lymphoma
New Perspectives in Immunopathology, Diagnosis, and Treatment

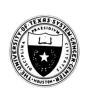
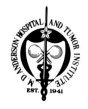

Published for
The University of Texas
M. D. Anderson Hospital and Tumor Institute at Houston
Houston, Texas, by Raven Press, New York

UT M. D. Anderson Clinical Conference
on Cancer
Volume 27

Hodgkin's Disease and Non-Hodgkin's Lymphoma
New Perspectives in Immunopathology, Diagnosis, and Treatment

Edited by

Richard J. Ford, Jr.,
M.D., Ph.D.
Associate Professor of Pathology
Department of Pathology

Lillian M. Fuller, M.D.
Professor of Radiotherapy
Department of Clinical Radiotherapy

Fredrick B. Hagemeister, M.D.
Associate Professor of Medicine
Department of Hematology

The University of Texas
M.D. Anderson Hospital and Tumor Institute at Houston
Houston, Texas

Raven Press ■ New York

Raven Press, 1140 Avenue of the Americas, New York, New York 10036

Made in the United States of America

Library of Congress Cataloging in Publication Data

Clinical Conference on Cancer (27th : 1983 : M. D.
    Anderson Hospital and Tumor Institute at Houston)
    Hodgkin's Disease and Non-Hodgkin's Lymphoma: New
    Perspectives in Immunopathology, Diagnosis, and Treatment

    Includes bibliographies and index.
    1. Lymphomas—Congresses. I. Ford, Richard J.,
1943-   . II. Fuller, Lillian M., 1923-   .
III. Hagemeister, Frederick B. IV. M. D. Anderson
Hospital and Tumor Institute at Houston. V. Title.
[DNLM: 1. Lymphoma—congresses. W3 C162H 27th 1983n /
WH 525 C641 1983n]
RC280.L9C48   1983   616.99′242   84-13429
ISBN 0-88167-039-1

This volume is a compilation of the proceedings of The University of Texas M. D. Anderson Hospital and Tumor Institute at Houston's 27th Annual Clinical Conference on Cancer, held November 9–12, 1983, in Houston, Texas.

The material contained in this volume was submitted as previously unpublished material, except in the instances in which credit has been given the source from which some of the illustrative material was derived.

Great care has been taken to maintain the accuracy of the information contained in the volume. However, the Editorial Staff, The University of Texas, and Raven Press cannot be held responsible for errors or for any consequences arising from the use of the information contained herein.

Preface

Malignant lymphomas have become the most intensively studied human cancers in recent years. Clinicians have used drugs and radiotherapy to treat lymphomas. We have had good results but have not had a good understanding of their basic biology. Now that we are beginning to understand some of the genetic and cellular interactions occurring in lymphomagenesis, we are also beginning to apply some of these concepts to the diagnosis and therapy of the lymphomatous diseases.

This conference was an important step not just for students of lymphoma but for all who are interested in cancer. Its purpose was to bring together the basic scientist and the clinical investigator who interact to provide an understanding of goals and resources in the search for better treatment for lymphoma patients.

A number of discoveries have been influential in clarifying newer concepts of lymphomagenesis. T- and B-cell markers on normal lymphoid cells, which can be used to distinguish between lymphoid malignancies, represent an important advance. Ultimately, these cell markers may be incorporated into a classification system that can be used for therapeutic selections and options. The study of oncogenes and other cytogenetic abnormalities that appear to be involved in intracellular functions, including the growth potential of tumor cells, may eventually explain cellular resistance to treatment. The discovery of the human T-cell leukemia virus, as a first definite link to an infectious etiology of human malignancy, may pave the way to finding other oncogenic viruses capable of tumor induction in humans. The acquired immune deficiency syndrome (AIDS), with its epidemiologic importance, has presented a unique opportunity to study lymphoid malignancy in the immunodeficient patient.

The study of lymphomas may yield further information about the causes of all malignancies. A number of major advances in the treatment of other cancers have followed developments in the treatment of hematologic malignancies. The development of combination chemotherapy, including MOPP, CHOP, alternating regimens, and combined modality programs, have prompted the development of similar approaches to treating other malignancies. It seems likely that newer therapies involving biologic response modifiers, with or without our current therapeutic modalities, also will be used first in lymphomas.

Our past has been marked by great advances in the treatment of patients with lymphatic malignancies; many patients currently enjoy long-lasting remissions and apparent cures. What the future holds in store will be based on directions we choose today. From what follows in this volume, it appears that the malignant lymphomas will continue to be in the forefront of contemporary cancer research. The lymphatic cancers today seem to offer the most instructive human tumor model systems where basic research findings can be translated into new therapeutic approaches. This cooperation, leading from the laboratory to the bedside, should make the next five years in the study and treatment of malignant lymphoma particularly exciting and rewarding.

Richard J. Ford, Jr.
Lillian M. Fuller
Fredrick B. Hagemeister

Acknowledgment

We would like to thank those who helped make the 27th Annual Clinical Conference possible. We are especially grateful to the Program Committee, Richard J. Ford, Jr., Lillian M. Fuller, and Fredrick B. Hagemeister, cochairpersons, Fernando F. Cabanillas, Evan M. Hersh, Luceil B. North, and Margaret P. Sullivan for organizing the conference and to the American Cancer Society, Texas Division, Inc.

In addition, we extend our appreciation for the generous support of Adria Laboratories, Inc., Atomic Energy of Canada, Ltd., Becton-Dickinson Monoclonal Center, Inc., Bristol-Myers Company, CGR Medical Corporation, Lederle Laboratories, Mead Johnson Pharmaceutical Division, Stuart Pharmaceuticals, The Upjohn Company, and Warner-Lambert Company.

Editorial Staff
Department of Scientific Publications

Carol K. Schappaugh, Managing Editor
Sally R. Hartline

Contents

Therapy for Advanced Hodgkin's Disease

NON-HODGKIN'S LYMPHOMAS
Etiology and Immunology

Diagnosis and Staging

Therapy of Non-Hodgkin's Lymphoma

**New Drugs and Modalities of Therapy for
Malignant Lymphomas**

Heath Memorial Award Lecture

The Jeffrey A. Gottlieb Memorial Lecture

Contributors

Kenneth C. Anderson
Division of Tumor Immunology
Dana-Farber Cancer Institute and the
Department of Medicine
Harvard Medical School
Boston, Massachusetts 02115

Andrew Arnold
Metabolism Branch and Laboratory of
    Pathology
National Cancer Institute
National Institutes of Health
Bethesda, Maryland 20205

Susan M. Azemove
Department of Therapeutic Radiology
University of Minnesota
Minneapolis, Minnesota 55455

Ajay Bakhshi
Metabolism Branch and Laboratory of
    Pathology
National Cancer Institute
National Institutes of Health
Bethesda, Maryland 20205

Robert Bargatze
Department of Pathology
Stanford University Medical Center
Stanford, California 94305 and
The Veterans Administration Medical
    Center
Palo Alto, California 94304

David Benjamin
Pediatric Branch and Laboratory of
    Pathology
National Cancer Institute
National Institutes of Health
Bethesda, Maryland 20205

Olav Behnke
Medical Anatomy Institute C
Panuminstituttet
DK-2200 Copenhagen, Denmark

Daniel E. Bergsagel
Department of Medicine
Princess Margaret Hospital
Toronto, Ontario M4X 1K9
Canada

Clara D. Bloomfield
Section of Medical Oncology
Department of Medicine
University of Minnesota Health Sciences
    Center
Minneapolis, Minnesota 55455

Andrew W. Boyd
Division of Tumor Immunology
Dana-Farber Cancer Institute and the
Department of Medicine
Harvard Medical School
Boston, Massachusetts 02115

Thomas C. Brown
Department of Pathology
Princess Margaret Hospital
Toronto, Ontario M4X 1K9
Canada

Raymond S. Bush
Director
Princess Margaret Hospital
Toronto, Ontario M4X 1K9
Canada

Eugene C. Butcher
Department of Pathology
Stanford University Medical Center
Stanford, California 94305 and
The Veterans Administration Medical
    Center
Palo Alto, California 94304

J. J. Butler
Department of Pathology
The University of Texas M. D. Anderson
    Hospital
and Tumor Institute at Houston
Houston, Texas 77030

Fernando Cabanillas
Department of Hematology
The University of Texas M. D. Anderson
Hospital
and Tumor Institute at Houston
Houston, Texas 77030

R. S. K. Chaganti
The Laboratory of Cancer Genetics and
Cytogenetics
Memorial Sloan-Kettering Cancer Center
New York, New York 10021

Theresa Chua
Department of Biostatistics
Princess Margaret Hospital
Toronto, Ontario M4X 1K9
Canada

Bayard D. Clarkson
Department of Medicine
Memorial Sloan-Kettering Cancer Center
New York, New York 10021

Robert D. Collins
Department of Pathology
Vanderbilt Medical Center
Nashville, Tennessee 37232

Geoffrey Cooper
Laboratory of Molecular Carcinogenesis
Dana-Farber Cancer Institute and the
Department of Pathology
Harvard Medical School
Boston, Massachusetts 02115

Jeffrey Cossman
Metabolism Branch and Laboratory of
Pathology
National Cancer Institute
National Institutes of Health
Bethesda, Maryland 20205

John B. Cousar
Department of Pathology
Vanderbilt Medical Center
Nashville, Tennessee 37232

Carlo M. Croce
The Wistar Institute of Anatomy and
Biology
Philadelphia, Pennsylvania 19104

Francesco d'Amore
Cancer Biology Laboratory
State University Hospital
DK-2100 Copenhagen, Denmark

Miguel da Cunha
Department of Experimental
Radiotherapy
The University of Texas M. D. Anderson
Hospital
and Tumor Institute at Houston
Houston, Texas 77030

Frances M. Davis
Department of Pathology
The University of Texas M. D. Anderson
Hospital
and Tumor Institute at Houston
Houston, Texas 77030

Joan Devine
Laboratory of Molecular Carcinogenesis
Dana-Farber Cancer Institute and the
Department of Pathology
Harvard Medical School
Boston, Massachusetts 02115

Vincent T. DeVita, Jr.
Medicine Branch
National Cancer Institute
National Institutes of Health
Bethesda, Maryland 20205

Marcus Diamant
Cancer Biology Laboratory
State University Hospital
DK-2100 Copenhagen, Denmark

Alan Diamond
Laboratory of Molecular Carcinogenesis
Dana-Farber Cancer Institute and the
Department of Pathology
Harvard Medical School
Boston, Massachusetts 02115

Karel Dicke
Department of Hematology
The University of Texas M. D. Anderson
    Hospital
and Tumor Institute at Houston
Houston, Texas 77030

Jan Erikson
The Wistar Institute of Anatomy and
    Biology
Philadelphia, Pennsylvania 19104

Donald I. Feinstein
Department of Medicine
University of Southern California School
    of Medicine and the
Los Angeles County University of
    Southern California
Medical Center
Los Angeles, California 90033

Alexandra H. Filopovich
Department of Pediatrics
University of Minnesota
Minneapolis, Minnesota 55455

Janet Finan
Department of Pathology and Laboratory
    Medicine
University of Pennsylvania School of
    Medicine
Philadelphia, Pennsylvania 19104

David Fisher
Division of Tumor Immunology
Dana-Farber Cancer Institute and the
Department of Medicine
Harvard Medical School
Boston, Massachusetts 02115

Richard I. Fisher
Section of Hematology/Oncology
Loyola University
School of Medicine
Maywood, Illinois 60153
formerly: Medicine Branch
National Cancer Institute
National Institutes of Health
Bethesda, Maryland 20205

Richard J. Ford, Jr.
Department of Pathology
The University of Texas M. D. Anderson
    Hospital
and Tumor Institute at Houston
Houston, Texas 77030

Emil Frei III
Department of Medicine
Dana-Farber Cancer Institute
Boston, Massachusetts 02115

Glauco Frizzera
Department of Laboratory Medicine and
    Pathology
University of Minnesota Health Sciences
    Center
Minneapolis, Minnesota 55455

Lillian M. Fuller
Department of Clinical Radiotherapy
The University of Texas M. D. Anderson
    Hospital
and Tumor Institute at Houston
Houston, Texas 77030

Kazimiera J. Gajl-Peczalska
Department of Laboratory Medicine and
    Pathology
University of Minnesota Health Sciences
    Center
Minneapolis, Minnesota 55455

Robert C. Gallo
Laboratory of Tumor Cell Biology
National Cancer Institute
National Institutes of Health
Bethesda, Maryland 20205

Kevin Gatter
Nuffield Department of Pathology
John Radcliffe Hospital
Oxford, England OX3 9DU

Edmund A. Gehan
Department of Biomathematics
The University of Texas M. D. Anderson
    Hospital
and Tumor Institute at Houston
Houston, Texas 77030

Johannes Gerdes
Institutes of Pathology and Biochemistry
Christian Albrecht University
D-2300 Kiel 1, West Germany

Mary Gospodarowicz
Department of Radiation Oncology
Princess Margaret Hospital
Toronto, Ontario M4X 1K9
Canada

Nancy M. Gutensohn
Department of Epidemiology
Harvard School of Public Health
Boston, Massachusetts 02115

Fredrick B. Hagemeister
Department of Hematology
The University of Texas M. D. Anderson
    Hospital
and Tumor Institute at Houston
Houston, Texas 77030

Shinji Harada
Department of Pathology and Laboratory
    Medicine
University of Nebraska Medical Center
Omaha, Nebraska 68105

Lynne Herron
Department of Pathology
Stanford University Medical Center
Stanford, California 94305 and
The Veterans Administration Medical
    Center
Palo Alto, California 94304

Elaine S. Jaffe
Metabolism Branch and Laboratory of
    Pathology
National Cancer Institute
National Institutes of Health
Bethesda, Marryland 20205

Sundar Jagannath
Department of Hematology
The University of Texas M. D. Anderson
    Hospital
and Tumor Institute at Houston
Houston, Texas 77030

Sirpa Jalkanen
Department of Pathology
Stanford University Medical Center
Stanford, California 94305 and
The Veterans Administration Medical
    Center
Palo Alto, California 94304

Stephen E. Jones
Department of Medicine
University of Arizona
University of Arizona Cancer Center and
The Veterans Administration Hospital
Tucson, Arizona 85724

Marshall E. Kadin
Departments of Laboratory Medicine and
    Pathology
University of Washington
Seattle, Washington 98105

Hagop Kantarjian
Department of Hematology
The University of Texas M. D. Anderson
    Hospital
and Tumor Institute at Houston
Houston, Texas 77030

Daniel S. Kapp
Department of Therapeutic Radiology
Yale University School of Medicine
New Haven, Connecticut 06510

John H. Kersey
Department of Laboratory Medicine/
    Pathology
University of Minnesota
Minneapolis, Minnesota 55455

Joseph S. Kong
Department of Clinical Radiotherapy
The University of Texas M. D. Anderson
    Hospital
and Tumor Institute at Houston
Houston, Texas 77030

Stanley J. Korsmeyer
Metabolism Branch and Laboratory of
Pathology
National Cancer Institute
National Institutes of Health
Bethesda, Maryland 20205

Nicola M. Kouttab
Department of Pathology
The University of Texas M. D. Anderson
Hospital
and Tumor Institute at Houston
Houston, Texas 77030

Benjamin Koziner
Department of Medicine
Memorial Sloan-Kettering Cancer Center
New York, New York 10021

Mary-Ann Lane
Laboratory of Molecular Immunobiology
Dana-Farber Cancer Institute and the
Department of Pathology
Harvard Medical School
Boston, Massachusetts 02115

Tucker W. LeBien
Department of Laboratory Medicine and
Pathology
University of Minnesota Health Sciences
Center
Minneapolis, Minnesota 55455

Burton J. Lee
Department of Medicine
Memorial Sloan-Kettering Cancer Center
New York, New York 10021

Hilmar Lemke
Institutes of Pathology and Biochemistry
Christian Albrecht University
D-2300 Kiel 1, West Germany

Alexandra M. Levine
Department of Medicine
University of Southern California School
of Medicine and the
Los Angeles County University of
Southern California Medical Center
Los Angeles, California 90033

Helen Lipscomb
Department of Pathology and Laboratory
Medicine
University of Nebraska Medical Center
Omaha, Nebraska 68105

Robert J. Lukes
Department of Pathology
University of Southern California School
of Medicine and the
Los Angeles County University of
Southern California Medical Center
Los Angeles, California 90033

Ian Magrath
Pediatric Branch
National Cancer Institute
National Institutes of Health
Bethesda, Maryland 20205

John Manning
Department of Pathology
The University of Texas M. D. Anderson
Hospital
and Tumor Institute at Houston
Houston, Texas 77030

George Manolov
Department of Pathology and Laboratory
Medicine
University of Nebraska Medical Center
Omaha, Nebraska 68105

Yanka Manolova
Department of Pathology and Laboratory
Medicine
University of Nebraska Medical Center
Omaha, Nebraska 68105

Moshe H. Maor
Department of Clinical Radiotherapy
The University of Texas M. D. Anderson
Hospital
and Tumor Institute at Houston
Houston, Texas 77030

David Y. Mason
Nuffield Department of Pathology
John Radcliffe Hospital
Oxford, England OX3 9DU

Beryl McCormick
Department of Radiation Therapy
Memorial Sloan-Kettering Cancer Center
New York, New York 10021

Peter McLaughlin
Department of Hematology
The University of Texas M.D. Anderson
Hospital
and Tumor Institute at Houston
Houston, Texas 77030

Shashi Mehta
Department of Pathology
The University of Texas M.D. Anderson
Hospital
and Tumor Institute at Houston
Houston, Texas 77030

Paul R. Meyer
Department of Pathology
Los Angeles County University of
Southern California Medical Center
Los Angeles, California 90033

Thomas P. Miller
Department of Medicine
University of Arizona
University of Arizona Cancer Center and
The Veterans Administration Hospital
Tucson, Arizona 85724

Jane Myers
Department of Medicine
Memorial Sloan-Kettering Cancer Center
New York, New York 10021

Lee M. Nadler
Division of Tumor Immunology
Dana-Farber Cancer Institute and the
Department of Medicine
Harvard Medical School
Boston, Massachusetts 02115

David M. Neville, Jr.
Laboratory of Neurochemistry
National Institute of Mental Health
National Institutes of Health
Bethesda, Maryland 20205

Lourdes Nisce
Department of Radiation Therapy
Memorial Sloan-Kettering Cancer Center
New York, New York 10021

Luceil B. North
Department of Diagnostic Radiology
The University of Texas M.D. Anderson
Hospital
and Tumor Institute at Houston
Houston, Texas 77030

Peter C. Nowell
Department of Pathology and Laboratory
Medicine
University of Pennsylvania School of
Medicine
Philadelphia, Pennsylvania 19104

K.K. Oh
Department of Internal Medicine
The University of Texas M.D. Anderson
Hospital
and Tumor Institute at Houston
Houston, Texas 77030

Lennart Olsson
Cancer Biology Laboratory
State University Hospital
DK-2100 Copenhagen, Denmark

Annlia Paganini-Hill
Department of Family and Preventive
Medicine
University of Southern California School
of Medicine and the
Los Angeles County University of
Southern California Medical Center
Los Angeles, California 90033

John W. Parker
Department of Pathology
University of Southern California School
of Medicine and the
Los Angeles County University of
Southern California Medical Center
Los Angeles, California 90033

Zdena Pavlova
Department of Pathology
University of Southern California School
of Medicine and the
Los Angeles County University of
Southern California Medical Center
Los Angeles, California 90033

Darleen R. Powars
Department of Pediatrics
University of Southern California School
of Medicine and the
Los Angeles County University of
Southern California Medical Center
Los Angeles, California 90033

Leonard R. Prosnitz
Division of Radiation Oncology
Duke University Medical Center
Durham, North Carolina 27710

David T. Purtilo
Department of Pathology and Laboratory
Medicine
The Eppley Institute for Research in
Cancer and Allied Diseases and the
Department of Pediatrics
University of Nebraska Medical Center
Omaha, Nebraska 68105

Irma Ramirez
Department of Pediatrics
The University of Texas M. D. Anderson
Hospital
and Tumor Institute at Houston
Houston, Texas 77030

K. Thomas Robbins
Department of Otolaryngology Head and
Neck Surgery
The University of Texas Medical School
at Houston
Houston, Texas 77030

Roger W. Rodgers
Department of Hematology
The University of Texas M. D. Anderson
Hospital
and Tumor Institute at Houston
Houston, Texas 77030

C. G. Sahasrabuddhe
Department of Pathology
The University of Texas M. D. Anderson
Hospital
and Tumor Institute at Houston
Houston, Texas 77030

Stuart F. Schlossman
Division of Tumor Immunology
Dana-Farber Cancer Institute and the
Department of Medicine
Harvard Medical School
Boston, Massachusetts 02115

Hauke Sieverts
Pediatric Branch and Laboratory of
Pathology
National Cancer Institute
National Institutes of Health
Bethesda, Maryland 20205

Bruce Slaughenhoupt
Division of Tumor Immunology
Dana-Farber Cancer Institute and the
Department of Medicine
Harvard Medical School
Boston, Massachusetts 02115

Christine C. B. Soderling
Department of Therapeutic Radiology
University of Minnesota
Minneapolis, Minnesota 55455

Gary Spitzer
Department of Hematology
The University of Texas M. D. Anderson
Hospital
and Tumor Institute at Houston
Houston, Texas 77030

Harald Stein
Institute of Pathology
Klinicum Steglitz
Free University of Berlin
1000 Berlin 45, West Germany
formerly: Nuffield Department of
Pathology
John Radcliffe Hospital
Oxford, England 0X3 9DU

David J. Straus
Department of Medicine
Memorial Sloan-Kettering Cancer Center
New York, New York 10021

Margaret P. Sullivan
Department of Pediatrics
The University of Texas M. D. Anderson
*   Hospital*
and Tumor Institute at Houston
Houston, Texas 77030

Simon Sutcliffe
Department of Pathology
Princess Margaret Hospital
Toronto, Ontario M4X 1K9
Canada

Nizar Tannir
Department of Hematology
The University of Texas M. D. Anderson
*   Hospital*
and Tumor Institute at Houston
Houston, Texas 77030

Eiji Tatsumi
Department of Pathology and Laboratory
*   Medicine*
University of Nebraska Medical Center
Omaha, Nebraska 68105

Timothy Triche
Pediatric Branch and Laboratory of
*   Pathology*
National Cancer Institute
National Institutes of Health
Bethesda, Maryland 20205

Jerry Tsao
Department of Pathology
The University of Texas M. D. Anderson
*   Hospital*
and Tumor Institute at Houston
Houston, Texas 77030

Susan Tucker
Department of Biomathematics
The University of Texas M. D. Anderson
*   Hospital*
and Tumor Institute at Houston
Houston, Texas 77030

Carlos Urmacher
Department of Pathology
Memorial Sloan-Kettering Cancer Center
New York, New York 10021

Daniel A. Vallera
Department of Laboratory Medicine and
*   Pathology*
University of Minnesota
Minneapolis, Minnesota 55455

William S. Velasquez
Department of Hematology
The University of Texas M. D. Anderson
*   Hospital*
and Tumor Institute at Houston
Houston, Texas 77030

Lijda Vellekoop
Department of Hematology
The University of Texas M. D. Anderson
*   Hospital*
and Tumor Institute at Houston
Houston, Texas 77030

Dharmvir Verma
Department of Hematology
The University of Texas M. D. Anderson
*   Hospital*
and Tumor Institute at Houston
Houston, Texas 77030

Mark C. Vlasak
Scott and White Memorial Hospital
Temple, Texas 76501

Thomas A. Waldmann
Metabolism Branch and Laboratory of
*   Pathology*
National Cancer Institute
National Institutes of Health
Bethesda, Maryland 20205

Sidney Wallace
Department of Diagnostic Radiology
The University of Texas M. D. Anderson
*   Hospital*
and Tumor Institute at Houston
Houston, Texas 77030

Flossie Wong-Staal
Laboratory of Tumor Cell Biology
National Cancer Institute
National Institutes of Health
Bethesda, Maryland 20205

Richard J. Youle
Laboratory of Neurochemistry
National Institute of Mental Health
National Institutes of Health
Bethesda, Maryland 20205

Charles W. Young
Developmental Chemotherapy Service
Memorial Sloan-Kettering Cancer Center
New York, New York 10021

Robert C. Young
Medicine Branch
National Cancer Institute
National Institutes of Health
Bethesda, Maryland 20205

Axel Zander
Department of Hematology
The University of Texas M. D. Anderson
  Hospital
and Tumor Institute at Houston
Houston, Texas 77030

Esmail D. Zanjani
Department of Medicine
University of Minnesota
Minneapolis, Minnesota 55455

John L. Ziegler
Associate Chief of Staff/Education
Veterans Administration Medical Center,
  and
Professor of Medicine
University of California
San Francisco, California 94143

HODGKIN'S DISEASE

Tumor Biology and Pathology

UT M.D. Anderson Clinical Conference on Cancer, Vol. 27, edited by R.J. Ford, L.M. Fuller, and F.B. Hagemeister. Raven Press, New York © 1984.

The Epidemiology of Hodgkin's Disease: Clues to Etiology

Nancy M. Gutensohn

Department of Epidemiology, Harvard School of Public Health, Boston, Massachusetts 02115

The biology of Hodgkin's disease (HD) presents a paradox. This paradox results from the coexistence of features of malignancy with the histologic appearance of chronic infection accompanied by immune dysfunction, all in the same syndrome. As Kaplan (1981, p. 813.) states: "Hodgkin's disease has long defied classification because it presents, in varying degree, a curious amalgam of the features of a malignant lymphoid neoplasm, a chronic granulomatous infection, and an immunologic disorder." The purpose of this paper is to attempt to reconcile these apparently conflicting features with the epidemiologic characteristics of the disease as a means of providing clues to its etiology.

THE BIOLOGIC PARADOX

HD has several clearly malignant properties, including aneuploidy, clonality, metastatic spread, and, most recently demonstrated, heterotransplantability (Kaplan 1980). However, unlike the histologic appearance of most malignancies, HD does not represent uncontrolled overgrowth of the transformed cell but rather a highly mixed cellular reaction in which the presumed malignant cell—the Reed-Sternberg cell—is only sparsely present. Further, the establishment of continuing cultures of Reed-Sternberg cells and their precursors, the Hodgkin's cells, has been a formidable task. Only a few apparently continuous cell lines have been reported (Diehl et al. 1982). Finally, although aneuploid clones have been clearly identified in chromosomal studies, the positivity rate has been much lower than for other lymphomas (Rowley 1982). Thus, as a malignancy, HD is exceptional in character.

The cellular milieu of involved lymph nodes of a reactive inflammatory cell admixture with a scattering of Reed-Sternberg cells tightly surrounded by helper T lymphocytes (Borowitz 1982) suggests the presence of a chronic infectious process. The clinical signs of lymphadenopathy, fever, and night sweats and the characteristic early splenic involvement are also suggestive of a granulomatous process. In fact, prior to 1948, HD was classified in the International Classification of Disease under "Other Infectious and Parasitic (communicable) Diseases" (Manual of Joint Causes of Death 1939).

Finally, inherent in HD is a functional immune disorder, primarily of T cells, that cannot be attributed to a reduction in cell populations. Kaplan (1980) reported that the disorder was characterized by a decreased responsiveness to both recall and new antigens by cell-mediated immunity as well as reduced ability to reject skin homografts. In vitro, lymphocytes from HD patients exhibit diminished lymphoblastic transformation after stimulation, reduced response to mixed lymphocyte reaction, reduced capacity to form E rosettes, reduced cap formation after lectin binding, and increased lectin agglutinability. There is evidence that these functional impairments are mediated by circulating inhibitors and suppressor cell effects. A blocking factor for E-rosette formation has been identified as a glycolipid (Bieber et al. 1979). Ford et al. (1982) have reported that HD splenic tissue grown in short-term culture secretes interleukin 1, a major immunoregulatory molecule, and a fibroblast-stimulating factor. Increased prostaglandin E levels have also been reported in association with suppression (Goodwin et al. 1977).

EPIDEMIOLOGIC CONSIDERATIONS

In economically advantaged populations, the age-incidence curve of HD is characterized by a peak in young adulthood that is not evident among economically disadvantaged populations. This distribution is reminiscent of the geographic distribution of paralytic polio in the prevaccine era. For polio, the risk of paralytic disease with infection increased with age at infection. In economically advantaged populations, improved hygiene and smaller families resulted in more older children and young adults being susceptible to late infection and, thus, greater risk of severe complications. These similarities between the two diseases suggest that HD may develop as a rare consequence of infection by a common virus and that the risk is markedly increased when infection occurs after childhood; early infection is generally mild and protective (Gutensohn and Cole 1977).

Accumulating evidence from analytic epidemiologic studies relating HD to social class and age at diagnosis supports this hypothesis. Briefly, in this country the incidence among children is quite low. However, those children who do develop the disease, particularly the very young, appear to be from lower social classes, which is consistent with early infection (Gutensohn and Shapiro 1982).

Among young adults, risk is associated with factors in childhood which inhibit early infections. Table 1 summarizes the findings for persons 15–39 years from a population-based case-control study conducted in the Boston and Worcester, Massachusetts metropolitan areas in the late 1970s (Gutensohn 1982). In this age group, risk of developing HD is associated with small family size, single family housing in childhood, and relatively high maternal education. Risk is also associated with a history of infectious mononucleosis (IM).

For middle-age persons (40–54 years), a similar pattern of social class risk factors is present, with maternal education being the strongest factor (Table 2). If the delayed age at infection hypothesis is correct, then the disease may occur among the remaining susceptible middle-age adults who are infected, perhaps by their children.

Table 1. *Percent Distribution of Young Adult Subjects and the Relative Risk of Hodgkin's Disease According to Childhood Social Class Risk Factor*

Risk factor	Subjects (number)		Relative risk	
	Cases (225)	Controls (447)	Crude	Adjusted
Sibship size				
1–2	34	23	1.00*	1.00†
3	26	27	0.64	0.64
4–5	27	31	0.60	0.72
6+	13	19	0.48	0.74
	100%	100%		
Housing				
1–family	67	57	1.00*	1.00‡
2–family	16	16	0.88	0.93
≥3-units	17	28	0.52	0.53
	100%	100%		
Maternal education				
≥13 years	32	29 ⎫	1.00*	1.00§
12 years	49	45 ⎭		
≤11 years	19	27	0.64	0.81
	100%	100%		

*Referent category.
†Adjusted for housing, religion, playmates, IM and birth order ($P_1 = 0.10$).
‡Adjusted for religion and mother's education ($P_1 = 0.006$).
§Adjusted for sibship size, housing, religion, and IM ($P_1 = 0.16$).
From Gutensohn, 1982.

Among older persons (≥55 years), the pattern of association seen among younger persons is not evident. As seen in Table 3, older patients come from larger families than expected; men, but not women, with HD were more likely to have lived in multiple-family housing as children, and no association is apparent with maternal education.

In summary, these findings imply that persons at risk of developing late childhood infections are also at increased risk of developing HD through the middle years. These risk factors were not associated with HD among the oldest persons. If a common viral infection does initiate the pathogenesis of HD, then the age-related host response appears to play a primary role.

The only other risk factor that has been consistently found is an occupational history of exposure to wood, as previously reviewed (Gutensohn and Cole 1980). In the Massachusetts study, we compared the lifetime occupational histories of patients to two control series; one consisting of controls drawn from the population base and a second consisting of siblings of the patients. We did not find a difference in terms of occupational exposure to wood; we did find that patients more frequently reported exposure to dust and sawdust at work. The association was only seen in patients with the lymphocyte predominance form of Hodgkin's disease (N. M. Gutensohn, unpublished observations).

Table 2. *Percent Distribution of Middle-Age Subjects and the Relative Risk of Hodgkin's Disease According to Childhood Social Class Risk Factors*

	Subjects (number)		Relative risk	
Risk factor	Cases (53)	Controls (106)	Crude	Adjusted
Sibship size				
1–2	40	29	1.00*	1.00†
3–5	49	45	0.80	1.21
6+	11	25	0.33	0.70
	100%	100%		
Housing				
1–family	38	33 }	1.00*	1.00‡
2–family	30	24 }		
≥3-units	32	43	0.62	0.69
	100%	100%		
Maternal/education				
≥13 years	16	7	1.00*	1.00§
12 years	44	25	0.80	0.99
9–11 years	16	15	0.47	0.47
≤8 years	24	53	0.21	0.15
	100%	100%		

*Referent category.
†Adjusted for maternal education and number of children sharing bedroom.
‡Adjusted for mother's education.
§Adjusted for sibship size and housing ($P_2 = 0.004$).
From Gutensohn, 1982.

MODEL OF PATHOGENESIS

These two sets of epidemiologic findings share a common feature. They both could represent exposure to chronic, low-grade antigenic stimulation. This could occur as an habitual exposure to aerosol dust at work or be induced by altered control of a latent oncogenic virus. Among children, such infection may be readily controlled, but among teenage or middle-age persons who are more likely to experience a severe infection the immune control may in some way be altered. For a latent lymphotrophic virus, such as a herpesvirus or retrovirus, the alteration could allow a continuing, low-grade viral expression. Among older persons, the disease may reflect a similar chronic antigenicity secondary to diminution of cellular immunity that occurs with age.

That chronic antigenic stimulation is relevant is suggested by the evolving understanding of the nature and source of the Reed-Sternberg cell. There appears to be a growing consensus that the cell derives from an Ia-positive macrophage lineage, perhaps from the newly described interdigitating reticulum cell (Kadin 1982). The primary function of an Ia-positive macrophage is antigen presentation, initiating the cascades of events in immune T-cell response.

Table 3. *Percent Distribution of Older Subjects and the Relative Risk of Hodgkin's Disease According to Childhood Social Class Risk Factors*

	Subjects (number)		Relative risk	
Risk factor	Cases (47)	Controls (93)	Crude	Adjusted
Sibship size				
1–2	11	17	1.0*	1.0†
3–5	47	51	1.5	1.4
6+	43	32	2.1	1.8
	100%	100%		
Housing			M F	M F
1–family	36	48 }		
2–family	21	24 }	1.0* 1.0*	1.0*‡ —
≥3-units	43	28	3.1 1.2	6.2 —
	100%	100%		
Maternal education				
≥9 years	39	37	1.0*	—
8 years	33	29	1.1	—
≤7 years	28	33	0.80	—
	100%	100%		

*Referent category.
†Adjusted for education and sex, $P_2 = 0.25$.
‡Adjusted for sibship size and education for 23 male cases, 46 controls; $P_2 = 0.008$.
From Gutensohn, 1982.

How can these observations be reconciled with the exceptional biologic character of HD? One explanation is suggested by the emerging information on the origin and expression of oncogenes in malignancy. It is becoming clear that, for a variety of lymphoid malignancies, oncogenesis involves an alteration in the expression of normal cellular genes controlling proliferation during differentiation. This alteration in expression can result from gene rearrangement, amplification, insertion, or deletion (Krontivis 1983). The probability that such translocations occur is likely to be proportional to the mitotic activity of the cells in question. The result is that inappropriate cell proliferation occurs.

Perhaps a similar alteration in normal gene expression occurs in HD. However, in this case it is not a gene controlling proliferation but rather a gene (or genes) controlling the expression of the normal, functionally active mediators released by antigen-stimulated macrophage-lineage cells. It may be that the alteration of gene expression is a quantitative change, resulting in a greatly amplified message. Alternatively, a gene, which normally shuts down the messages by feedback inhibition, may be translocated and underexpressed. The result in either case could be an immune system that is perpetually mobilized in response to a chronic antigen and cannot then respond to others. The mechanism underlying such an alteration in gene expression could be triggered by the continuing antigenic stimulation of the cells, and there would have to be a selective advantage for the altered cells to remain viable. In any case, the result is not the immortalization of the target cells but rather of its message, hence the many failures to establish cell cultures.

If this hypothesis is true, it could explain the biologic paradox of HD: the malignant properties reflecting the underlying genetic changes, the histologic features reflecting the response of normal immune cells to the perpetual message, and the immune defect reflecting the resulting imbalance in the immune response system. A parallel might be drawn to the biology of the acquired immune deficiency syndrome (AIDS). In AIDS, the immune system is in a profound state of suppression because of the selective loss of helper T cells. In HD, the immune defect may result from a more subtle imbalance caused by its being in a continual state of response.

Evaluation of this hypothesis would involve both cell biology and epidemiologic investigation. The consistency between the in vitro biologic behavior of Reed-Sternberg cells with that of Ia-positive macrophages should be evaluated. Further, suppressive mediators in HD patients, both in vivo and in vitro, should be completely characterized. Finally, evidence should be sought to evaluate whether the quality of immune response to candidate viruses varies with age at infection. Such information could be obtained from serial serum collections from relatively young populations for whom age at seroconversion can be documented.

In summary, the conflicting biologic features of HD involving malignant, granulomatous, and immunologic qualities may be reconciled in light of a model of altered gene expression provided by our present knowledge of oncogenes. The model suggests that in HD, the gene that is amplified is one that normally controls the production of chemical mediators in immune response. The fact that the epidemiologic features of the disease are consistent with chronic antigenic stimulation and that the Reed-Sternberg cell apparently derives from an antigen-processing cell supports the analogy. If such a hypothesis is true, then the appropriate definition of HD may be the one offered in 1973 by Berard (Berard 1973, p 261), which simply states, "HD is a malignant cellular immune process."

ACKNOWLEDGMENT

This investigation was supported by grant 19619, awarded by the National Cancer Institute, US Department of Health and Human Services. Dr. Gutensohn's research is also supported by a grant from the Mellon Foundation.

REFERENCES

Berard CW. 1973. Synthesis and implications for the etiology, pathogenesis, and spread of Hodgkin's disease. Natl Cancer Inst Monogr 36:261–263.

Bieber MM, King DP, Strober S, Kaplan HS. 1979. Characterization of an E-rosette inhibitor (ERI) in the serum of patients with Hodgkin's disease as a glycolipid. (Abstract) Clin Res 27:81A.

Borowitz MJ, Croker BP, Metzgar RS. 1982. Immunohistochemical analysis of the distribution of lymphocyte subpopulations in Hodgkin's disease. Cancer Treat Rep 66:667–674.

Diehl V, Kirchner HH, Burrichter H, Stein H, Fonatsch C, Gerder J, Schaadt M, Heit W, Uchanska-Ziegleir B, Ziegler A, Heintz F, Suenok K. 1982. Characteristics of Hodgkin's disease-derived cell lines. Cancer Treat Rep 66:615–632.

Ford RJ, Mehta S, Davis F, Maizel AL. 1982. Growth factors in Hodgkin's disease. Cancer Treat Rep 66:633–638.

Goodwin JS, Messner RP, Bankhurst AD, Peake GT, Saiki JH, Williams RC. 1977. Prostaglandin-producing suppressor cells in Hodgkin's disease. N Engl J Med 297:963–968.

Gutensohn NM, Cole P. 1977. Epidemiology of Hodgkin's disease in the young. Int J Cancer 19:595–604.

Gutensohn N, Cole P. 1980. Epidemiology of Hodgkin's disease. Semin Oncol 7:92–102.

Gutensohn N, Shapiro DS. 1982. Social class factors among children with Hodgkin's disease. Int J Cancer 30:433–435.

Gutensohn N. 1982. Social class and age at diagnosis of Hodgkin's disease: New epidemiologic evidence on the "two-disease" hypothesis. Cancer Treat Rep 66:689–695.

Kadin ME. 1982. Possible origin of the Reed-Sternberg cell from an interdigitating reticulum cell. Cancer Treat Rep 66:601–608.

Kaplan HS. 1980. Hodgkin's disease: Unfolding concepts concerning its nature, management and prognosis. Cancer 45:2439–2474.

Kaplan HS. 1981. Hodgkin's disease: Biology, treatment, prognosis. Blood 57:813–822.

Krontivis TG. 1983. The emerging genetics of human cancer. N Engl J Med 309:404–409.

Manual of the Joint Causes of Death. 1939. United States Printing Office. Washington DC p. 62.

Rowley JD. 1982. Chromosomes in Hodgkin's disease. Cancer Treat Rep 66:639–644.

UT M.D. Anderson Clinical Conference on Cancer,
Vol. 27, edited by R.J. Ford, L.M. Fuller, and
F.B. Hagemeister. Raven Press, New York © 1984.

Phenotypic Attributes of the Malignant Cell Population in Hodgkin's Disease

Lennart Olsson, Francesco d'Amore, Marcus Diamant, and Olav Behnke*

*Cancer Biology Laboratory, State University Hospital, and *Medical Anatomy Institute C, Panuminstituttet, Copenhagen, Denmark*

An unambiguous histopathological diagnosis of Hodgkin's disease is based on identification of one or more characteristic Reed-Sternberg cells in the appropriate pleomorphic stromal background. The Reed-Sternberg cells appear in formalin-fixed tissue sections stained with hematoxylin-eosin, typically as binucleate cells with densely stained nuclear membranes, vacuolated or clear nucleoplasm, large nucleoli, and abundant, slightly amphophilic or pale-blue cytoplasm (Rappaport 1966). Multinucleate cells or cells with hyperlobated nuclei, but otherwise with features like the typical Reed-Sternberg cells, may also be components in the giant-cell population, which is considered pathognomonic for Hodgkin's disease. However, cells indistinguishable from Reed-Sternberg cells have been demonstrated in tissue sections from patients with infectious mononucleosis (Lukes et al. 1969) and from patients with non-Hodgkin's lymphomas (Strum et al. 1970).

It has been suggested that the Reed-Sternberg cells constitute the neoplastic cell population in Hodgkin's disease. This is difficult to reconcile with the sparse number of these cells (<0.01–1.0%) in most tissue specimens that contain lesions of Hodgkin's disease, in particular considering the abundance of tumor cells in other types of neoplastic lesions. The stromal cell population consists of varying proportions of small and medium-size lymphocytes, eosinophils, plasma cells, fibroblasts, and benign histiocytes. However, in addition to the above-mentioned cell types, large amounts of mononuclear cells with nuclear morphology like the Reed-Sternberg cells are found in Hodgkin's disease lesions. These cells are often referred to as Hodgkin's cells but may be encountered in other types of malignant lymphomatous lesions.

The natural origin and phenotypic characteristics of the neoplastic cells in Hodgkin's disease have been one of the major enigmas of this disease but have, on the other hand, been considered crucial for the understanding of the many peculiar features that may be associated with its clinical expression. The rather extensive literature on studies of fresh biopsy specimens and cultured cells clearly demonstrates the sometimes vivid discussion of the natural biology of the malignant cells

11

in Hodgkin's disease. It is beyond the scope of this paper to review extensively this literature (for reviews see Kaplan 1980, Kaplan et al. 1982). Instead, we will first briefly describe the conclusions derived from studies of fresh biopsy material, and then, in more detail, discuss the information derived from in vitro studies that recently have provided very strong evidence for a macrophage–monocyte origin of the neoplastic cell population in Hodgkin's disease.

STUDIES OF FRESH BIOPSY MATERIAL

Two types of populations have been identified by cytogenetic studies. One population has a diploid (46) chromosome content and is believed to belong to the nonmalignant, stromal cell population. The other population seems variable in number but is typically sparse and clearly aneuploid and often hypotetraploid. Abnormal marker chromosomes are often observed in multiple mitotic figures as an indication of the clonal origin of these cells (Seif and Spriggs, 1967). Chromosome analysis indicates that most Hodgkin's disease lesions seem to be of monoclonal origin at the time of diagnosis (Kaplan 1980), which obviously does not exclude an oligo- or polyclonal nature of the disease in preclinical stages (Olsson 1983).

The proliferative capacity of the Reed-Sternberg cells and the Hodgkin's cells has been analyzed by tritiated thymidine incorporation. These investigations failed to reveal the proliferative capacity of the Reed-Sternberg cells but revealed mitotic activity in the Hodgkin's cells (Marmount and Damasio 1967, Peckham and Cooper 1969), leading to the assumption that the Reed-Sternberg cells constitute end-stage products of the truly neoplastic cells. This opinion was later challenged by studies on cultured cells from Hodgkin's lesions that demonstrated Reed-Sternberg cells are capable of incorporating tritiated thymidine as an indication of DNA-synthesis activity (Kaplan and Gartner, 1977). However, our very recent experiments again support the assumptions that although Reed-Sternberg cells may go into mitosis, they have a very limited proliferative potential—only a few cell divisions—and they probably are end-stage products of the malignant cells.

The morphological appearance and cell-surface markers have been the basis for debate on the natural history of Hodgkin's cells. Their size and light microscopic morphology indicated a reticulum cell–histiocytic morphology (Ackerman et al. 1952, Rappaport 1966), but the otherwise characteristic nonspecific esterase enzyme for histiocytes could not be detected in the Reed-Sternberg cells or Hodgkin's cells using cytochemical techniques (Dorfman 1961). Lymphoid cells undergo remarkable morphological and cytochemical changes during mitogen-induced blastogenic transformation. When this was first observed, suggestions emerged that the malignant cells in Hodgkin's disease were derived from lymphoid cells that had undergone blastogenic transformation in vivo as a result of inappropriate antigenic stimulation (Order and Hellman 1972, Lukes and Collins 1974). Some investigators proposed a T-lymphocyte origin (Order and Hellman 1972, Biniaminov and Ramot 1974). However, the majority of the reports favoring a lymphoid cell origin suggested that the giant Hodgkin's cells were derived from B lymphocytes, mainly based on the observation that such cells may contain cytoplasmic immunoglobulin (Ig) or even express cell surface Ig (Leech 1973, Garvin et al. 1974, Boecker et al. 1975). These early reports were soon followed by several studies reporting that such giant cells could contain both kappa and lambda Ig-light chains (Taylor 1976, Poppema et al. 1978, Kadin et al. 1978). In contrast, B lymphocytes contain either kappa or lambda chains because they only encode for one type of Ig (Gearhart et al. 1975). The Ig in the giant cells is, therefore, probably a result of either active or passive uptake of exogenous Ig. Moreover, Reed-Sternberg cells are consistently negative for immunoperoxidase reactions for the J chain of Ig, although this is a marker consistently associated with B-lymphocyte malignancies (Isaacson 1979).

Ultrastructural studies of the giant cells in Hodgkin's disease have also failed to reveal the nature of the cell of origin. Some investigators have stressed structural similarities to lymphocytes (Dorfman et al. 1973); others have considered that structures like lysosomes and certain cytoplasmic processes favor a macrophage origin (Carr 1975).

Altogether, the studies on fresh biopsy material in Hodgkin's disease lesions have provided little information on the cell type of origin of the giant, malignant cells. The major suggestions are outlined in Table 1. However, the knowledge of lymphocytic phenotypes and the malignant tumors that may occur from such lymphocytes confirms that Hodgkin's cells are not derived from lymphoid cells. This leaves the macrophage–monocyte as the most probable candidate.

STUDIES ON IN VITRO CULTURES OF HODGKIN'S CELLS

Early Studies and Pitfalls

Cultivation of Hodgkin's cells was attempted very early after the introduction of nodern in vitro tissue culturing techniques as well as cultivation of cells in diffusion

Table 1. *Various Proposals for the Cellular Origin of Hodgkin's and Reed-Sternberg Cells as Based on Studies on Fresh Biopsies*

Proposed cellular origin	Parameter	Reference
Reticulum cell– histiocyte	Morphology	Ackerman et al. 1952
T lymphocyte	Morphology/ surface markers	Order and Hellman 1972 Biniaminov and Ramot 1974
B lymphocyte	Cytoplasmic and surface Ig	Leech 1973 Garvin et al. 1974 Boecker et al. 1975
Non-B lymphocyte	Polyclonal Ig	Taylor 1976 Poppema et al. 1978 Kadin et al. 1978
Lymphocyte	Ultrastructure	Dorfman et al. 1973
Macrophage	Ultrastructure	Carr 1975

chambers in vivo, most often in the peritoneal cavities of mice. These early studies have been reviewed extensively elsewhere (Kaplan 1980). The present paper will, therefore, be restricted to more recent reports, most of which can now be rejected as having described other types of cells than Hodgkin's cells. At the same time, it demonstrates the many pitfalls that surround attempts to establish cell lines of Hodgkin's cells.

Several early reports described cultures of Hodgkin's cells, but reconsideration of these reports seems to indicate that most of the cultures consisted of Epstein-Barr virus (EBV)–transformed B-lymphoblastoid cells that had overgrown the other cell types in the cultures and were thereby erroneously identified as the neoplastic cell population (Ito et al. 1968, Sykes et al. 1962, Ponten 1967); another example of this was reported by Friend et al. (1978).

Contamination of cell cultures with extraneous cell lines confuses attempts to establish the phenotypic characteristics of Hodgkin's cells. Four lines were thus reported to be derived from Hodgkin's lesions (Long et al. 1977), but three of these lines were later identified as consisting of owl monkey kidney cells, and the fourth line was derived from a spleen free of Hodgkin's disease lesions (Harris et al. 1981).

Erroneous histopathological diagnosis of the cultivated cells also contributed to the problems in cultivating Hodgkin's cells. Thus, one report (Boecker et al. 1975) was far more consistent with a diagnosis of diffuse histiocytic lymphoma than Hodgkin's disease. Likewise, the report by Ben-Bassat et al. (1980) probably described a T-lymphoblastic lymphoma.

More Recent Studies

A review of the attempts to establish cell lines from more than 100 specimens of tissue of Hodgkin's disease lesions was recently reported by Kaplan et al. (1982). In it, the criteria for considering a cell line established are underscored. The report of Kaplan and Gartner (1977) described a culture with a modal chromosome number of 53. It grew intracerebrally in nude mice, and the cells displayed cell-surface markers and lysozyme patterns compatible with an origin from macrophages. However, this culture eventually died out.

Roberts et al. (1978) described a highly pleomorphic cell line (HUT$_{11}$) that, even after cloning, consisted of some cells with macrophagic characteristics and other cells with features more like B lymphocytes. The cells of this line did not resemble either the L428 line or the SU/RH-HD-1 line.

The L428 cell line was established by Diehl's group (Schaadt et al. 1980, Diehl et al. 1981) from a pleural effusion in a patient with advanced Hodgkin's disease. The cells lack phagocytic activity and do not secrete lysozyme, are negative for lymphocyte and monocyte–macrophage markers, express HLA-DR antigens, and are capable of acting as stimulators in human mixed lymphocytic cultures, of secreting interleukin-1 and colony-stimulating factors, and of being nonspecific esterase positive (Fisher et al. 1983, Burrichter et al. 1983). We recently examined the L428 cells (kindly provided by Dr. V. Diehl) with a panel of monoclonal antibodies (Olsson et al. unpublished data) against T lymphocytes, B lymphocytes, monocytes, macrophages, and myeloid cells. It was found that the cells only bound the antibodies against myeloid cells, which supports a recent report from Diehl's group (Ziegler et al. 1981). Altogether, these results indicate that the L428 cells may be a myelomonocytic phenotypic variant of the neoplastic cells in Hodgkin's disease. A summary of the earlier in vitro studies is given in Table 2.

THE SU/RH-HD-1 CELL LINE

Establishment of the Culture

A spleen specimen was obtained in August 1980 from a patient with Hodgkin's disease, nodular sclerosis type. Several irregular, grey nodules of Hodgkin's disease lesions could be identified. One of these nodules was dissected free of surrounding spleen tissue, cut into small pieces, and seeded into 24-well plates in RPMI-1640 medium with 15% fetal calf serum.

Two types of cells could be identified one to two weeks after initiation of the cultures, very thin, adherent giant cells and fibroblasts mixed with macrophages. The giant cells grew more slowly than the fibroblasts and were easily detached from the plastic surface. After six to eight months, the fibroblasts gradually died out, whereas the giant cells continued to grow expansively. Initial attempts to clone the cells in semisolid medium (agar, agarose, methylcellulose) failed, and the line was therefore cloned by limiting dilution. Two years after initiation of the line, we have been successful in cloning the giant cells in methylcellulose. The line is designated SU/RH-HD-1 and has been described extensively elsewhere (Olsson et al. 1984). Some of the major features are outlined below.

Table 2. *Previous Studies on In Vitro Established Cell Lines from Lesions of Hodgkin's Disease*

Cellular origin of the line	Expansive growth properties	Reference
EBV-transformed lymphoblastoid line	+	Sykes et al. 1962
	+	Ito et al. 1968
	+	Pontén, 1967
	+	Friend et al. 1978
Owl monkey kidney cells	+	Long et al. 1977 (for review, Harris et al. 1981)
Diffuse histiocytic lymphoma	+	Boecker et al. 1975
T-lymphoblastic lymphoma	+	Ben-Bassat et al. 1980
Hodgkin's disease	+	Kaplan and Gartner 1977
Hodgkin's disease	+	Diehl et al. 1981

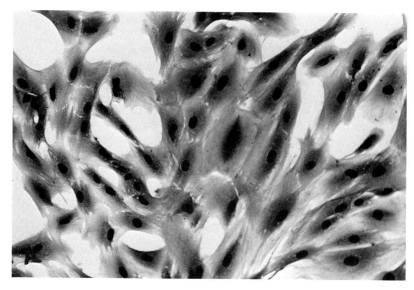

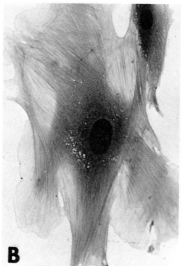

Figure 1. Light micrographs of the cloned giant cell line, stained with hematoxylin and eosin. **A.** The polymorphism of the very scattered cells. Reduced from × 150. **B.** Some vacuoles in the basophilic and perinuclear area and stress fibers diverging into broad pseudopods. Reduced from × 400.

Light Microscopy and Ultrastructure

Cytocentrifuge slides of the trypsinized, otherwise adherent cell population revealed large, round cells with a diameter of 35-60 μm. The cytoplasm was pale, and the nuclei were large with one or several prominent nucleoli. Most of the cells were mononuclear but about 1% were bi- or multinucleate. The morphology of the cells as they adhered to a plastic surface (Figure 1) was quite different from that

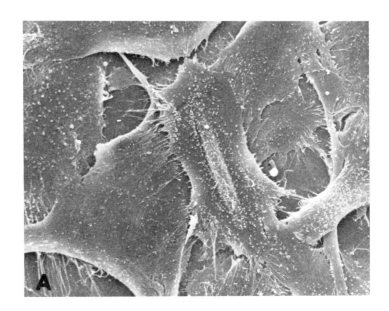

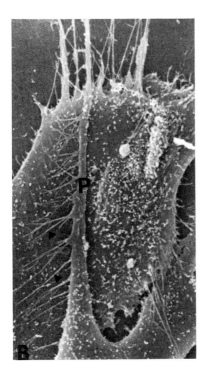

Figure 2. Scanning electron micrographs of the culture. **A.** Cells growing in multiple layers and filopodia anchoring cells to one another and to the plastic dish. Reduced from ×1200. **B.** A slender pseudopod (P) of one cell extends filopodia (arrow heads) from one edge but not from the other. The small protuberances seen at the surfaces of the cells are microvilli. Reduced from ×2200.

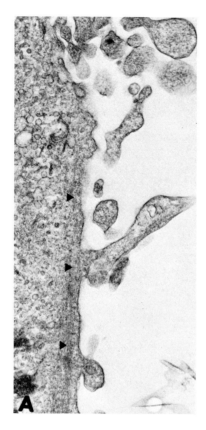

Figure 3. A. Part of peripheral cytoplasm showing subcortical filaments (arrow heads) and filopodia. Reduced from ×24,500. **B.** and **C.** Golgi areas of two cells showing vesicles and some granules with an electron-dense content. The granular endoplasmic reticulum is rich in polysomal configurations. Reduced from ×30,000.

of the cytocentrifuge preparations and, in fact, more representative of the morphology of the growing culture.

Scanning electron microscopy clearly demonstrated the highly pleomorphic nature of the cloned SU/RH-HD-1 culture. The cells were frequently observed to form multiple layers and possessed slender, sometimes forked or branching pseudopodia 10-100 μm long (Figure 2).

Transmission electron microscopy showed large and flattened nuclei, often indented with one or several prominent nucleoli. Distended Golgi areas, vacuoles, and networks of microfilaments were observed in the cytoplasm (Figure 3). At zones of overlapping cells, densities could be found along the cytoplasmic sides of the membrane (Figure 4), but these densities were not desmosomes; rather, they were zonula adherens-like structures. Many cells had smooth pits and a few had coated pits (Figure 5). The cytoplasm often exhibited a maze of smooth endoplasmic membranes between loose bundles of intermediate filaments and microtubules (Figure 6).

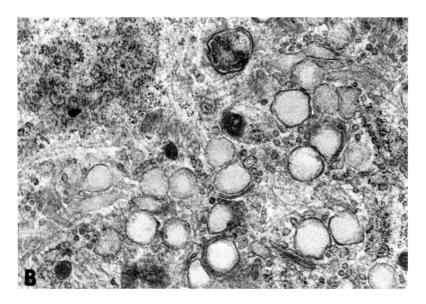

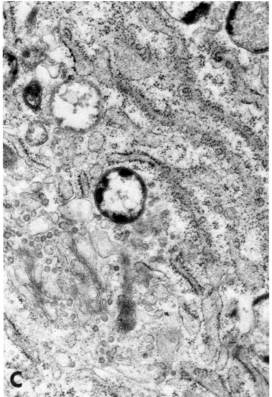

Figure 3. Cont.

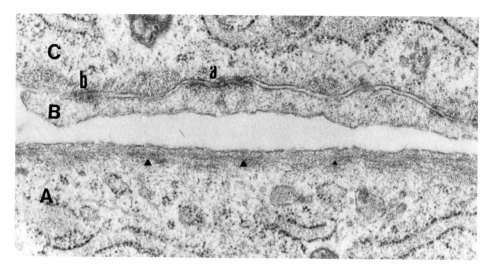

Figure 4. Part of peripheral cytoplasm of three cells (A,B,C). Cells A and C contain prominent cortical mats of fine filaments (arrow heads) seen in longitudinal and transverse section respectively. Two zonula adherenslike contact areas are seen between cells B and C (a,b). Reduced from ×30,000.

Proliferative Activity

The mitotic activity in the early cultures could not be estimated because of their contamination with fibroblasts and macrophages–monocytes. However, 12 months after initiation of the culture, the mitotic index was estimated to be 0.11% and has been at that level for the past two years. Fluorescence-activated cell sorter analysis revealed that the DNA content of isolated nuclei from the SU/RH-HD-1 was slightly higher than in diploid fibroblasts.

Cytochemical and Membrane Marker Characteristics

The cloned SU/RH-HD-1 cells were nonspecific esterase positive and were negative for lysozyme, EBV-associated nuclear virus, and reverse transcriptase. The cells expressed both HLA class I and HLA class II antigens, were negative for T-lymphocytic and B-lymphocytic markers but have Fc and C′ receptors and bind a monoclonal antibody, reportedly specific for macrophages–monocytes (Table 3).

Karyologic analysis indicated a variable chromosome content with a modal chromosome number of 47, including a marker chromosome.

The cells grew, only with difficulty, in nude mice. Only 1 out of 14 mice got detectable tumor upon grafting of SU/RH-HD-1 cells. Very recently, the graft-take rate of the SU/RH-HD-1 cells in nude mice increased significantly when the cells were grafted in a nest of human foreskin fibroblasts.

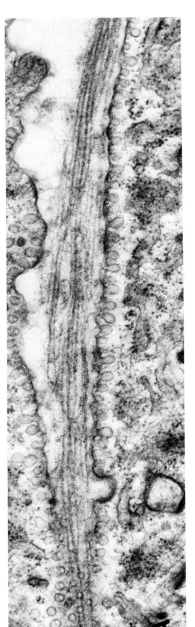

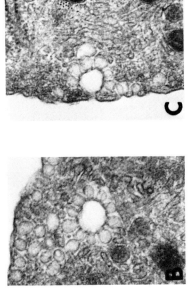

Figure 5. **A.** Cells possessing an abundance of smooth pits on the plasma membrane. The filaments seen in the intercellular space are of unknown composition (possibly fibronectin). ×37,500. **B.** Vesicles studded with smooth pits appear in the cytoplasm. ×37,000. **C.** Vesicles studded with small pits and in continuity with the plasma membrane. ×37,500.

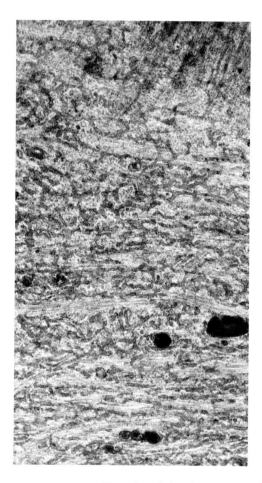

Figure 6. Cytoplasmic area with a maze of smooth endoplasmic reticulum with interspersed bundles of filaments. Reduced from ×37,000.

Functional Attributes of SU/RH-HD-1 Cells

Both latex particles and ink were taken up by the SU/RH-HD-1 cells. A pronounced heterogeneity among the cells was observed; some cells phagocytosed the particles and others apparently had no phagocytic activity. The cell-surface marker studies indicated that the SU/RH-HD-1 cells originated from monocytes–macrophages, which also was substantiated by the demonstration of phagocytic activity by the cells. Another important functional attribute of macrophages–monocytes is their ability to present antigen to immunocompetent, HLA-DR–compatible T lymphocytes, which resulted in blastogenic transformation of the T cells. The HLA type of the SU/RH-HD-1 cells is A10;19;B5;Cw6;DR1,4. T lymphocytes were obtained from a person highly responsive to PPD (purified protein derivative of tuberculin) and with a HLA-DR–type identical to the SU/RH-HD-1 cells (HLA-DR1,4), and the ability of SU/RH-HD-1 cells to present the PPD antigen to these T lymphocytes was analyzed (Table 4). The cultured SU/RH-HD-1 cells could

Table 3. *Immunological Markers of the SU/RH-HD-1 Hodgkin's Cell Lines*

Marker	Normal cell type	Negative	Positive	% Positive
		Expression on the cultured cells >24 months after establishment		
Leu-1	All mature lymphocytes	√		
Leu-2a	T_S-T_C lymphocytes	√		
Leu-3a	T_H lymphocytes	√		
Leu-7	Large granular lymphocytes	√		
Leu-10	B lymphocytes	√		
SmIg	B lymphocytes	√		
IgG-EA	B lymphocytes, monocytes, macrophages		√	>90
IgM-EA	(Control)	√		
IgM-EAC$_{3b}$	B lymphocytes, macrophages		√	>80
IgM-EAC$_{3d}$	B lymphocytes	√		
HLA-Class I[a]	All		√	>95
HLA-DR(Class II)[a]	Lymphocytes, monocytes, macrophages		√	>95
Leu M1	Granulocytes/monocytic	√		
Leu M2	Monocytes (subset)		√	>95
1.9A.10E[b]	Myeloid leukemia	√		
2.3A.11D[b]	Myeloid leukemia	√		
Nonspecific esterase	Monocytes, macrophages		√	>95

Table 4. *Antigen Presentation by SU/RH-HD-1 to HLA-DR–Compatible Immune T Lymphocytes*

Type	Amount	Pulsed with		Response of immune T cells* $(\text{cpm} \times 10^{-3}(^3\text{H})\text{TdR}$ incorporation/culture)
CAC	10^4	PBS		16.1 ± 6.0
CAC	10^4	PPB	$2.7 \pm 1.2‡$	$31.8 \pm 6.3§$
CAC	2×10^4	PBS		17.0 ± 1.9
CAC	2×10^4	PPD	$4.6 \pm 1.5‡$	$48.5 \pm 8.2§$
SU/RH-HD-1	10^4	PBS		7.6 ± 3.0
SU/RH-HD-1	10^4	PPD	$1.4 \pm 0.6‡$	$12.7 \pm 3.8§$
SU/RH-HD-1	2×10^4	PBS		4.4 ± 1.8
SU/RH-HD-1	2×10^4	PPD	$1.5 \pm 0.7‡$	$23.8 \pm 7.2§$

Header for Table 4 accessory cells: Accessory cells (AC)

*2×10^5/well.

†immune T cells pulsed with PPD and cultured in RPMI-FCS at 37°C in the absence of AC.

‡AC pulsed with PPD and cultured in RPMI-FCS at 37°C in the absence of immune T cells.

§Significantly different ($P < .05$) from the corresponding control value.

CAC—irradiated MNC autologous to T cells; PBS—phosphate-buffered saline; PPD—purified protein derivative.

present antigen to compatible T lymphocytes, although not to the same extent as normal monocytes. Also, the SU/RH-HD-1 cells could stimulate a mixed leukocytic reaction but were negative for interleukin-1 production assays. The tests described indicate, therefore, that the SU/RH-HD-1 have functional attributes as macrophages–monocytes.

CONCLUSION

The SU/RH-HD-1 cell line was established from a young man with Hodgkin's disease, nodular sclerosis type. The capacity of the cells to grow in semisolid medium, their aneuploid chromosome pattern, and their ability (although low) to form tumors in nude mice all indicate the malignant nature of the SU/RH-HD-1 cell line. Furthermore, the phagocytic capacity, the content of nonspecific esterase, and their immunological cell-surface markers all indicate a macrophage–monocyte origin of these cells. This was further substantiated by the ability of the cells to present antigen (PPD) to HLA-DR–compatible T lymphocytes. Monoclonal antibodies with a high degree of specificity for the SU/RH-HD-1 cells have recently been generated, and their reactivity to cells in fresh biopsies of Hodgkin's disease lesions are currently under investigation. If such antibodies react specifically with Hodgkin's cells, it is a further indication that the SU/RH-HD-1 cells are representative of the malignant Hodgkin's cells in vivo. However, it should be stressed that such antibodies cannot be used as direct proof that SU/RH-HD-1 cells (or any other cells) originate from Hodkgin's lesions but only that the cells share epitopes. Substantiation of our findings of a macrophage–monocyte origin of the Hodgkin's cells will require establishment and analyses of more cell lines from Hodgkin's cells in line with this analysis.

ACKNOWLEDGMENT

This work has been supported by grants from the Danish Medical Research Council, The Danish Cancer Society, NIH grant Ca-35227, and research contract 1-CP-91044 from the National Institute of Health.

REFERENCES

Ackerman GA, Knouff RA, Hoster HA. 1951. Cytochemistry and morphology of neoplastic and non-neoplastic human lymph nodes with special reference to Hodgkin's disease. JNCI 12:465–489.

Ben-Bassat HS, Mitrani-Rosenbaum S, Gamliel H, Naparstek E, Leizerowitz R, Korkesh A, Sagi M, Voss R, Kohn G, Polliack A. 1980. Establishment in continuous culture of a T-lymphoid cell line (HD-MAR) from a patient with Hodgkin's lymphoma. Int J Cancer 25:583–590.

Biniaminov M, Ramot B. 1974. Possible T-lymphocyte origin of Reed-Sternberg cells. Lancet I:368.

Boecker WR, Hossfield DK, Gallmeier WM, Schmidt CG. 1975. Clonal growth of Hodgkin cells. Nature 258:235–236.

Burrichter H, Heit W, Schaadt M, Kirchner H, Diehl V. 1983. Production of colony-stimulating factors by Hodgkin cell lines. Int J Cancer 31:269–274.

Carr I. 1975. The ultrastructure of the abnormal reticulum cells in Hodgkin's disease. J Pathol 115:45–50.

Diehl V, Kirchner HH, Schaadt M, Fonatsch C, Stein H, Gerdes J, Boie C. 1981. Hodgkin's disease: Establishment and characterization of four in vitro cell lines. J Cancer Res Clin Oncol 101:111–124.

Dorfman RF. 1961. Enzyme histochemistry of the cells in Hodgkin's disease and allied disorders. Nature 190:925–926.

Dorfman RF, Rice DF, Mitchell AD, Kempson RL, Levine G. 1973. Ultrastructural studies of Hodgkin's disease. Natl Cancer Inst Monogr 36:221–238.

Fisher RI, Bostick-Bruton F, Sauder DN, Scala G, Diehl V. 1983. Neoplastic cells obtained from Hodgkin's disease are potent stimulators of human primary mixed lymphocyte cultures. J Immunol 130:2666–2670.

Friend C, Marovitz W, Henle G, Henle W, Tsuel D, Hirsschhorn K, Holland JG, Cuttner J. 1978. Observations on cell lines derived from a patient with Hodgkin's disease. Cancer Res 38:2581–2591.

Garvin AJ, Spicer SS, Parmley RT, Munster AM. 1974. Immunohistochemical demonstration of IgG in Reed-Sternberg and other cells in Hodgkin's disease. J Exp Med 139:1077–1083.

Gearhart PJ, Sigal NH, Klinman NR. 1975. Production of antibodies of identical idiotype but diverse immunoglobulin classes by cells derived from a single stimulated B cell. Proc Natl Acad Sci USA 72:1707–1711.

Harris NL, Gaug DU, Quay SC, Poppema S, Zamecnik PC, Nelson-Rees WA, O'Brien SJ. 1981. Contamination of Hodgkin's disease cell cultures. Nature 289:228–230.

Isaacson P. 1979. Immunochemical demonstration of J chain: a marker of B-cell malignancy. J Clin Pathol 32:802–807.

Ito Y, Shiratori O, Kurita S, Takahashi T, Kurita Y, Ota K. 1968. Some characteristics of a human cell line (AICHI-4) established from tumorous lymphatic tissue of Hodgkin's disease. JNCI 41:1367–1375.

Kadin ME, Asbury AK. 1973. Long term cultures of Hodgkin's tissue. A morphologic and radioautographic study. Lab Invest 28:181–184.

Kadin ME, Stites DP, Levy R, Warnke R. 1978. Exogenous immunoglobulin and the macrophage origin of Reed-Sternberg cells in Hodgkin's disease. N Engl J Med 299:1208–1214.

Kaplan HS, 1980. Hodgkin's disease. Harvard University Press, Cambridge, MA

Kaplan HS, Gartner S. 1977. Sternberg-Reed giant cells of Hodgkin's disease: Cultivation *in vitro*, heterotransplantation, and characterization as neoplastic macrophages. Int J Cancer 19:511–525.

Kaplan HS, Olsson L, Burke JS, Osserman EF, Henle W, Henle G. 1982. In vitro cultivation of the giant neoplastic cells of Hodgkin's disease: some unsolved problems. In Rosenberg SA, Kaplan HS, eds., Advances in Malignant Lymphomas: Etiology, Immunology, Pathology, Treatment. Academic Press, New York, pp. 1–34.

Leech J. 1973. Immunoglobulin positive Reed-Sternberg cells in Hodgkin's disease. Lancet 2:265–266.

Long JC, Zamecnik PC, Aisenberg AC, Atkins L. 1977. Tissue culture studies in Hodgkin's disease: Morphologic, cytogenetic, cell surface, and enzymatic properties of cultures derived from splenic tumors. J Exp Med 145:1484–1500.

Lukes RJ, Tindle BH, Parker JS. 1969. Reed-Sternberg-like cells in infectious mononucleosis. Lancet 1:1003–1004.

Marmont AM, Damasio EE. 1967. The effects of two alkaloids derived from Vinca Rosea on the malignant cells of Hodgkin's disease, lymphosarcoma and acute leukemia in vivo. Blood 29:1–21.

Order SE, Hellman S. 1972. Pathogenesis of Hodgkin's disease. Lancet 1:571–573.

Olsson L. 1983. Phenotypic diversity of leukemia cell populations. Cancer Metastasis Review 2:153–163.

Olsson L, Behnke O, Kaplan HS. 1984. Establishment and characterization of a permanent cell line from a patient with Hodgkin's disease. JNCI (Submitted).

Peckham MJ, Cooper EH. 1969. Proliferation characteristics of the various classes of cells in Hodgkin's disease. Cancer 24:135–146.

Pontén J. 1967. Spontaneous lymphoblastoid transformation of long-term cell cultures from human malignant lymphoma. Int J Cancer 2:311–325.

Poppema S, Elema JD, Halie MR. 1978. The significance of intracytoplasmic proteins in Reed-Sternberg cells. Cancer 42:1793–1803.

Rappaport H. 1966. Tumors of the hematopoietic system. In Atlas of Tumor Pathology. Section III, Fascicle 8. Armed Forces Institute of Pathology, Washington, D.C. pp. 97–161.

Roberts AN, Smith KL, Dowell BL, Hubbard AK. 1978. Cultural, morphological, cell membrane, enzymatic, and neoplastic properties of cell lines derived from a Hodgkin's disease lymph node. Cancer Res 38:3033–3043.

Schaadt M, Diehl V, Stein H, Fonatsch C, Kirchner HH. 1980. Two neoplastic cell lines with unique features derived from Hodgkin's disease. Int J Cancer 26:723–731.

Seif GSF, Spriggs AI. 1967. Chromosome changes in Hodgkin's disease. JNCI 39:557–570.

Strum SB, Park JK, Rappaport H. 1970. Observation of cells resembling Sternberg-Reed cells in conditions other than Hodgkin's disease. Cancer 26:176–190.

Sykes JA, Dmochowski L, Shullenberger CC, Howe CD. 1962. Tissue culture studies on human leukemia and malignant lymphoma. Cancer Res 22:21–26.

Taylor CR. 1977. Upon the nature of Hodgkin's disease and the Reed-Sternberg cell. In: Mathe G, Seligmann M, Tubiana M, eds. Proceedings of the CNRS International Colloquium. Vol. 64. Berlin: Springer-Verlag, pp. 214–231.

Ziegler A, Diehl V, Uchaviska-Ziegler B, Kirchner H, Burrichter H, Wernet P. 1981. Cell surface antigens on a Hodgkin's disease derived cell line, L428 cells, and 5 subclones as detected by monoclonal antibodies. Immunobiology 160:137–138

UT M.D. Anderson Clinical Conference on Cancer,
Vol. 27, edited by R. J. Ford, L. M. Fuller, and
F. B. Hagemeister. Raven Press, New York © 1984.

Hodgkin's Disease in Immunologic Perspective

Richard J. Ford, Jr., Jerry Tsao, Frances M. Davis,
C. G. Sahasrabuddhe, and Shashi Mehta

Department of Pathology, The University of Texas M. D. Anderson Hospital and Tumor Institute at Houston, Houston, Texas 77030

Hodgkin's disease (HD) is one of the success stories in modern cancer therapy (Kaplan 1980a). Although our treatment strategies are quite effective, we still know relatively little about the biology or pathophysiology of the disease process itself (Kaplan 1980b). Three major questions, in fact, that remain unanswered may hold the key to our understanding of HD; they are:

What is the nature of the malignant cell? From which normal cellular lineage are the Reed-Sternberg cell and its mononuclear variant Hodgkin's cell derived?

What immunobiologic or pathophysiologic factors control the histopathologic appearance of the Hodgkin's disease lesion? Do such factors provide clues to the etiology of the disease process?

What is the cause of the characteristic T-cell immune defect seen in Hodgkin's disease patients, and what is the relationship, if any, to the pathologic processes involved in Hodgkin's disease?

These questions relate to the nature of the malignant cell, factors controlling the histopathologic appearance of the HD lesion, and the cause of the immunologic defect in HD.

THE NATURE OF THE MALIGNANT CELL

HD is a pleomorphic lymphoreticular neoplasm composed of cells of several lineages. The Reed-Sternberg cell (RSC), a binucleate giant cell with prominent usually eosinophilic nucleoli, is the hallmark of the Hodgkin's lesion (Figure 1). The presence of this cell is necessary but is not sufficient alone for definitive diagnosis, as many other pathologic conditions, including infectious mononucleosis, can display cells that are morphologically indistinguishable from RSC (Lukes et al. 1967). The RSC must be observed in the presence of the other cellular background components of the Hodgkin's lesion before the diagnosis can be made. The other cellular components include the mononuclear variants of RSC, usually termed Hodgkin's cells (HC) and a mixture of acute and chronic inflammatory cells such

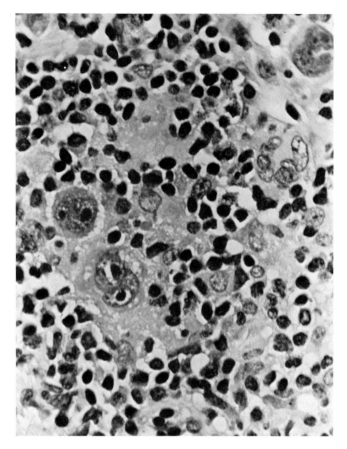

Figure 1. Photomicrograph of a typical Hodgkin's disease lesion, showing several Reed-Sternberg cells and mononuclear variant Hodgkin's cells admixed with apparently normal lymphoid cells. × 100.

as lymphocytes, granulocytes, eosinophils, and plasma cells. If we assume that RSC and HC represent the tumor cell populations that are supported by both histopathologic and in vitro proliferative studies (Lukes and Butler 1966, Peckman and Cooper 1980) and that the other cellular components of the lesion are reactive rather than neoplastic, then we wonder what is the lineage of the RSC? This question has been historically elusive and remains the center of intense controversy.

Virtually every known cell type of the hematopoietic and lymphoid system has been impugned as in the normal counterpart of the RSC. Evidence has been presented in the literature for T-cell (Order and Hellman 1972), B-cell (Taylor 1978), monocyte-macrophage (Kaplan and Gartner 1977), and even dendritic cell (Kadin 1982) origin for the RSC. Our own studies on the malignant cell in HD (Ford et al. 1982) suggest that the RSC and HC are related to the monocyte-macrophage lineage because the malignant cells usually express some degree of nonspecific esterase positivity, weak phagocytic properties, DR antigens (Table 1), and the production of interleukin-1 (IL-1) activity in culture cell supernatants (Table 2). These cell cultures were obtained from fragments of histologically proven HD tissue derived from biopsy specimens. We have also used the human malignancy-associated nucleolar antigen (HMNA), which discriminates between neoplastic and normal lymphoid cells in the non-Hodgkin's lymphomas (NHL) (Ford et al. 1984a), to identify RSC and HC both in histopathologic sections and in in vitro-cultured cells.

Table 2 shows that the original HD lesion contains a relatively small number of cells that morphologically appear to be RSC or HC and express the HMNA but that the number increases with culture time in vitro, presumably because of the loss of nonadherent reactive or normal cells. The cultures are composed of large monocytoid cells that after two to three weeks are esterase positive and are weakly phagocytic for latex particles, bacteria, or opsonized red cells. Virtually all of the cells express the HMNA and morphologically resemble RSC or HC.

These cultures do not, however, develop into permanent cell lines but are usually terminated by fibroblastic overgrowth after protracted culture periods. This has also been the experience of other workers (Kaplan et al. 1982) who have tried similar approaches to culturing RSC and HC. Diehl's group, who have reported the establishment of continual cell lines from pleural effusions from HD patients, is the exception (Schaadt et al. 1980).

Table 1. *Characteristics of Hodgkin's Disease Cultured Cells*

Morphologic appearance	
Large binucleate and mononucleate monocytoid cells resembling Reed-Sternberg cells and mononuclear variant Hodgkin's cells	
Immunologic markers	
Surface Ig	−
Cytoplasmic Ig	+ (polyclonal λ + κ chains)
E_n rosettes	−
Anti-MØ monoclonal antibodies	+/−
Enzyme activities	
Nonspecific esterase	+
Acid phosphatase	+
Lysozyme	−
Phagocytic activity	
Latex particles	weakly +
Zymosan	weakly +
Opsonized RBC	weakly +
Functional activities in culture supernatants	
IL-1 activity	+
IL-2 activity	−

RBC, red blood cells.

Table 2. *Cellular Phenotype in Hodgkin's Disease Cell (HDC) Cultures*

Day	Patient	M∅*	T†	B†	Null†	HMNA‡
0	1	15	68	5	10	12
	2	22	60	2	14	18
10	1	82	3	2	12	80
	2	88	1	0	6	76
22	1	91	1	2	3	88
	2	86	0	2	10	79

Patient 1: HDC were derived from a cervical lymph node biopsy from a patient with stage III nodular sclerosing Hodgkin's disease (NSHD). Initial cell viability was 82% by trypan blue exclusion.

Patient 2: HDC were derived from splenic nodules from a patient with stage IIIB NSHD. Initial cell viability was 78%.

*M∅ is the generic term used here for nonspecific esterase-positive cells including cells with Reed-Sternberg cells and HDC morphology, as well as normal monocytes and macrophages. The number presented reflects the percentage of viable cells present in a lab-Tek slide chamber. (Miles Laboratories, Elkhart, IN)

†T-cells percentages were determined by E_n rosettes or OKT-11 monoclonal antibody and B cells by SIg^+ cells by immunofluorescence. Null cells reflect the E_n^-, SIg^-, and NSE^- cell population.

‡Human malignancy-associated nucleolar antigen (HMNA) was determined by indirect immunofluorescence.

This inability to establish primary neoplastic cell cultures from explanted HD tissues raises several important questions regarding differences between the in vivo and in vitro microenvironments vis-à-vis malignant cell growth. It also appears to contradict the older concepts that tumor cells show unrestrained growth without the intrinsic cellular regulatory mechanisms characteristic of normal cell proliferation. Diehl's cell lines, which were apparently established with no special culture techniques (Diehl et al. 1982) but which might have been derived from an in vivo "culture system" (i.e. a pleural effusion), may reflect the need for an in vitro transformation process of some type to occur before the establishment of immortal or continuous cell lines is possible.

FACTORS CONTROLLING THE HISTOPATHOLOGIC APPEARANCE OF THE HD LESION

The well-known pleomorphic appearance of the HD lesion has long fascinated pathologists, who are used to seeing rather monomorphic expansions of tumor cells as in the nonlymphoid neoplasms. While some morphologic heterogeneity is usually expressed in these types of tumors, the presence of large numbers of cells of different lineages is distinctly unusual, making the histopathologic pattern in HD particularly interesting. The often prodigious growth observed in HD lesions that are composed of a relative minority of apparent tumor cells raises a number of questions regarding the relationship of the tumor cells to the other nonneoplastic cells present in the lesion.

Finding that HD tumor cell (RSC and HC) culture supernatants contain the monokine IL-1 (Ford et al. 1982) suggests that the tumor cells are retaining at least some of the functional capabilities of their putatively normal counterparts. The most likely candidates for these normal precursor cells are the monocyte-macrophage or perhaps one of the other cell types that secrete factors with IL-1-like activity (e.g. epidermal T-cell activating factor). Our hypothesis has been that most, if not all, of the histopathologic features of the HD lesion can be explained on the basis of known biologic activities of IL-1 or related soluble factors (Ford et al. 1982). This view focuses on products secreted by the RSC and HC that influence the activities of the normal and reactive accessory cells present in the lesion. Possibly, these accessory cells, primarily T cells, which appear to be immunologically competent in standard assays for mitogen stimulation and growth factor [interleukin-2 (IL-2) and B-cell growth factor] production, can influence the biologic behavior of the RSC and HC.

NATURE OF THE IMMUNOLOGIC DEFECT IN HD

Dorothy Reed, the codiscoverer of the Reed-Sternberg cell, was the first person to report an immunologic defect, anergy to purified protein derivative (PPD) in HD over 80 years ago (Reed 1902). Since then, and most recently with the rapid advances in cellular immunology, the nature of this immunologic defect has begun to unfold. Soon after the discovery that human lymphocytes could be separated into functional subsets of T- or B-cell lineage, it was demonstrated that the abnormalities in HD occurred primarily in the T-cell–mediated responses, such as phytohemagglutinin (PHA) reactivity, mixed lymphocyte culture response, and delayed hypersensitivity (Ziegler et al. 1975, Young et al. 1972). In the past twenty years, a variety of immunologic suppressor mechanisms that involve monocytes (Twomey et al. 1980), suppressor T cells (Fisher 1982), and serum factors (Fuks et al. 1976) have been described in HD. It has been hypothesized that they are the cause of the T-cell defect. The fact that so many possible suppressive mechanisms can be experimentally demonstrated suggests that either a multifactorial etiology in the pathogenesis of the defect exists or that the in vitro assays utilized may be somewhat artifactual relative to the in vivo disease process.

The advent of growth factor technology in cellular immunology has provided a new framework for understanding human T-cell regulation and function (Morgan et al. 1976). The identification of soluble factors (lymphokines and monokines) that mediate these processes and the target cells for their action has delineated the series of events that appear to be necessary for human T-cell activation (Smith et al. 1980). Using this framework, we have studied HD patients' T-cell systems to ascertain where a defect might be found. Such a defect could then explain the hyporesponsiveness observed in HD patients' T-cell responses and thus provide clues as to how the defect might be treated, possibly by biologic response modification.

Our initial studies on 14 untreated nodular sclerosing Hodgkin's disease (NSHD) patients indicated that they were virtually all immunodeficient as demonstrated by skin test reactivity to recall antigens and hyporesponsiveness to PHA stimulation. The patients' ages ranged from 17 to 36 years and they represented the entire clinical staging spectrum from stage IA to IVB. When standard in vitro assays were used to measure growth factor activities, we found that the HD patients' IL-1 responses were normal compared to age- and sex-matched controls (Ford et al. 1984b). The HD patients' peripheral blood T cells, after activation with PHA, were also equally responsive when compared to the normal controls. IL-2 (T-cell growth factor) responses in the Hodgkin's patients were, however, significantly decreased (Table 3). The relative inability of HD patients' peripheral blood mononuclear cells to make IL-2 could therefore account for at least some of the T-cell deficiency noted in these patients. This finding apparently identifies at least one site of T-cell abnormality in HD but not the cause of the defect.

This type of T-cell abnormality might stem from several types of abnormalities within the T-cell system, which now needs to be systematically studied. For instance, such an IL-2 production defect could result from an absolute loss of the IL-2-producing T-cell subset, a failure of IL-1 to stimulate that T-cell subset responsible for IL-2 production, or an active suppressor mechanism mediated by either suppressor T cells or by monocytes. This latter mechanism, through the secretion of prostaglandin E_2, is active in HD (Twomey et al. 1980, Goodwin et al. 1977).

Table 3. *Growth Factor Assays on Hodgkin's Disease Patients Peripheral Blood Mononuclear Cells (PBMC)*

Patient	PHA* response CPM	IL-1† generation CPM	Response‡ to exogenous IL-2 CPM	IL-2** generation CPM
MM	8425	21741	45435	8965
Control	17605	25843	83184	20296
JR	ND	17970	4546	1461
Control	ND	14536	17440	11710
BA	16053	34529	32072	3029
Control	19181	36378	19677	6210

*Stimulation with 0.75% phytohemagglutinin (PHA) for 72 hr, with labeling with 0.5 μci ³H-Tdr for final 24 hr.

†IL-1 was generated from adherent PBMC after 24 hr stimulation with 1 μg/ml lipopolysaccharide at 37°C. Dialyzed supernatants were assayed on thymocytes from six to eight week C3H/HeJ mice in mitogenic assays with concanavalin A (ConA) for 72 hr in vitro. ³H-Tdr was added for the final 24 hr.

‡PHA-stimulated T-cell blasts, after 7-10 days in vitro, were stimulated with partially purified IL-2 preparations from lymphocyte-conditioned media. After 48 hr in culture ³H-Tdr incorporation was measured during the final 24 hr in culture.

**PBMC were stimulated with 1.25 μg/ml ConA for 48 hr at 37°C. Dialyzed supernatants were then assayed on long-term human T-cell lines for IL-2 activity in 72-hr in vitro assays.

In summary, HD appears to be biologically, immunologically, and clinically different from the constellation of B- and T-cell neoplasms known as the non-Hodgkin's lymphomas. The neoplastic cell in HD still has not been definitely identified, but our studies favor a cell related to the monocyte-macrophage cell lineage. We feel that this cell is also functionally similar to a macrophage in that it secretes a molecule with IL-1 activity, which can account for many, if not all, of the histopathologic characteristics of the disease (Ford et al. 1982). We also hypothesize that secretory products from the nonneoplastic reactive cellular components of the HD may influence the growth characteristics of the RSC and HC. The connection between the primary pathologic process in HD and the characteristic T-cell defect remains elusive. The IL-2 production deficiency probably accounts for some of this defect that may also prove to be multifactorial. What we learn from these studies is that even though our understanding of many of the pathophysiologic processes in HD is still incomplete, the methodologies needed to dissect the intricate immunopathologic and ultimately molecular biologic processes involved are rapidly becoming available.

ACKNOWLEDGMENT

This investigation was supported by grants CA31479 and CA36243 awarded by the National Cancer Institute, United States Department of Health and Human Services.

REFERENCES

Diehl V, Kirchner H, Burrichter H, Stein H. 1982. Characteristics of Hodgkin's disease-derived cell lines. Cancer Treat Rep 66:613–632.

Fisher RI. 1982. Implications of persistent T cell abnormalities for the etiology of Hodgkin's disease. Cancer Treat Rep 66:601–608.

Ford RJ, Cramer M, Davis F. 1984a. Identification of human lymphoma cells by antisera to malignancy-associated nucleolar antigens. Blood 63:559–565.

Ford RJ, Mehta S, Davis F, Maizel AL. 1982. Growth factors in Hodgkin's disease. Cancer Treat Rep 66:633–638.

Ford RJ, Tsao J, Kouttab N, Sahasrabuddhe CG, Mehta S. 1984b. The association of interleukin abnormalities with the T cell defect in Hodgkin's disease. Blood (In press).

Fuks Z, Strober S, Kaplan HS. 1976. Interaction between serum factors and T lymphocytes in Hodgkin's disease. N Engl J Med 295:1273–1278.

Goodwin JS, Messner RP, Bankhurst AD, Peake GT, Saiki JH, Williams RC. 1977. Prostaglandin producing suppressor cells in Hodgkin's disease. N Engl J Med 297:963–968.

Kadin ME. 1982. Possible origin of the Reed-Sternberg cell from an interdigitating reticulum cell. Cancer Treat Rep 66:601–608.

Kaplan HS. 1980a. Hodgkin's Disease. Cambridge, Mass, Harvard University Press.

Kaplan HS. 1980b. Hodgkin's Disease. Unfolding concepts concerning its nature, management, and prognosis. Cancer 45:2439–2474.

Kaplan HS, Gartner S. 1977. "Sternberg-Reed" giant cells of Hodgkin's disease. Cultivation in vitro, heterotransplantation and characterization as neoplastic macrophages. Int J Cancer 19:511–525.

Kaplan HS, Ohlsson L, Burke JS, Osserman E, Henle W, Henle G. 1982. In vitro cultivation and characterization of giant neoplastic cells of Hodgkin's disease: Some unresolved problems. In Rosenberg SA, Kaplan HS, eds., Malignant Lymphomas Academic Press, New York, pp. 2–32.

Lukes RJ, Butler JJ. 1966. The pathology and nomenclature of Hodgkin's disease. Cancer Res 26:1063–1081.

Lukes RJ, Tindle BH, Parker JW. 1967. Reed-Sternberg-like cells in infectious mononucleosis. Lancet 2:1003–1004.

Morgan D, Ruscetti F, Gallo RC. 1976. Selective in vitro growth of T lymphocytes from normal human bone marrows. Science 193:1007–1008.

Order SE, Hellman S. 1972. Pathogenesis of Hodgkin's disease. Cancer 1:571–573.

Peckman MJ, Cooper EH. 1980. Proliferation characteristics of the various classes of cells in Hodgkin's disease. Cancer 45:2439–2474.

Reed DM. 1902. On the pathologic changes in Hodgkin's disease with especial reference to its relationship to tuberculosis. Johns Hopkins Hospital Report 10:133–196.

Schaadt M, Diehl V, Stein H, Fonatsch C, Kirchner H. 1980. Two neoplastic cell lines with unique features derived from Hodgkin's disease. Int J Cancer 26:723–731.

Smith KA, Lachman LB, Oppenheim JJ, Favata M. 1980. The functional relationship of the interleukins. J Exp Med 151:1551–1556.

Taylor CR. 1978. A history of the Reed-Sternberg cell. Biomedicine 28:196–203.

Twomey J, Laughter A, Rice L, Ford RJ. 1980. Spectrum of immunodeficiencies in Hodgkin's disease. J Clin Invest 66:629–637.

Young RC, Corder MP, Haynes HA, DeVita VT. 1972. Delayed hypersensitivity in Hodgkin's disease: A study of 103 patients. Am J Med 52:63–72.

Ziegler JB, Hansen P, Penny R. 1975. Intrinsic lymphocyte defect in Hodgkin's disease: Analysis of PHA dose response. Cellular Immunology and Immunopathology 3:451–460.

UT M.D. Anderson Clinical Conference on Cancer,
Vol. 27, edited by R.J. Ford, L.M. Fuller, and
F.B. Hagemeister. Raven Press, New York © 1984.

Immunohistological Classification of Hodgkin's Disease and Malignant Histiocytosis

Harald Stein, Johannes Gerdes,* Hilmar Lemke,* Kevin Gatter, and David Y. Mason

*Nuffield Department of Pathology, John Radcliffe Hospital, Oxford, England OX3 9DU, and *Institutes of Pathology and Biochemistry, Christian Albrecht University, D-2300 Kiel 1, West Germany*

The origin and identity of the tumor cells in Hodgkin's disease, i.e. Hodgkin's and Reed-Sternberg cells, are still controversial, in contrast to non-Hodgkin's lymphomas and acute lymphoblastic leukemias.

Many theories have been propounded in the past. The most recent have suggested that Hodgkin's and Reed-Sternberg cells are related to B cells, macrophages, follicular dendritic reticulum cells, interdigitating reticulum cells, myelomonocytic precursor cells and, very recently, to dendritic cells of the Steinman type.

To test these possibilities we have immunostained tissue biopsies affected with Hodgkin's and other diseases using a large panel of monoclonal antibodies raised against B cells, T cells, macrophages, and others. None of these antibodies were selectively reactive with Hodgkin's and Reed-Sternberg cells, and we have therefore raised antibodies, first polyclonal (Stein et al. 1981) and subsequently monoclonal (Schwab et al. 1982, Stein et al. 1982b) against the Hodgkin's disease-derived cell line L428 (Schaadt et al. 1980, Diehl et al., 1981). The results obtained led to the detection of a hitherto unidentified lymphoid cell type, designated Ki-1 cell, which appears likely to be the normal counterpart of the Hodgkin's and Reed-Sternberg cells. Our study provided evidence suggesting that the Ki-1 cell gives rise not only to Hodgkin's disease but also to large-cell lymphomas. These were frequently misinterpreted in the past as being malignant histiocytosis.

MATERIALS AND METHODS

Tissue Samples

The source and processing of the tissue samples were described in detail elsewhere (Stein et al. 1982b).

Antibodies and Anti-Immunoglobulin Enzyme Conjugates

The source and reactivities of the polyclonal and monoclonal antibodies are described in Table 1. Peroxidase-conjugated rabbit anti-mouse immunoglobulin and peroxidase-conjugated swine-anti-rabbit immunoglobulin were purchased from Dakopatts a/s, Copenhagen, Denmark.

Immunoenzyme Staining

The two- and three-stage immunoperoxidase method and the mouse alkaline phosphatase anti-alkaline phosphatase (APAAP) technique have been described in several other articles (Stein et al. 1980, 1982b, Cordell et al. 1984).

Enzyme Cytochemical Staining

Peroxidase staining was performed on unfixed sections of cytospines using the methods of Graham and Karnovsky (1966). Chloroacetate esterase was demonstrated with the method of Leder (1967).

RESULTS AND DISCUSSION

The results of our multiple marker analysis, presented in Table 2, clearly show that the antigen and enzyme profiles of Hodgkin's and Reed-Sternberg cells do not correspond to those of any of the known cell types of the hematolymphoid system. This means that none of the concepts of the origin of Hodgkin's and Reed-Sternberg cells mentioned above are likely to be correct. We concluded, from our findings, that Hodgkin's and Reed-Sternberg cells represent a new, as yet unidentified, cell population or alternatively an as yet unrecognized differentiation stage of a known cell type.

To throw light on this question, we raised polyclonal and, later, monoclonal antibodies against a Hodgkin's disease-derived cell line L428 (Schaadt et al. 1980, Diehl et al. 1981, 1982, 1983). As can be seen from the Table 2, the antibody reactivity pattern of the L428 cell line was identical to that of Hodgkin's and Reed-Sternberg cells in tissue sections, suggesting that this cell line is derived from Hodgkin's and Reed-Sternberg cells and not from other cell types.

Among the large number of hybridomas we obtained by immunizing mice with this cell line, we could select three that produced antibodies reactive with the L428 cell line and with Hodgkin's and Reed-Sternberg cells in tissue sections but not with normal B cells, T cells, macrophages, follicular dendritic reticulum cells, or interdigitating reticulum cells (Table 3) (Stein et al. 1982a). Two of these monoclonal antibodies, designated Ki-24 and Ki-27, were not restricted in their reactivity to the cell line L428 and Hodgkin's and Reed-Sternberg cells. Ki-24 reacted with a number of non-Hodgkin's lymphomas of clear-cut B- or T-cell type but, interestingly, not with any cells of normal lymphoid tissue, while Ki-27 recognized, in addition to Hodgkin's and Reed-Sternberg cells, endothelial cells, smooth muscle cells, and a proportion of epithelial cells (Stein et al. 1983).

Table 1. *Polyclonal and Monoclonal Antibodies Used in the Present Study*

Antibody	Specificity	Molecular weight	Reference	Equivalent or identical antibodies
Tü35	HLA-DR	28,000/34,000	Ziegler et al. 1982	L243 Becton Dickinson (B-D) Dako-HLA-DR
To15	All B cells	150,000	Stein et al. 1982	Dako-pan-B
Anti-IgM	IgM	900,000		Dako-IgM, anti-IgA, Bethesda Research Laboratory (BRL)
Anti-IgD	IgD			Dako-IgD
C3RTo5	C3b receptor	205,000	Gerdes et al. 1982	Dako-C3b receptor
Leu-1	All T cells, B-CLL, centrocytic lymphoma and follicular mantle lymphocytes weakly	65–69,000	Engleman and Levy 1980, Stein et al. 1984	Dako-T1, OKT1
T11/Lyt3	Sheep erythrocyte receptor	55,000	Verbi et al. 1982, Kamoun et al. 1981	Leu-5 B-D
UCHT1	All T cells	19,000	Beverley and Callard 1981	OKT3, Leu-4
Leu-7	Natural killer cells		Abo and Balch 1981	
T-ALL 2	Interdigitating reticulum cells, cortical thymocytes		BRL	
NA1/34	Interdigitating reticulum cells, cortical thymocytes, Langerhans cells		McMichael et al. 1979	OKT6
Antimonocyte 2	Monocytes, macrophages		BRL	
OKM1	Granulocytes, monocytes, macrophages, natural killer cells		Breard et al. 1980	
S-HCL 3	Macrophages, hairy cell leukemia cells, granulocytes (weakly)	90,000/150–160,000	Schwarting et al. 1984	
R4/23	Follicular dendritic reticulum cells, splenic marginal zone cells (weakly)		Naiem et al. 1982	Dako-DRC1
Antilysozyme	Lysozyme		Dakopatts	
Anti-α_1-antitrypsin	α_1-antitrypsin		Dakopatts	
Ki-1	See text		Schwab et al. 1982	
Ki-24	See text	120–130,000	Stein et al. 1982	
Ki-27	See text		Stein et al. 1982	
3C4	Cells of granulopoietic origin and Reed-Sternberg cells		Schienle et al. 1982, Stein et al. 1982	

B-CLL—chronic lymphocytic leukemia of B-cell type.
T-ALL—acute lymphoblastic leukemia.

Table 2. Comparison of the Antigenic and Enzymatic Profile of the Most Important Cell Types of the Lymphoid Tissue with That of Hodgkin's (H) and Reed-Sternberg (RS) Cells and the Hodgkin's Disease-Derived Cell Line L428 as Detected by Immuno-Peroxidase Staining of Frozen and Paraffin Tissue Sections or Cytocentrifuge Slides

Markers used	H and RS cells	B cells	T cells	Monocytes/ macrophages	IRC*	FDRC†	Granulopoietic cells	Cell line L428
Surface Ig	−	+	−	−‡	−	+	−	−
To15 (pan B cell)	−	+	−	−	−	−	−	−
C3RTo5 (C3bR)	−	+	−	+	−	+	+	−
OKT11/Lyt3	−	−	+	−	−	−	−	−
UCHT1/T3	−	−	+	−	−	−	−	−
OKM1	−	−	−	+	−	(+)	+	−
Antimonocyte 2	−	−	−	+	−	+	(+)	−
S-HCL 3	−	−§	−§	+	−	−	+	−
Lysozyme	−	−	−	+	+	−	+	−
α₁-Antitrypsin	−/+	−	−	+	+	(+)	+	−
NA1/34 / T-ALL2	−	−	−	−‖	+	−	−	−
3C4	+/−	−	−	−	−	−	+	+
Peroxidase	−	−	−	−/+	−	−	+	−
Chloroacetate esterase	−	−	−	−/+	−	−	+	−

*Interdigitating reticulum cells.
†Follicular dendritic reticulum cells of lymphoid follicles.
‡Sometimes weakly positive.
§Reacts with a very small percentage of lymphoid cells, probably of B cell type.
‖Weakly stains macrophage-derived epitheliod cells and other macrophage subsets.

Table 3. *Reactivity of Three Monoclonal Antibodies That were Raised Against the Hodgkin's Disease-Derived Cell Line L428 and were Found to be Reactive with the L428 Cell Line Cells but not with Normal B Cells, T Cells, or Macrophages*

Antibody	Reactive cells (other than H and RS cells)	L428	H and RS cells* in tissue sections
Ki-1	Large lymphoid cells around B cell follicles	+ (100%)	+
Ki-24	Cells of various non-Hodgkin's lymphomas, e.g. of centroblastic type but no normal cells of lymphoid tissue	+ (100%)	+/−
Ki-27	Endothelial cells, smooth muscle cells, epidermal cells but no normal B or T cells, macrophages, or dendritic or interdigitating reticulum cells or non-Hodgkin's lymphomas with a clear-cut B- or T-cell phenotype	+ (30-50%)	+/−

*H and RS cells—Hodgkin's and Reed-Sternberg cells.

Monoclonal antibody Ki-1, in contrast to the other two reagents, labeled Hodgkin's and Reed-Sternberg cells in all cases of Hodgkin's disease investigated but appeared initially to be unreactive with all other cell types or tissues (Figure 1). This latter finding was based on immunostaining representative samples from all normal tissue and organs using a two-stage direct immunoperoxidase method.

When the sensitivity of the immunohistological labeling system was enhanced, however, by application of multilayer procedures and by the use of alkaline phosphatase in place of peroxidase as a marker, sheets of strongly stained large cells around lymphoid follicles became visible (Figure 2).

Adjacent tonsil sections were stained with monoclonal antibodies that were reactive with immunoglobulin, macrophages, follicular dendritic reticulum cells, interdigitating reticulum cells, natural killer cells, and others. The Ki-1–positive cell population did not show labeling with any of these antibodies, indicating that normal Ki-1–positive cells differ from all other known cell types not only by their expression of Ki-1 and absence of macrophage and accessory cell markers but also by their large size and their typical distribution around lymphoid follicles. No other cell type described in the literature shows a similar distribution pattern.

Having defined the typical distribution of Ki-1 cells in normal tissue, we studied the distribution of Hodgkin's and Reed-Sternberg cells (i.e. neoplastic Ki-1–positive cells) in Hodgkin's disease and found that these cells were also preferentially localized around follicles (Figure 1). The similarity of tissue distribution of non-neoplastic and neoplastic Ki-1–positive cells, together with the observation that the perifollicular region is a site in lymphoid tissue were earliest involvement by Hodgkin's disease is seen (Lukes et al. 1971), strongly suggests that the Ki-1 cells found in normal lymphoid tissue represent the physiological counterpart of Hodgkin's and Reed-Sternberg cells.

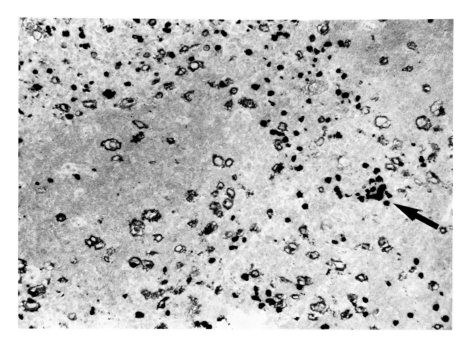

Figure 1. Hodgkin's disease, mixed cellularity, frozen section stained with the monoclonal antibody Ki-1, using a three-stage immunoperoxidase method. Hodgkin's and Reed-Sternberg cells show a ringlike surface labeling. Smaller, dark, stained clumps (arrow) represent eosinophils containing endogenous peroxidase. × 150.

When we routinely used the Ki-1 antibody for characterizing non-Hodgkin's lymphomas, especially those that were morphologically difficult to classify, it became evident that the Ki-1 antigen was not restricted to the tumor cells of Hodgkin's disease since a minority of non-Hodgkin's lymphomas showed strong labeling. All of these Ki-1–positive lymphomas were of large-cell type and had been classified morphologically as polymorphic immunoblastic lymphomas (Figure 3), anaplastic carcinomas or, most frequently, as malignant histiocytosis.

Table 4 summarizes some of the data we obtained by determining the immunophenotypes of 29 Ki-1–positive large cell lymphomas. The data in Table 4 show that the antigen profile of the Ki-1 cell tumors is not homogenous. Only seven of the Ki-1–positive lymphomas lacked T-cell–associated and B-cell–associated antigens, whereas 13 expressed T-cell–associated antigens alone, 4 expressed the B-cell–associated antigen Tol5, and 3 expressed both Tol5 and T-cell–associated antigens. Two cases expressed surface immunoglobulin. All cases had in common a very strong expression of HLA-DR and the absence of macrophage-associated antigens, with the exception of α_1 antitrypsin.

These unexpected findings should be interpreted in the light of results obtained when determining the immunophenotype of the Hodgkin's disease-derived cell lines that are currently available. As Table 5 reveals, all three Hodgkin's disease-derived

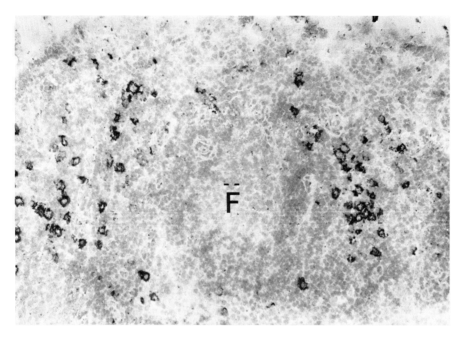

Figure 2. Normal lymph node frozen section stained with the monoclonal antibody Ki-1, using the three-stage immunoperoxidase method. Large cells around the periphery of a B-cell follicle (F) are labeled. ×200.

cell lines (L428, L540, and L591) express the Ki-1 antigen and two of these cell lines also express the 3C4 antigen (an antigen that is shared by Hodgkin's and Reed-Sternberg cells and cells of granulopoietic origin). The two newly established Hodgkin's disease-derived cell lines express T-cell antigens either alone (L591) or in association with the B-cell–associated antigen Tol5 (L540). Among the various other cell lines tested, only Epstein-Barr virus–positive lymphoblastoid cell lines proved to be Ki-1–positive. These cell lines also expressed the granulocytic antigen 3C4. This is of interest since nearly all non-Hodgkin's lymphomas of clear-cut B- or T-cell type lack this antigen. The Ki-1–positive lymphoblastoid cell lines differed from the Hodgkin's disease-derived cell lines by the expression of surface immunoglobulin and the consistent absence of T-cell antigens.

These results, in conjunction with the data obtained with the large lymphomas, suggest that the Ki-1 antigen may be expressed by cells of at least two lineages, namely, surface Ig-positive B cells and surface Ig-negative, HLA-DR–positive cells, which often express T-cell–associated antigens with or without the B-cell–associated antigen Tol5.

The observation that a proportion of Ki-1–positive lymphomas and of Hodgkin's derived cell lines express T- or B-cell associated antigens or both implies that the same may be true of Hodgkin's and Reed-Sternberg cells. We, therefore, reinves-

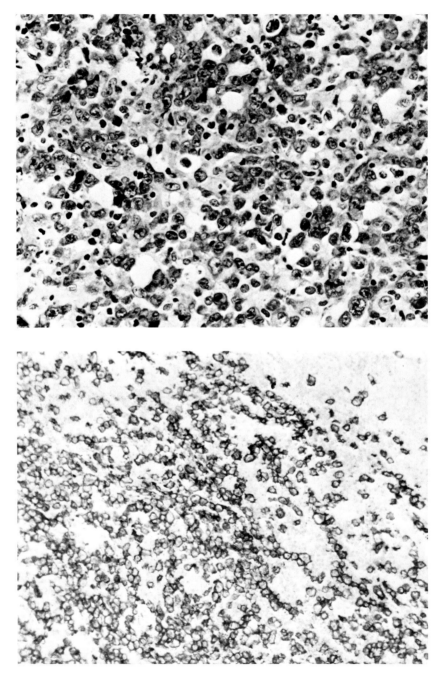

Figure 3. Top. Large-cell lymphoma diagnosed morphologically as malignant histiocytosis. Hematoxylin and eosin-stained paraffin section. × 700. **Bottom.** Frozen section stained with the monoclonal antibody Ki-1. The large tumor cells are strongly labeled. × 200.

Table 4. Immunohistological Labeling Reactions of 29 Ki-1-Positive Large Cell Lymphomas

No. of cases	Reed-Sternberg cell–associated antigens			Granulocyte-associated antigens 3C4	T-cell-associated antigens T11/UCHT1	HLA-DR Tü35	B-cell–associated antigens To15	SIg	Macrophage-associated antigens*	α_1-AT†
	Ki-1	Ki-24	Ki-27							
7	+	−/+	−/+	−/+	−	+	−	−	−	−/+
13	+	−/+	−/+	−/+	+	+	−	−	−	−/+
4	+	−/+	−/+	−/+	−	+	+	−	−	−/+
2	+	−/+	−	−/+	−	+	+	+	−	−
3	+	−/+	−/+	−/+	+	+	+	−	−	−/+

*Antimonocyte 2, OKM1, S-HCL 3, lysozyme.
†α_1-Antitrypsin.

Table 5. *Reactivity of Hodgkin's Disease-Derived Cell Lines (L428, L540 and L591), EBNA⁺ Lymphoblastoid Cell Lines (LCL), the Burkitt's Lymphoma-Derived Cell Line DAUDI and Histiocytic Cell Line U937*

	L428	L540	L591	LCL	DAUDI	U937
Ki-1	+	+	+	+	−	−
Ki-24	+	−	−	+	−	−
Ki-27	+	−	−	−	−	−
3C4	+	+	−	+	−	−
OKT11/Lyt 3	−	+	+	−	−	−
HLA-DR	+	+	+	+	+	−
To15	−	+	−	+	+	−
Surface Ig	−	−	−	+	+	−
Antimonocyte 2	−	−	−	−	−	+
S-HCL 3	−	−	−	−	−	+
Lysozyme	−	−	−	−	−	+

Table 6. *Surface Antigen Pattern on Hodgkin's and Reed-Sternberg Cells as Revealed with Immunoenzyme Histological Methods with Increased Sensitivity*

Antigens	Common phenotype	Variant		
		I	II	III
Surface Ig	−	−	−	−
HLA-DR	+	+	+	+
B-cell–associated antigen To15	−	−	+	+
T11 and/or UCHT1/T3	−	+	−	+

This phenotypical variant was also found in the cells of a polymorphic large-cell lymphoma that developed from a case of nodular type of Hodgkin's disease with lymphocyte predominance (nodular paragranuloma).

tigated a large number of Hodgkin's disease samples for their reactivity with antibodies against T-cell–associated antigens, B-cell–associated antigens, and other antigens, using optimized immune enzyme histological methods.

Table 6 summarizes the results of our second study. With the antibodies listed in this table, we found four different phenotypes of Hodgkin's and Reed-Sternberg cells. The most common phenotype was the one we had described previously (Stein et al. 1982a), i.e. negative for all markers except HLA-DR. However, in addition, three rarer phenotypic variants were observed, a finding that had been overlooked in our initial study, principally because of the presence of numerous reactive T cells in the vicinity of the Hodgkin's and Reed-Sternberg cells.

It is evident that the phenotypic variants of Hodgkin's and Reed-Sternberg cells are similar or identical to the phenotypic variants of Ki-1–positive and surface Ig-negative large-cell lymphomas. The overlap in markers substantiates our concept that the tumor cells of the Ki-1 cell lymphomas expressing T-cell–associated or B-cell–associated antigen Tol5 or both are also identical to Hodgkin's and Reed-

Sternberg cells. There are several other lines of evidence favoring this view. First, a significant number of the Ki-1–cell lymphomas express additional markers that we found to be very characteristic for Hodgkin's and Reed-Sternberg cells. These markers are Ki-24, Ki-27, granulocytic antigen 3C4, and α_1 antitrypsin. It has been shown by Payne et al. (1982) and by us (Stein et al. 1982b) that Hodgkin's and Reed-Sternberg cells in approximately one-third of the cases contain granules of α_1 antitrypsin in the cytoplasm. α_1 antitrypsin granules were also detectable in approximately one-third of the Ki-1–cell lymphomas.

Second, in both Hodgkin's disease and Ki-1–positive large-cell lymphomas, the tumor cells showed similar homing properties. This could be particularly well demonstrated in lymph nodes that were only partly infiltrated by Ki-1–positive large-cell lymphomas, since in such lymph nodes the tumor cells show a preferential tendency to localize around B-cell follicles in a similar way to Hodgkin's and Reed-Sternberg cells.

Third, in both Hodgkin's disease and Ki-1–positive large cell lymphomas, the tumor cells tend to spread into the marginal sinuses of lymph nodes, a pattern not seen in non-Hodgkin's lymphomas of clear-cut B-cell and T-cell type.

Taken together, the results of our studies suggest that Ki-1 antigen is present on two cell types: (a) a B-cell subset that gives rise to lymphoblastoid cell lines and rarely to large cell lymphomas, and (b) a surface Ig-negative and Ki-1–positive perifollicular lymphoid cell population that we designate as Ki-1 cells, for the time being. This Ki-1 cell population regularly expresses HLA-DR and may also express T-cell–associated antigens, B-cell–associated antigens, or both. If the perifollicular Ki-1 cell population becomes neoplastic, it may give rise to at least two morphological types of neoplasms: Hodgkin's disease and solid large-cell tumors. Here arises the question of why a single-cell population produces two such different types of tumor following malignant transformation. To clarify this question we have first to look at the differences between Hodgkin's disease and solid Ki-1–positive large-cell lymphomas. According to our results, the only consistent difference between these two types of lymphomas is the presence of an abundant admixture of various nonmalignant cells among the tumor cells in Hodgkin's disease. It is widely believed that in Hodgkin's disease this admixture of nonmalignant cells is the result of a host reaction against the tumor cells. However, if this were true, other neoplasms might also be expected to show a similar admixture of numerous nonmalignant cells, in which the tumor cells would represent only a small minority. Such neoplasms do not, to the best of our knowledge, exist, indicating that the concept of the florid host versus tumor reaction is unlikely to be correct. It is more logical to assume that the presence of the nonmalignant cells is due to a secretion of soluble factors by the Hodgkin's and Reed-Sternberg cells.

If this hypothesis were correct, the question as to why Hodgkin's disease is characterized by the presence of an abundant admixture of nonmalignant cells, whilst these cells are virtually absent in Ki-1–positive lymphomas, could be answered by assuming that in Hodgkin's disease, proliferating Ki-1 cells release a mixture of biological factors that attract numerous nonmalignant cells to the vicinity of the tumor cells. In Ki-1–positive large-cell lymphomas, however, the proliferating Ki-1 cells do not secrete significant amounts of such biological factors. The results are solid tumors containing only a minor infiltrate of nonmalignant cells.

The concept presented above clearly requires further evidence to prove or disprove its validity, including the production of new antibodies reactive with Hodgkin's cells, the analysis of soluble factors liberated by Hodgkin's-derived cell lines, and the characterization of the Ki-1 antigen in molecular terms. However, there is reason to hope that the mystery that has long surrounded the nature and origin of Hodgkin's and Reed-Sternberg cells will finally begin to dissipate.

ACKNOWLEDGMENT

We thank Miss Heinke Asbahr and Miss Kirsten Tiemann for skillful technical assistance.

This investigation was supported by grants from the Deutsche Krebshilfe and the Leukaemia Research Fund.

REFERENCES

Abo T, Balch CM. 1981. A differentiation antigen of human NK and K cells identified by a monoclonal antibody HNK-1. J Immunol 127:1024–1029.

Beverley PCL, Callard RE. 1981. Distinctive functional characteristics of human 'T' lymphocytes defined by E rosetting and a monoclonal anti-T cell antibody. Eur J Immunol 11:329–334.

Breard JM, Reinherz EL, Kung PC, Goldstein G, Scholossman SF. 1980. A monoclonal antibody reactive with human peripheral blood monocytes. J Immunol 124:1943.

Cordell J, Falini B, Erber WN, Ghosh AK, Abdulaziz Z, MacDonald S, Pulford KAF, Stein H, Mason DY. 1984. Immunoenzymatic labelling of monoclonal antibodies using immune complexes of alkaline phosphatase and monoclonal anti-alkaline phosphatase (APAAP complexes). J Histochem Cytochem 32:219–229.

Diehl V, Burrichter H, Schaadt M, Kirchner HH, Fonatsch C, Stein H, Gerdes J, Heit W, Ziegler A. 1983. Hodgkin's Disease cell lines: Characteristics and biological activities. Hamatol Bluttransfus 28:411–417.

Diehl V, Kirchner HH, Burrichter H, Stein H, Fonatsch C, Gerdes J, Schaadt M, Heit W, Uchanska-Ziegler B, Ziegler A, Heintz H, Sueno K. 1982. Characteristics of Hodgkin's disease-derived cell lines. Cancer Treat Rep 66:615–632.

Diehl V, Kirchner HH, Schaadt M, Fonatsch C, Stein H, Gerdes J, Boie C. 1981. Hodgkin's Disease: Establishment and characterisation of four *in vitro* cell lines. J Cancer Res Clin Oncol 101:111–124.

Engleman EG, Levy R. 1980. Immunologic studies of a human T lymphocyte antigen recognised by a monoclonal antibody. Clinical Research 28:502A.

Gerdes J, Naiem M, Mason DY, Stein H. 1982. Human complement (C3b) receptors defined by a mouse monoclonal antibody. Immunology 45:645–653.

Graham RC Jr, Karnovsky MJ. 1966. The early stages of absorption of injected horseradish peroxidase in the proximal tubules of mouse kidney: ultrastructural cytochemistry by a new technique. J Histochem Cytochem 14:291–302.

Kamoun M, Martin PJ, Hansen JA, Brown MB, Siadek AW, Nowinski RC. 1981. Identification of a human T lymphocyte surface protein associated with the E-rosette receptor. J Exp Med 153:207–212.

Leder LD. 1967. Die fermentcytochemische Erkennung normaler und neoplastischer Erythropoesezellen in Schnitt und Ausstrich. Blut 15:289–293.

Lukes RJ. 1971. Criteria for involvement of lymph node, bone marrow, spleen and liver in Hodgkin's disease. Cancer Res 31:1755–1767.

McMichael AJ, Pilch JR, Galfre G, Mason DY, Fabre JW, Milstein C. 1979. A human thymocyte antigen defined by a hybrid myeloma monoclonal antibody. Eur J Immunol 9:205–210.

Naiem M, Gerdes J, Abdulaziz Z, Stein H, Mason DY. 1983. Production of a monoclonal antibody reactive with human dendritic reticulum cells and its use in the immunohistological analysis of lymphoid tissue. J Clin Pathol 36:167–175.

Payne SV, Newell DG, Jones DB, Wright DH. 1982. The macrophage origin of Reed-Sternberg cells. An immunohistologic study. J Clin Pathol 35:159–166.

Schaadt M, Diehl V, Stein H, Fonatsch C, Kirchner H. 1980. Two neoplastic cell lines with unique features derived from Hodgkin's disease. Int J Cancer 26:723–731.

Schienle HW, Stein H, Müller-Ruchholtz W. 1982. Neutrophil granulocytic cell antigen defined by a monoclonal antibody—its distribution within normal haemic and non-haemic tissue. J Clin Pathol 35:959–966.

Schwab U, Stein H, Gerdes J, Lemke H, Kirchner H, Schaadt M, Diehl V. 1982. Production of a monoclonal antibody specific for Hodgkin and Sternberg-Reed cells of Hodgkin's lymphoma and a subset of normal lymphoid cells. Nature 299:65–67.

Schwarting R, Stein H, Wang CY. 1984. The monoclonal antibodies S-HCL-1 and S-HCL3 allow the diagnosis of hairy cell leukaemia. Blood (In press).

Stein H, Bonk A, Tolksdorf G, Lennert K, Rodt H, Gerdes J. 1980. Immunohistologic analysis of the organisation of normal lymphoid tissue and non-Hodgkin's lymphomas. J Histochem Cytochem 28:746–760.

Stein H, Gerdes J, Mason DY. 1982a. The normal and malignant germinal centre. Clin Haematol 11:531–559.

Stein H, Gerdes J, Schwab U, Lemke H, Diehl V, Mason DY, Bartels H, Ziegler A. 1983. Evidence for the detection of the normal counterpart of Hodgkin and Sternberg-Reed cells. Haematological Oncology 1:21–29.

Stein H, Gerdes J, Kirchner H, Schaadt M, Diehl V. 1981. Hodgkin Sternberg-Reed cell antigen(s) detected by an antiserum to a cell line (L428) derived from Hodgkin's disease. Int J Cancer 28:425–429.

Stein H, Gerdes J, Schwab U, Lemke H, Mason DY, Ziegler A, Schienle W, Diehl V. 1982b. Identification of Hodgkin and Sternberg-Reed cells as a unique cell type derived from a newly-detected small-cell population. Int J Cancer 30:445–459.

Stein H, Lennert K, Feller A, Mason DY. 1984. Immunohistological analysis of human lymphoma: Correlation of histological and immunological categories. Adv Cancer Res (In press).

Verbi W, Greaves MF, Schneider C, Koubek K, Janossy G, Stein H, Kung P, Goldstein G. 1982. Monoclonal antibodies OKT 11 and OKT 11A have pan-T activity and block sheep erythrocyte "receptors." Eur J Immunol 12:81–86.

Ziegler A, Uchonska-Ziegler B, Zeutheu J, Wernet P. 1982. HLA-antigen expression at the single cell level on a K562 and B cell hybrid: an analysis with monoclonal antibodies using bacterial binding assays. Somatic Cell Genet 8:775–789.

Therapy for Hodgkin's Disease

UT M. D. Anderson Clinical Conference on Cancer,
Vol. 27, edited by R. J. Ford, L. M. Fuller, and
F. B. Hagemeister. Raven Press, New York © 1984.

Initial Staging of Lymphoma Using Chest and Abdominal Radiographic Techniques

Luceil B. North and Sidney Wallace

Department of Diagnostic Radiology, The University of Texas M. D. Anderson Hospital and Tumor Institute at Houston, Houston, Texas 77030

CHEST

Radiographic imaging of the chest and abdomen is a primary clinical method of staging lymphomas. Appropriate management of the patient depends on accurate detection of the presence and extent of disease.

Choice of the proper radiographic method of staging is facilitated by detailed knowledge of the characteristic distribution of adenopathy for each type of lymphoma. For instance, excluding stage IV, untreated patients with Hodgkin's disease are very likely to have masses in the mediastinum but not in the mesentery, whereas in the non-Hodgkin's lymphomas, mediastinal masses are less common but mesenteric masses are frequent.

In the chest, selection of the proper imaging examination requires understanding of lymph node anatomy of the mediastinum and knowledge of typical sites of involvement. In general, the masses of lymphoma are seen in the upper half of the mediastinum in the middle and anterior portions. Nodal groups most commonly involved have been described by Filly et al. (1976), Bragg (1978), and Burgener (1981) and include the paratracheal, tracheobronchial, anterior mediastinal, aortopulmonic, subcarinal, and bronchopulmonary (hilar) lymph nodes. In the untreated patient, lymph nodes in the lower mediastinum are involved in Hodgkin's disease only if the upper mediastinal nodes are also enlarged. In general, this is true in non-Hodgkin's lymphoma, but occasionally discrepancy in nodal enlargement with large lower or posterior mediastinal nodes with minimal or no obvious upper mediastinal adenopathy may be seen.

A typical configuration of mediastinal lymphoma is familiar to all who treat this disease. Large masses are easily detectable by standard chest radiography, and standard radiography may be the only examination required for evaluation (Figure 1).

In the patient with minimal evidence of disease in the mediastinum, further studies may be necessary for accurate staging. Until recent years, tomography was the only imaging modality available for such further study and is adequate for identification of disease, particularly projecting toward the lung. In a patient with

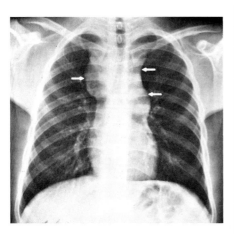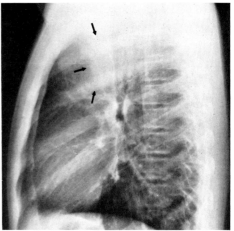

Figure 1. Nodular sclerosing Hodgkin's disease. **Left:** Frontal radiograph shows masses projecting laterally involving paratracheal, tracheobronchial and aortopulmonic (ductus) lymph nodes. **Right:** Lateral radiograph shows anterior mediastinal mass.

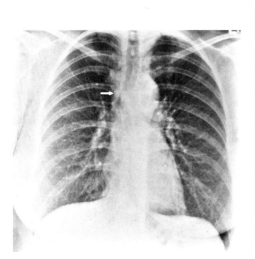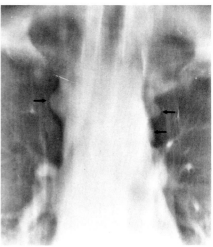

Figure 2. Diffuse large cell lymphoma. **Left:** Frontal radiograph shows minimal mediastinal abnormality. **Right:** Standard tomography demonstrates multiple bilateral mediastinal masses.

minimal disease, tomography frequently detects considerably more disease in the mediastinum than expected (Figure 2). Standard tomography has been extremely valuable for identifying enlarged lymph nodes, airway narrowing, and lung lesions.

For staging and treatment planning, it may be important to determine whether or not disease projecting toward the lung represents enlarged lymph nodes alone or whether there is actual lung invasion. If the use of computed tomography (CT) is not anticipated, standard tomography may be done to evaluate the borders of the mass lesion. An irregular border suggests lung invasion. If CT scanning is done, however, this modality is extremely useful in determining the nature of the borders of a mass and in evaluating abnormal densities seen in the lung (Figure 3).

Defining the extent of known disease may be important in setting up appropriate radiation therapy fields. In the patient illustrated in Figure 4, there is mediastinal widening typical of paratracheal adenopathy in the frontal radiograph of the chest. The CT scan of this patient shows that the disease extends far more posteriorly than expected; it extends beyond the vertebral body and into the concavity of the rib.

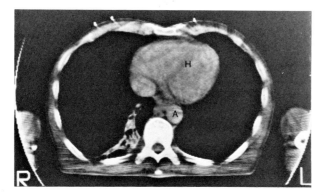

Figure 3. Nodular sclerosing Hodgkin's disease. Pulmonary density seen on routine radiography represents collapsed lung secondary to nodal obstruction shown on a more cephalad cut. There is no evidence of lung invasion by lymphoma (arrow). Radiotherapy localization markers are present on the anterior chest. A–aorta; H–heart.

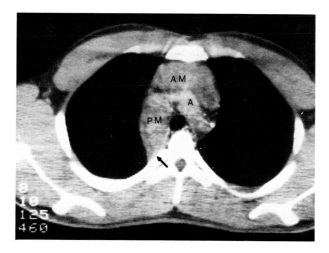

Figure 4. Nodular sclerosing Hodgkin's disease. Computed tomography (CT) shows anterior mediastinal mass noted on routine radiography. A right paratracheal mass also noted is shown by means of CT to extend far more posteriorly than expected (arrow). Left pleural effusion is also present. A–aorta; AM–anterior mediastinal mass; PM–paratracheal mass.

In Hodgkin's disease patients with low neck and supraclavicular disease, examination with CT is extremely valuable. Because of the continuity of the cervical and mediastinal lymph nodes, mediastinal involvement in Hodgkin's disease is probably the rule rather than the exception in these patients.

The extent of disease seen in the chest by means of CT is sometimes unsuspected, as seen in Figure 5. This patient presented with a right pleural effusion and a normal mediastinum seen on the chest radiograph. CT scans through the mediastinum show multiple enlarged pretracheal lymph nodes. These nodes cannot be imaged by standard chest radiography or standard tomography because of the position of the nodes and their small size. This patient also had enlarged subcarinal and diaphragmatic lymph nodes shown at the lower levels.

Enlarged lymph nodes may be encountered about the diaphragm and pericardium as described by Jochelson et al. (1983). This type of adenopathy cannot be detected by means of plain radiography or standard tomography unless the nodes become massively enlarged. The patient illustrated in Figure 6 shows a nodal mass at the level of the diaphragm, anterior to the heart. Detection of these lower lymph nodes is important because this area may be outside of the radiation field and marginal relapse in this area may occur, as described by Carmel et al. (1976) and North et al. (1982).

Enlarged nodes may also be identified in the retrocrural area. This area is not imaged by any technique other than CT scan, except occasionally by lymphangiography, and is not uncommonly involved with either abdominal or chest disease (Figure 7). This area will be seen either on chest or upper abdominal CT scan.

Pleural abnormalities are best detected by CT scan. Frequently, if they are small or flat, they may not be seen by means of standard chest radiography. Pulmonary

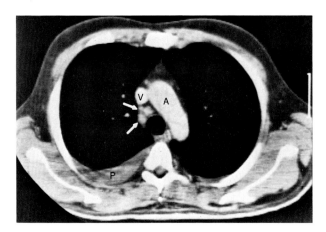

Figure 5. Nodular sclerosing Hodgkin's disease. CT scan taken at the level of the aortic arch shows multiple enlarged lymph nodes anterior and lateral to the trachea (arrows). These do not project laterally enough to indent the lung and were not detectable on standard radiographs. Bilateral pleural effusions are present, the left one was not detected on standard radiographs. A–aorta, V–vena cava; P–right pleural effusion.

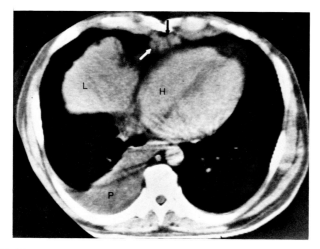

Figure 6. Nodular sclerosing Hodgkin's disease. CT scan taken more caudad of same patient in Figure 5 shows enlarged lymph nodes anterior to the pericardium (arrows). Right pleural effusion is again evident. H–heart; L–liver; P–pleural effusion.

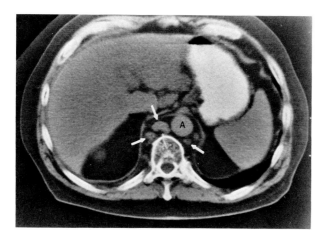

Figure 7. Nodular poorly differentiated lymphoma. CT at the thoracoabdominal level shows multiple enlarged lymph nodes in the retrocrural area. A–aorta.

nodules are occasionally seen unexpectedly on CT scan. In general, standard chest radiographs will be sufficient for evaluation of pulmonary nodules. Since the yield of nodule detection is so low, in our experience, whole lung tomography or CT scan is not done in patients with normal chest radiographs. Castellino et al. (1976) have pointed out that in only 1.2% of 243 patients in their study was staging changed as a result of whole lung tomography.

In summary, the chest radiograph, in frontal and lateral projections, is the basic screening study in the lymphoma patient. This should be followed by CT scan of the mediastinum, if there is suspicious evidence that there are enlarged nodes in the mediastinum, if there is low neck or supraclavicular disease, particularly in a patient with Hodgkin's disease, or if it is necessary to outline the extent of disease for planning or follow up. CT is also the best method for evaluating the presence of pleural masses. Standard tomography is most useful for evaluating airway narrowing and may be as good as the CT scan in evaluating the hilar areas. Evaluation for lung extension or pulmonary nodules can be done by either method.

ABDOMEN

The chief radiographic staging modalities for the abdomen include lymphangiography and CT. Intravenous pyelography is not necessary with CT, since the study is generally done using intravenous contrast material, and if kidney localization is necessary for radiation therapy, an abdominal radiograph may be obtained at the completion of the scan. Evaluation of the stomach is now done, to a large extent, by means of endoscopy. The gastrointestinal tract is outlined by contrast material for CT, which may obviate the need for separate small bowel examination.

In determining the appropriate method of staging, it is necessary to know the probabilities of disease localization. In the abdomen, Hodgkin's disease involves predominantly the para-aortic, common iliac, and external iliac nodes, or the areas well evaluated by lymphangiography. It is unusual to find disease outside of these nodal groups if the lymphangiogram is negative.

In our experience, staging is changed in 35% of stages I and II Hodgkin's disease patients who had negative lymphangiogram, as described by Gamble et al. (1975). Data collected by Dr. J. J. Butler, Department of Pathology UT M. D. Anderson Hospital (personal communication 1983) show that 30% of these patients have their disease upstaged because of involvement in the spleen. Only 5% are upstaged because of disease missed on lymphangiography and only 1% have mesenteric disease.

In the untreated patient with Hodgkin's disease, mesenteric adenopathy is uncommon, even with a positive lymphangiogram. In a small unpublished preliminary series of 28 patients with positive lymphangiograms evaluated in our department, only 2 patients had mesenteric disease as seen on CT, and both had mixed cellularity histopathology.

On the other hand, in our experience, and that of others, patients with non-Hodgkin's lymphoma, particularly nodular lymphoma, had a high incidence of intra-abdominal disease even if they had negative lymphangiograms (Goffinet et al. 1977, Heifetz et al. 1980). In the Heifetz report, 28 patients with stages I and II nodular lymphomas as determined by lymphangiogram had staging laparotomies, and in this series disease in 17 (61%) of these patients was upstaged. There were seven incidences of para-aortic lymph node involvement in spite of the negative lymphangiogram, probably because of the small size of the nodes and the type of distribution of disease within the nodes. Eight of these patients had mesenteric, nine celiac, and three porta hepatis lymph node enlargement indicating disease outside of the lymphangiogram-imaged area. Eleven patients also had splenic involvement.

In the same study, there were 40 patients with lymphangiogram-staged I and II diffuse lymphomas, and disease in 9 of these patients was upstaged at laparotomy. Three of these had disease in the para-aortic nodes, and otherwise, their disease was rather evenly distributed, including mesenteric, celiac, and porta hepatis nodes, and in one patient, splenic lymphoma.

Since CT can be used to visualize nodes inside and outside of a lymphangiographic area, the question arises as to the more appropriate method of assessing abdominal disease. Since both modalities are expensive, time-consuming, and involve considerable radiation exposure, it would be desirable to rely on one modality or the other. However, in many instances, the examinations are complementary. A recent review of the merits of these two modalities is detailed by Castellino and Marglin (1982).

It is important to understand the advantages and limitations of each examination. Lymphangiography generally outlines only those nodes along the external and common iliac arteries and the aorta to about the L2 level. Mesenteric nodes, which are commonly involved by the non-Hodgkin's lymphomas, are not imaged (Figure 8). The procedure is tedious and time-consuming and requires considerable experience and expertise to interpret. However, since the contrast material is absorbed very slowly from the lymph nodes, this allows follow-up examination to be done by means of a single abdominal radiograph only. The internal architecture of the opacified nodes can be evaluated by this method, which may be important because an enlarged lymph node may be merely hyperplastic and not involved by lymphoma. On the other hand, small nodes may have lymphomatous foci that are visible by lymphangiography but are too small to be seen by means of CT (Figure 9).

CT criteria for identifying abnormal nodes are limited by somewhat arbitrary designation of nodal size. Any node smaller than a certain measurement, e.g., 1.5 cm in the retroperitoneum, is considered normal, and nodes larger than this diameter are considered abnormal and, thus, probably involved by lymphoma. Nodal architecture cannot be evaluated. On the other hand, there is enormous advantage to examination by this method because all abdominal nodal groups can be imaged, as can the solid organs, gastrointestinal tract, abdominal wall, and regional skeleton. Liver and spleen size can be determined and lesions of sufficient size can be detected by appropriate contrast enhancement.

In addition, CT is useful for judging the status of intra-abdominal organs. Retroperitoneal masses frequently obstruct the kidney and, on occasion, they may actually invade the kidney (Figure 10). Enlarged lymph nodes in the porta hepatis may obstruct the common bile duct or pancreatic duct. These lesions can be well evaluated by using CT. Bowel involvement is occasionally seen, particularly in patients with large mesenteric masses. Such a patient is shown in Figure 11; the large mesenteric mass is entrapping some of the small bowel.

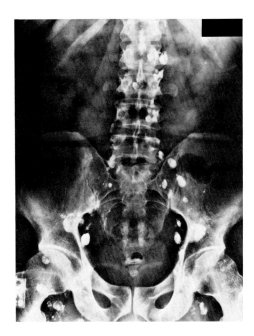

Figure 8. Nodular poorly differentiated lymphoma. **A.** Lymphangiogram is normal and no abdominal mass is suspected. **B.** CT scan shows no retroperitoneal adenopathy, but there is a large mesenteric mass. A–aorta; M–mesenteric mass.

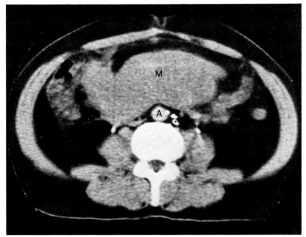

In the liver and spleen, CT has provided a means of localizing focal defects that are large enough to be detected. This is possible because of intravenous contrast enhancement of normal tissue.

Development of newer pharmaceutical agents that enhance visualization of liver and spleen defects will soon be generally available. These will be of special value in staging because of the incidence of splenic lesions now found only at staging laparotomy, particularly in patients with Hodgkin's disease and nodular lymphomas. In a cooperative study with the National Institutes of Health, we have evaluated

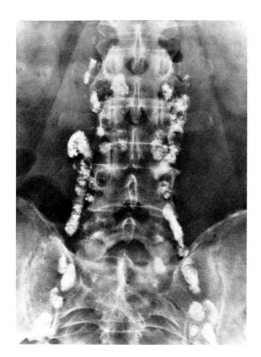

Figure 9. Nodular poorly differentiated lymphoma. **A.** Lymphangiogram shows para-aortic lymph nodes with defects consistent with lymphoma. **B.** CT scan showed no enlarged retroperitoneal nodes. Small nodes opacified by contrast material from lymphangiogram are seen in the retroperitoneum (arrows). A–aorta; V–vena cava; K–kidneys.

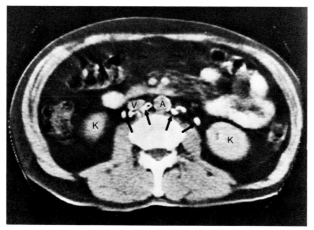

the usefulness of such a contrast agent, Ethiodol Oil Emulsion 13 (EOE 13) (Savage Laboratories, Houston, TX), for the detection of liver and splenic involvement with tumor, and the results have been published by Vermess et al. (1981). This technique holds the promise of improved detection of lesions, but the numbers of patients examined thus far have been too few to justify a definitive statement.

In summary, abdominal evaluation varies for patients with Hodgkin's disease and non-Hodgkin's lymphomas because of the differing distribution of disease. In the

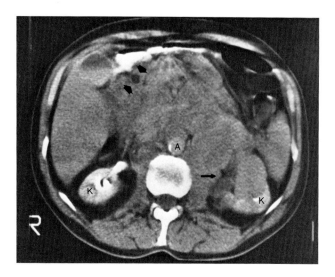

Figure 10. Diffuse poorly differentiated lymphoma. Huge retroperitoneal and mesenteric masses are seen with invasion of the left kidney (arrow). The mesenteric mass obstructs the common bile duct (arrowheads). A–aorta; K–kidneys.

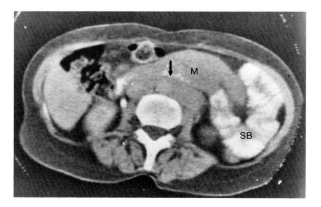

Figure 11. Nodular poorly differentiated lymphoma. Small bowel entrapment (arrow) and obstruction by a large mesenteric mass is shown by means of CT utilizing oral contrast material. SB–small bowel; M–mesenteric mass.

Hodgkin's disease patient, lymphangiography is probably the screening procedure of choice, since the nodes in the area imaged by this technique are the ones typically involved by Hodgkin's disease, and nodal architecture can be evaluated. Since the incidence of disease outside of these abdominal nodes is unusual in the face of a negative lymphangiogram, CT is probably not needed for nodal evaluation. However, when special contrast agents that will greatly improve visualization of disease in the liver and spleen become available, CT, at least of the upper abdomen, will be an important tool in staging.

In the patient with non-Hodgkin's lymphomas, CT and lymphangiography may be complementary. Because a large number of patients with non-Hodgkin's lymphomas present with adenopathy outside of the lymphangiogram-imaged area, CT is probably the screening method of choice. In a patient with a normal CT evaluation, lymphangiography might be helpful to determine if there is disease in small lymph nodes that cannot be imaged by CT. Also, the contrast-filled lymph nodes serve as markers for future follow-up studies using abdominal radiograph alone.

ACKNOWLEDGMENT

Acknowledgment is made of the contributions by Drs. Bao-shan Jing and Errol Lewis.

REFERENCES

Bragg D. 1978. The clinical, pathologic and radiographic spectrum of the intrathoracic lymphomas. Invest Radiol 13:2–11.

Burgener F, Hamlin D. 1981. Intrathoracic histiocytic lymphoma. AJR 136:499–504.

Carmel R, Kaplan H. 1976. Mantle irradiation in Hodgkin's disease: An analysis of technique, tumor eradication, and complications. Cancer 37:2813–2825.

Castellino R, Filly R, Blank N. 1976. Routine full-lung tomography in the initial staging and treatment planning of patients with Hodgkin's disease and non-Hodgkin's lymphoma. Cancer 38:1130–1136.

Castellino R, Marglin S. 1982. Imaging of abdominal and pelvic lymph nodes—lymphography or computed tomography? Invest Radiol 17:433–443.

Filly R, Blank N, Castellino R. 1976. Radiographic distribution of intrathoracic disease in previously untreated patients with Hodgkin's disease and non-Hodgkin's lymphoma. Radiology 120:277–281.

Gamble J, Fuller L, Martin R, Sullivan M, Jing B, Butler J, Shullenberger C. 1975. Influence of staging celiotomy in localized presentations of Hodgkin's disease. Cancer 35:817–825.

Goffinet D, Warnke R, Dunnick N, Castellino R, Glatstein E, Nelsen T, Dorfman R, Rosenberg S, Kaplan H. 1977. Clinical and surgical (laparotomy) evaluation of patients with non-Hodgkin's lymphomas. Cancer Treat Rep 61:981–992.

Heifetz L, Fuller L, Rodgers R, Martin R, Butler J, North L, Gamble J, Shullenberger C. 1980. Laparotomy findings in lymphangiogram-staged I and II non-Hodgkin's lymphomas. Cancer 45:2778–2786.

Jochelson M, Balikian J, Mauch P, Liebman H. 1983. Peri and paracardial involvement in lymphoma: A radiographic study of 11 cases. AJR 140:483–488.

North L, Fuller L, Hagemeister F, Rodgers R, Butler J, Shullenberger C. 1982. Importance of initial mediastinal adenopathy in Hodgkin disease. AJR 138:229–235.

Vermess M, Bernardino M, Doppman J, Fisher R, Thomas J, Velasquez W, Fuller L, Russo A. 1981. Use of intravenous liposoluble contrast material for the examination of the liver and spleen in lymphoma. J Comp Assist Tomogr 5:709–713.

UT M.D. Anderson Clinical Conference on Cancer, Vol. 27, edited by R. J. Ford, L. M. Fuller, and F. B. Hagemeister. Raven Press, New York © 1984.

Modulated Therapy of Hodgkin's Disease in Children

Margaret P. Sullivan

Department of Pediatrics, The University of Texas M. D. Anderson Hospital at Houston, Houston, Texas 77030

Physicians at a number of institutions who are experienced in the care of children with Hodgkin's disease have achieved long-term survival for approximately 90% of patients. This is usually accomplished through the use of radiotherapy alone for disease stages IA and IIA and combined modality therapy for stages IB, IIB, and more advanced, except stage IVB, which might be treated with chemotherapy alone (Tan, et al. 1983, Lange and Littman 1983). Other investigators used radiotherapy alone (Mauch et al. 1983), both radiotherapy and chemotherapy with radiation volume being the variable among the stages (Donaldson 1980), chemotherapy and low-dose total nodal radiotherapy in clinically staged patients (Jenkin et al. 1982), and chemotherapy alone (Ziegler et al. 1972, Olweny et al. 1974). No particular chemotherapeutic regimen has emerged as being the regimen of choice, although a preference has often been shown for MOPP (mechlorethamine, vincristine, pro- carbazine, prednisone) on the basis of seniority and performance but ignoring patient acceptability. The radiotherapy fields and doses have not been uniform among investigators; current trends have been in the direction of decreasing the tumor dose, the irradiated volume, or both (Tan et al. 1983, Donaldson 1980, Jenkin et al. 1982, Thompson 1982).

Treatment options are now available that do not jeopardize results. End results in young children may well be unacceptable when a regimen designed for adults, and highly acceptable in terms of cure and late effects in a mature individual, is employed for children. Figure 1 shows the spectrum of late effects at age 14 that followed total nodal therapy (mediastinum excluded) delivered when the patient was 5½ years of age. The child, cured of Hodgkin's disease at age 8, has some 65 years of life yet to live. Accordingly, treatments must be devised that miminize, in so far as possible, the most harmful and debilitating effects of therapy in the young.

Probably neither the patients nor members of the treatment team could agree on which side effects of therapy are most undesirable. Table 1 lists late effects of most concern to physicians and those of greatest concern to patients. The risk of increased susceptibility to overwhelming infection with encapsulated gram-negative organ- isms, primarily *Streptococcus pneumococci* and *Hemophilus influenzae*, following

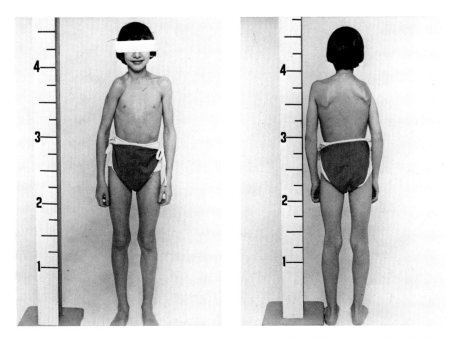

Figure 1. Front and back view of a 14-yr-old boy given total nodal radiotherapy (mediastinum excluded) at age 5½ yrs.

Table 1. *Late Effect of Therapy for Hodgkin's Disease: Concerns of Physicians and of M.D. Anderson Pediatric Patients <8 Years of Age with Hodgkin's Disease*

Physician concerns	Patient concerns
Overwhelming infection following splenectomy	Hair loss
Second malignant tumors	Vomiting
Sterility	"Being different" from peers and considered "weird"
Break(s) in latency of Herpes zoster infection	Avoidance of sunburn to irradiation fields
Growth retardation and other specific organ system irradiation effects	Change in musculature and soft tissues of the upper chest and neck following local irradiation
Cuspal and cervical caries from radiation scatter	Failure of faculties to consider the patient as a serious candidate for advanced degrees

splenectomy is now tempered by commercial availability of the 14-valent pneumococcal vaccine and the acceptance of prophylactic oral penicillin therapy by both physicians and patients.

The occurrence of second malignant tumors is an important treatment risk factor in children with Hodgkin's disease. The proportion of children, thus far, who develop second malignant tumors is much smaller than in adults (Coltman and Dixon 1982). Also, the type of second malignancies in children differ from those found in adults (Sullivan and McNeese 1980). The future must be viewed with skepticism, however, because of the length of the risk period that the child faces.

The sterilizing effects of therapy in girls are minimized by relocation, at the time of surgical staging, of the ovaries to a position outside the boundaries of an inverted "Y" field. Avoiding sterility in boys, at present, depends on identifying new chemotherapeutic regimens that will not cause testicular aplasia.

Additional concerns include the occurrence of herpes zoster, growth retardation of irradiated tissues, effects of irradiation on specific organs, such as heart and lungs, and the indirect effect that incidental irradiation of the salivary glands has on the teeth.

The nature and outcome of therapy given Hodgkin's disease patients less than eight years of age at the UT M. D. Anderson Hospital is the subject of this report.

STUDY MATERIAL

Since 1967, the staging laparotomy has been a part of the staging procedure for children with Hodgkin's disease at the UT M. D. Anderson Hospital, and chemotherapeutic regimens have utilized multiple rather than single agents. Since that time, we have given children younger than eight years of age with Hodgkin's disease "modulated" therapy for the express purpose of reducing late effects of treatment (Sullivan and McNeese 1980). Modulations employed include: (1) omission of splenectomy from the diagnostic work-up of children younger than five years of age; (2) routine employment of involved field (IF) radiotherapy rather than extended field or total nodal radiotherapy; (3) use of moderate radiotherapeutic doses in the 3000-3500 rad range; (4) use of IF radiotherapy only in treating upper neck stage IA disease, all histologies other than lymphocyte depletion (LD); (5) use of supervoltage radiotherapeutic sources and employment of the electron beam when suitable and available; and (6) protection of the hip joint from radiotherapy when stage IA disease is present in the inguinal-femoral or iliac regions.

Since July 1967, 39 children younger than eight years of age have been treated at the UT M. D. Anderson Hospital. Twelve children were younger than five years of age and 27 were five to eight years old. Twenty-eight were boys and 11 were girls (male:female ratio, 1:0.25).

Disease stages and splenectomy status for the patients are shown in Table 2. Nine patients did not have splenectomy and were thus clinically staged; six patients had splenectomy delayed until their fifth birthdays; some received IF radiotherapy to upper-torso disease in the interval from diagnosis to staging laparotomy.

Table 3 correlates disease stages and specific histologies of the study patients. The absence of disease with lymphocyte depletion is noteworthy.

The proposed modulations of therapy were actually employed in the treatment of the 39 children as follows. Splenectomy was not performed on any child who was younger than five years of age. Five children had IF upper-torso radiotherapy

Table 2. *Correlation of Disease Stage and Splenectomy Status, M.D. Anderson Pediatric Patients <8 Years of Age with Hodgkin's Disease*

	Splenectomy (# pts)		
Disease stage	Not done	Prior to therapy	Delayed
I (N = 14)	4	9	1
II (N = 10)	3	5	2
III (N = 13)	1	10	2
IV (N = 02)	1	1	0
Total (N = 39)	9	25	5

Table 3. *Correlation of Disease Stage and Specific Histology, M.D. Anderson Pediatric Patients <8 Years of Age with Hodgkin's Disease*

	Specific histology (# pts)				
Disease stage	Lymphocyte predominance	Nodular sclerosis	Mixed cellularity	Lymphocyte depletion	Unclassified
I (N = 14)	2	4	8	0	0
II (N = 10)	1	6	3	0	0
III (N = 13)	0	3	9	0	1
IV (N = 02)	0	0	2	0	0
Total (N = 39)	3	13	22	0	1

on the basis of clinical staging and subsequently underwent staging laparotomy with splenectomy after their fifth birthdays. No changes in stage occurred as a result of delayed splenectomy. Six children had no staging laparotomy. Protection to the splenectomized patients was afforded by pneumococcal vaccine, available to us since Novemeber 1975, and by the use of prophylactic penicillin or erythromycin.

The type of therapy given each patient is correlated with stage of disease in Table 4. IF therapy was frequently augmented in cases of lower and more extensive neck disease; of the 10 children with stages I and II disease who had unilateral neck disease, 5 had radiotherapy to both sides of the neck and 5 had radiotherapy to the involved side of the neck. The limitation to 3500 rad tumor dose was exceeded in 10 of the 29 patients given radiotherapy. Basic tumor dose to one or more fields ranged from 3700 to 4500 rad tumor dose in 6 patients; 4 patients received "boosts" of 950-1300 rad given dose to the basic dose, achieving a total dose in excess of 3500 rad tumor dose. Electrons were used in treating 7 children. In two instances, electrons were the only energy delivered to a field; electrons were used as a "boost" to other megavoltage sources in five instances. Two children with lower-torso disease were treated with chemotherapy alone to avoid irradiation of the femoral head and hip joint. The pretreatment extent of disease in each child, as demonstrated by lymphangiogram, is shown in Figure 2.

Table 4. *Correlation of Disease Stage and Initial Treatment Regimen, M.D. Anderson Pediatric Patients <8 Years of Age with Hodgkin's Disease*

Disease stage	Radiotherapy alone (# pts)	Involved field radiotherapy plus chemotherapy (# pts)	Chemotherapy alone (# pts)
I (N = 14)	3	5, XRT-chemotherapy 1, sandwich chemotherapy-XRT	5
II (N = 10)	4	3, XRT-chemotherapy* 1, alternating XRT-chemotherapy	2
III (N = 13)	0	6, sandwich chemotherapy-XRT† 2, sequential chemotherapy-XRT 5, sequential XRT-chemotherapy	0
IV (N = 02)	0	0	2
Total (N = 39)	7	23	9

XRT–Radiotherapy.
*One patient, Intergroup Hodgkin's Disease in Children Study, (POG 7660).
†Six study patients, (POG 7612); Sandwich chemotherapy-XRT–2 courses chemotherapy followed by involved field XRT, followed by 4 courses chemotherapy.

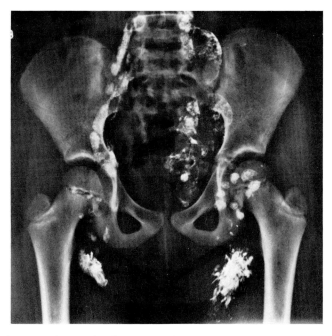

Figure 2. Lymphangiogram showing extensive Hodgkin's disease of the pelvis that was treated successfully with chemotherapy to avoid irradiation of hip joint as well as ovaries.

Results of Therapy

Complete remissions were attained by all of the 39 patients. Six, or 15%, have relapsed; no relapses have occurred since February, 1979. Number and percentage

of relapses by stage and therapy were as follows: stage I—2 of 14 patients (14%),
1 following IF radiotherapy 4000 rad to the neck and 1 following IF plus 6 MOPP;
stage II—2 of 10 patients (20%), 1 following alternating radiotherapy and chemotherapy, and 1 following IF plus 6 MOPP; stage III—2 of 13 patients (15%) relapsed,
1 following sandwich ACOPP (doxorubicin, cyclophosphamide, vincristine, procarbazine, and prednisone) plus IF therapy and 1, a noncompliant patient, following
sequential ACOPP-MOPP therapy; stage IV—0 of 2 patients (0).

Thirty-seven of the 39 patients (95%) are alive. No deaths have occurred since
November, 1971. Disease-free survival and survival are shown graphically in Figure
2.

Late Effects of Treatment

Eight patients have had late effects of considerable consequence. With one
exception, these late effects have occurred in patients receiving chemotherapy and
radiotherapy. The exception was a patient, given chemotherapy alone, whose bowel
perforated as a consequence of obstruction from adhesions following second-look
exploratory surgery.

Late effects among the seven patients receiving radiotherapy and chemotherapy
are as follows per patient: glioblastoma of the brain; exophytic osteochondroma of
the clavicle; herpes zoster, gynecomastia and hypothyroidism; herpes zoster; goiter;
preexcitation syndrome, herpes zoster; and cardiac enlargement with pericardial
effusion, pneumococcal sepsis in a splenectomized patient (sepsis due to a pneumococcal capsular type not included in the vaccine), encephalitis, and extensive
verruca vulgaris.

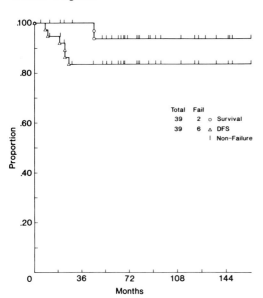

Figure 3. Survival and disease-free survival—UT M. D. Anderson Hospital pediatric patients with Hodgkin's disease younger than 8 years of age.

CONCLUSIONS

Therapy has been modulated for children with Hodgkin's disease who were younger than eight years of age at the time of diagnosis. The disease-free survival and overall survival are comparable to that being obtained with the most effective regimens now being reported. Serious side effects were limited, with one exception, to patients receiving both radiotherapy and chemotherapy; the single fulminate infection occurred in a splenectomized patient who appeared, on the basis of other infections, to have an immunologic deficiency. The incidence of zoster infections (7.7%) is less than the 25% reported for broader-based treatment groups (Donaldson and Kaplan 1982). Other complications were so infrequent as to make comparisons with other series meaningless.

ACKNOWLEDGMENT

This study was supported in part by grant CA-03713 from the National Institutes of Health, United States Department of Health and Human Services.

REFERENCES

Coltman CA Jr, Dixon DO. 1982. Second malignancies complicating Hodgkin's disease: A Southwest Oncology Group 10-year followup. Cancer Treat Rep 66:1023–1033.

Donaldson S. 1980. Pediatric Hodgkin's disease: Focus on the future. *In* Van Eys J, Sullivan MP, eds., Status of the Curability of Childhood Cancer. Raven Press, New York, pp. 235–249.

Donaldson SS, Kaplan HS. 1982. Complications of treatment of Hodgkin's disease in children. Cancer Treat Rep 66:977–989.

Jenkin D, Chan H, Freedman M, Greenburg M, Gribbin M, McClure P, Saunders F, Sonley M. 1982. Hodgkin's disease in children: Treatment results with MOPP and low-dose extended-field radiotherapy. Cancer Treat Rep 66:949–959.

Lange B, Littman P. 1983. Management of Hodgkin's disease in children and adolescents. Cancer 51:1371–1377.

Mauch PM, Weinstein H, Botnick L, Belli J, Cassady JR. 1983. An evaluation of long-term survival and treatment complications in children with Hodgkin's disease. Cancer 51:925–932.

Olweny CLM, McBiddle EK, Nkwocha J, Magrath I, Ziegler JL. 1974. Chemotherapy of Hodgkin's disease. Lancet 2:1397.

Sullivan MP, McNeese M. 1980. Therapeutic modulations for very young children with Hodgkin's disease (HD). Proceedings of the American Society of Clinical Oncology 21:387.

Tan C, Jereb B, Chan KW, Lesser M, Mondora A, Exelby P. 1983. Hodgkin's disease in children: Results of management between 1970-1981. Cancer 51:1720–1725.

Thompson EI, Wilimas JA, Smith KL, Vogel R, Sklar M, Hustu HO. 1982. Decreased therapy in childhood Hodgkin's disease (HD). Proceedings of the American Society of Clinical Oncology 24:159.

Ziegler JL, Bluming AZ, Fass L, Magrath IT, Templeton AC. 1972. Chemotherapy of childhood Hodgkin's disease in Uganda. Lancet 2:679–682.

UT M.D. Anderson Clinical Conference on Cancer,
Vol. 27, edited by R. J. Ford, L. M. Fuller, and
F. B. Hagemeister. Raven Press, New York © 1984.

Treatment of Laparotomy-Staged I and II Hodgkin's Disease

Lillian M. Fuller, Fredrick B. Hagemeister,* and
Miguel da Cunha†

*Departments of Clinical Radiotherapy, *Hematology, and †Experimental Radiotherapy,
The University of Texas M. D. Anderson Hospital at Houston, Houston, Texas 77030*

A 30-year record of continuous improvement in results for all stages of Hodgkin's disease has been achieved, mostly as a result of increasing the amounts of treatment. Unfortunately, during this time, the quality of life sometimes suffered from adverse effects of overly aggressive therapy. In the mid-1960s, complications were a calculated risk of curative radiotherapy. While the major complications of pneumonitis and pericarditis have been virtually eliminated through modifications and refinements in treatment techniques, sterility and acute myelogenous leukemia continue to be major risks of combination chemotherapy with or without radiotherapy.

For most patients, Hodgkin's disease develops at a critical age when treatment interruptions threaten plans for education, sports, budding careers, and parenthood. For them, options that offer effective minimum treatment are particularly attractive.

Selection of the minimum amount of treatment that is compatible with optimal results depends on both the investigative procedures that are used in determining the extent and the stage of the disease and on the results of previous treatment programs.

Sequential staging with lymphangiography followed by staging laparotomy has demonstrated that at least 50% of patients have generalized disease at the time of diagnosis. Management policies among major institutions differ significantly for all stages of Hodgkin's disease. Controversies on staging center on whether staging laparotomy is necessary and on whether computed tomography (CT) can be substituted for lymphangiography. Oncologists who feel that laparotomy is not necessary, regardless of the initial presentation of the disease, argue that negative surgical findings are not used for treatment decisions.

The extent to which laparotomy findings are used for treatment decisions usually depends on the surgical stage. As a result of reports on prognostic factors both for stage III and stage IV disease, there is a growing trend to give less treatment to patients with relatively favorable characteristics, including surgical findings, and to give more treatment to patients with poor prognostic factors.

Based on the rationale that staging laparotomy is only a sampling procedure, most investigators continue to give prophylactic radiotherapy to the para-aortic nodes and splenic bed despite negative staging laparotomy findings (Hoppe 1983). Very little has been reported on lesser amounts of treatment for patients with laparotomy-staged I and II disease.

Our policy for staging laparotomy and subsequent treatment is based on the status of the lymphangiogram. When the lymphangiogram is negative, we recommend a staging laparotomy, except for patients with lower torso disease presentations and those with very high upper cervical stage IA disease (Vlasak et al. 1983). Laparotomy is not done for patients with positive lymphangiograms regardless of the stage because our treatment decisions would seldom be influenced by either positive or negative findings.

Whether we can rely on a negative laparotomy to confirm the wisdom of effective minimal treatment decisions depends on whether the percentage of abdominal findings approximates the incidence of abdominal relapses in patients with negative lymphangiograms who were treated with only involved field (IF) or mantle radiotherapy. In our experience, patients with negative lymphangiograms had about a 40% incidence of abdominal relapses (Ibrahim et al. 1972). By comparison, our incidence of positive laparotomy findings in 360 patients was 33%. However, the incidence of positive findings from the para-aortic region was only 3% as compared with a 30% incidence of occult disease in the celiac portal nodes and the spleen (Figure 1) (Vlasak et al. 1983).

During the 1970s, we collaborated in two clinical trials for patients with laparotomy-staged I and II upper torso disease. The first study compared IF radiotherapy, including treatment to the mantle only, with extended field (EF) treatment to the mantle and para-aortic nodes. The second study compared EF radiotherapy with IF plus 6 MOPP (mechlorethamine, vincristine, procarbazine, and prednisone) (Hagemeister et al. 1982b).

The conclusions from this study were that mantle radiotherapy alone is effective minimum treatment for most categories of patients with laparotomy-staged I and II disease. IF radiotherapy was less effective in achieving long-term disease-free survivals because of the disease's tendency for spread to the immediately adjacent nodes of the upper torso. There were three categories of patients for whom radiotherapy alone was inadequate even when the treatment was EF. These consisted of patients with large mediastinal masses, patients with hilar disease, and those with constitutional B symptoms, regardless of the status of the mediastinum. Results of IF radiotherapy plus six MOPP were excellent for these categories of patients; the treatment is not acceptable because it causes long-term sterility in most males and prolonged menstrual problems in women older than 30 years. This is in contrast to our experience in using two cycles of MOPP with radiotherapy in stage III disease. Recovery of spermatogenesis was relatively prompt in men who did not undergo pelvic irradiation (da Cunha et al. 1983). As a result of these findings, we have modified our program for effective minimum treatment for these three categories of patients.

Our current program for patients with favorable upper torso disease presentations is to irradiate the mantle only. Patients with B symptoms receive two MOPP prior

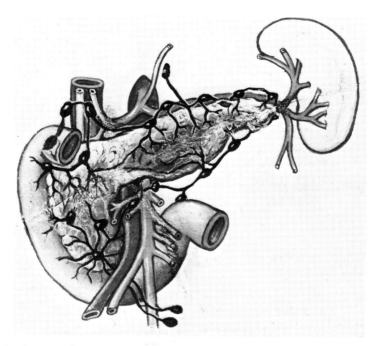

Figure 1. Anastomatic complex of lymphatic vessels and nodes associated with celiac portal complex. (Reproduced from Vlasak et al. 1983, with permission of Medical Arts Publishing Foundation).

to radiotherapy. Those with unfavorable mediastinal disease are treated with two MOPP followed by definitive radiotherapy to the mantle and low-dose irradiation to one or both lungs. Treatment of patients with lower torso disease is based on the presentation. Those with stage IA inguinal disease receive IF radiotherapy to the hemipelvis, while patients with extensive abdominal disease receive two MOPP followed by radiotherapy to the entire abdomen and subsequently, the pelvis.

In the remainder of this chapter we will review the pertinent background data from our previous studies including data on sterility associated with MOPP chemotherapy. Preliminary results of our new study will be presented.

INFORMATION FROM PREVIOUS STUDIES

We have published separate reports on patients with mediastinal (Hagemeister et al. 1981) and nonmediastinal (Hagemeister et al. 1982a) laparotomy-staged I and II disease in which we compared results for IF or mantle only, EF, and EF followed by six cycles of MOPP.

Mediastinal Disease

There were 101 patients with mediastinal disease; 44 had large disease according to criteria established in 1966. At that time, we found that the incidence of pulmonary relapse was significantly greater for patients who had mediastinal masses with transverse diameters of more than 7.5 cm. In this series, the incidence of both hilar adenopathy and constitutional symptoms was approximately the same for patients with small or large mediastinal masses. However, the effect of these factors on results was more significant for patients with large masses who were treated with either IF or EF radiotherapy.

The overall five-year survival figures for the three regimens was not significantly different due to effective rescue programs for patients with relapse of disease (Figure 2). The survival figures were 98% for IF plus six MOPP, 90% for EF, and 88% for IF. However, the disease-free survival rate for patients treated with IF plus six MOPP was significantly better, 98%, than the results for the other two treatments, 55% for EF, and 62% for IF. These differences were largely explained by an increased incidence of intrathoracic relapse in patients with large mediastinal masses who were treated with radiotherapy alone. For those with large mediastinal masses, the incidence was 38% as compared with 15% for patients with small masses. This was largely due to lymphogenous spread throughout the lungs and pleura.

When the results of radiotherapy alone were analyzed according to the extent of mediastinal disease, hilar adenopathy, and constitutional symptoms, the disease-free survival figures were satisfactory for patients with small mediastinal masses (82%) and no constitutional symptoms regardless of the status of the hila (Table 1). Disease-free survival rates were unsatisfactory for other categories of patients. Rates for patients with large mediastinal masses and hilar adenopathy were translated into a poor survival of 63%. For patients with no constitutional symptoms, the survival rate was 75%, and three of five patients with B symptoms died.

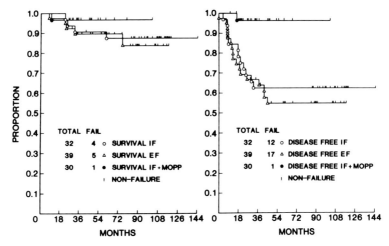

Figure 2. Patients with laparotomy-staged I and II mediastinal disease: Comparative survival and disease-free interval rates for involved fields (IF), extended fields (EF) and IF plus six MOPP. (Reproduced from Hagemeister et al. 1981, with permission of *Radiology*.)

Table 1. *Results for Patients Treated with Radiotherapy Alone According to Disease at Presentation**

Presentation	Patients			Survival (%)			Disease-free survival (%)		
	All	Without symptoms	B symptoms	All	Without symptoms	B symptoms	All	Without symptoms	B symptoms
Mediastinal									
Small	32	22	10	94	95	90	72	82	50
Large without hila	22	17	5	96	94	5/5†	58	71	1/5†
Large with hila	17	12	5	63	75	3/5†	35	42	1/5†
Nonmediastinal									
Stage I	60	59	1	98	98	1/1†	80	80	1/1†
Stage II	24	21	3	100	100	3/3†	62	67	1/3†

*For values connected by vertical lines, $P < .05$; all other comparisons are not significant.
†No. of patients rather than %.
Reproduced from Hagemeister et al. 1982b.

To summarize, small mediastinal masses with no constitutional symptoms can be treated effectively with radiotherapy alone, and results for IF compare very favorably with those for EF. However, neither EF nor IF radiotherapy alone is sufficient treatment for patients with large masses. While IF plus six MOPP was extremely effective in terms of survival, other approaches are needed because of complications associated with this treatment.

Nonmediastinal Disease

Ninety-five patients had negative chest radiographs. Eight-five presented with upper torso disease (65 had stage I and 20 had stage II). Ten patients with lower torso disease did not have staging laparotomies. Of the 85 patients with upper torso disease, 11 were treated with IF irradiation followed by six MOPP, 36 received IF radiotherapy alone, 17 received treatment to the mantle only, and 21 were treated with EF radiotherapy. The results for these 95 patients were compared in terms of survival and disease-free survival. All 11 patients who were treated with IF radiotherapy and six MOPP are surviving. However, two developed new disease and underwent subsequent rescue therapy. Also, all of the patients who underwent mantle or EF radiotherapy only are surviving. The five-year survival rate for IF treatment was 97%. The disease-free survival figures were 94% for mantle treatment only, 78% for EF, and 67% for IF (Figure 3). However, the only statistically significant difference was between results for the mantle and IF treatments. Also, for patients with stage I disease, the disease-free survival for treatment to the mantle or EF was 96%, as compared to only 61% for stage II. Of the 15 patients with stage II disease, 5 developed new disease. In four patients, the relapse occurred in an extranodal site. This would suggest that the patients with stage II upper torso

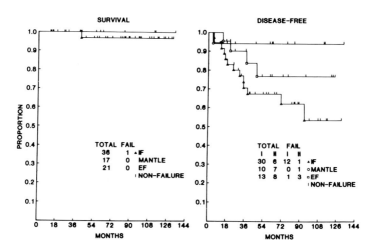

Figure 3. Influence of treatment for Hodgkin's disease patients with laparotomy-staged I and II nonmediastinal, upper torso disease presentations. Treatment includes IF, mantle, and EF. (Reproduced from Hagemeister et al. 1982b, with permission of *Cancer Treatment Reports*.)

disease should receive both chemotherapy and radiotherapy. All patients with lower torso involvement are disease free.

While there were no complications secondary to radiotherapy itself, one patient who received only radiotherapy to the neck, which was followed by six MOPP for stage I disease, developed acute myelogenous leukemia five years after treatment.

To reiterate, in keeping with our policy of effective minimal treatment, we feel that in the light of disease-free survival results for mantle treatment being equal or better than those of EF, treatment for patients with upper torso disease presentations should be limited to mantle radiotherapy, with the possible exception of a minority of patients with stage II disease presentations.

Sterility Due to MOPP

We have recently published a comprehensive summary on what is known about the effects of cytotoxic agents on gonadal tissue and the possible blocking mechanisms (da Cunha et al. 1983). Here, we will limit our discussion to information on MOPP that is pertinent to our current combined modality program for patients with unfavorable presentations of laparotomy-staged I and II Hodgkin's disease.

Our experience with MOPP and its effect on spermatogenesis is somewhat unique in that we have comparative data for men who received six cycles of MOPP and for those who received only two cycles. However, approximately half of the latter group also received radiotherapy to the pelvis. The effects of these different treatments on spermatogenesis were significantly different for a minimum follow-up of 30 months and a maximum of 128 months.

Our findings for six MOPP were in keeping with those of other centers in that 91% of the patients were azospermic. By contrast, 60% of men who received two MOPP but no pelvic irradiation were normospermic, and only 12% were azospermic. The results for those who received two MOPP and pelvic radiotherapy were in between. While only 20% of them were azospermic, only 28% were normospermic. The remainder were oligospermic at the time of last follow up.

While we do not have specific documentation for women, our impression is that recovery from menstrual disturbances after two cycles of MOPP has been prompt, and there have been no known instances of early menopause.

At the present time, we are investigating the use of testosterone in men and a combination of estrogen and progesterone in women to determine whether hormonal manipulation may be useful in preserving gonadal function in patients who are scheduled to receive cytotoxic agents. The possible mechanism for this approach are discussed in our review article (da Cunha et al. 1983).

EFFECTIVE MINIMUM TREATMENT

Our current program for stages I and II Hodgkin's disease was designed to give only the minimum amounts of treatment that are necessary to produce maximum disease-free survival rates and the best possible quality of life. In developing this program, we recognized that patients with favorable disease features clearly require less treatment than those with poor prognostic factors. Because the least amounts of treatment that can be given for upper torso disease are dependent on negative findings of sequential staging, we continue to use lymphangiography and staging laparotomy for all patients with upper torso presentations, with one exception. This is stage IA disease in the high upper neck located in the region of the tail of the parotid or the submaxillary gland. As previously stated, we do not use staging laparotomy for patients with lower torso disease presentations because laparotomy findings seldom change our treatment decisions, which have provided 100% disease-free survival rates.

Our current program for patients with laparotomy-staged I and II upper torso disease is based on: (1) patterns of spread after mantle radiotherapy, particularly for patients with unfavorable mediastinal disease; (2) information on MOPP-induced sterility; (3) information on the effect of two MOPP on the incidence of pulmonary relapse; and (4) information on the effect of low-dose lung irradiation on the incidence of pulmonary relapse. Since the first two factors have been considered previously, only the effect of two MOPP and that of low-dose pulmonary radiation will be discussed.

Our experience in using only two cycles of MOPP has been in a multimodality program of chemotherapy and radiotherapy for the treatment of stage III disease (Rodgers et al. 1981). In this study, we used two cycles of MOPP followed by radiotherapy to the mantle and the entire abdomen, with or without radiotherapy to the pelvis. When we compared our results for patients with stage III mediastinal disease with patients who had stages I and II mediastinal disease and who received only radiotherapy to the mantle or to EF, we found that the incidence of pulmonary relapse for those with stage III disease was approximately half of that for patients with stage II disease. We found no evidence that including irradiation to the hila, with generous margins, helps to prevent pulmonary relapse in patients with mediastinal masses, except for those with actual hilar involvement. We have been impressed, however, with reports from other institutions on low-dose lung irradiation given in combination with definitive treatment to the mantle for patients with prognostically unfavorable mediastinal disease (Lee et al. 1982).

Our current program for patients with laparotomy-staged I and II upper torso disease is to treat those with favorable presentations with mantle irradiation only. This includes all patients with stage I disease with peripheral presentations and patients with small mediastinal masses and no evidence of hilar involvement or constitutional symptoms. However, patients with constitutional B symptoms and those with stage II nonmediastinal upper torso disease, received two MOPP prior to radiotherapy.

Our approach to management of patients with unfavorable mediastinal masses that measure 7.5 cm or more in transverse diameter or have associated hilar disease depends on local symptoms such as cough, pain, or vascular distention. Patients who have no contraindications to an immediate staging laparotomy receive two cycles of MOPP one to two weeks after surgery followed by definitive radiotherapy to the mantle with low-dose radiotherapy to one or both lungs. However, patients with local symptoms or very large mediastinal or neck masses who are deemed unsuitable for immediate surgery receive radiotherapy prior to staging laparotomy. If laparotomy results are negative, the patient is scheduled to receive two MOPP to complete the treatment. Sperm banking is offered to men with adequate sperm counts prior to initiating MOPP.

Management of patients with lower torso disease is based on clinical or diagnostic laparotomy findings. Patients with localized femoral or inguinal presentations and negative lymphangiograms receive hemipelvic radiotherapy only. Those with external iliac disease are treated with the inverted Y field irradiation. (Treatment to the pelvis is followed in one month by radiotherapy to the para-aortic nodes.) Patients with more extensive disease receive two cycles of MOPP followed by sequential radiotherapy to the abdomen and pelvis. Again, a rest of approximately one month is allowed between courses of radiotherapy.

Radiotherapy Techniques

Mantle

The choice of treatment to the mantle alone or to the mantle and one or both lungs depends on the status of the mediastinum as determined by the posterior-anterior and lateral radiographs and CT scanning. Patients with negative findings or small mediastinal masses receive definitive irradiation to the mantle only. Those with disease greater than 7.5 cm or with hilar involvement receive low-dose radiotherapy to one or both lungs in addition to definitive treatment to the mantle.

The dose of radiation to the mediastinum is based on mediastinal disease status at initiation of radiotherapy. Patients with no mediastinal disease, either initially or after two MOPP, as seen on CT scan, receive a tumor dose of 3,500 rad in three and one-half weeks. This is calculated in the coronal plane of the upper mediastinum. Those with mediastinal adenopathy received 4,000 rad in four weeks.

The decision to treat one or both lungs prophylactically is based on the status of the hila and the projection of the mediastinal disease. Treatment to the lungs is delivered at a rate of 80 rad per fraction for a total tumor dose of 1,200 rad, which includes a 10% correction for the pulmonary parenchyma.

To minimize the possibility of complications, as much of the lungs and the left lateral heart border as possible are excluded from definitive treatment. When the disease is confined to the anterior mediastinum and the paratracheal nodes, the major portion of the treatment is delivered through an anterior mantle field at a rate of 200 rad given dose per fraction for a total given dose of 4,000 rad. Separate posterior mediastinal, axillary, and neck fields are irradiated to supplement the doses from the anterior field. This technique provides dose gradients between both the anterior and posterior and the upper and lower mediastinum. However, when the disease extended posteriorly to the paravertebral gutter, treatment is delivered through equally loaded anterior and posterior mantle fields with appropriate shielding to limit the dose to the spinal cord and the heart.

Lower Torso Fields

Techniques for treating the pelvis and para-aortic nodes (inverted Y field) are fairly standard. Our policy is to deliver 150 rad per fraction for a total of 3,000 rad in four weeks.

Our technique for treating the entire abdomen is to use parallel opposed anterior and posterior fields that extend from the dome of the diaphragm to the level between the fourth and fifth lumbar vertebrae.

Treatment is given at a rate of 150 rad tumor dose per day for a total of 3,000 rad in four weeks. From the beginning of treatment, the kidneys are posteriorly shielded with two half-value layers (HVL) of lead to limit the dose they receive to 1,800 rad. The right lobe of the liver is anteriorly and posteriorly shielded with one HVL to reduce the dose it receives to 1,500 rad. We reduce the dose to the liver because of our experience with a significant incidence of hepatitis that occurred when we began using two cycles of MOPP prior to radiotherapy (Rodgers et al. 1981).

Population and Results

To date, we have entered 59 patients in our new study. Of 41 patients with mediastinal disease involvement, 26 were classified as having favorable presentations and 15 as having adverse features. Among the nonmediastinal group, 12 had upper torso disease presentations and 6 had lower torso disease. These patients have been followed up for a maximum of three years (Figure 4). All 59 patients are surviving. The projected five-year disease-free survival figure is 89%. Three patients each had a solitary relapse. In two patients with mediastinal involvement, the disease recurred in the lung in one and the abdomen in the other. One nonmediastinal patient suffered a relapse in bone.

To date, there have been no major complications, including pericarditis, pneumonitis, or acute myelogenous leukemia.

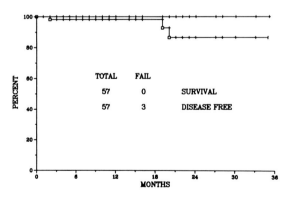

Figure 4. Survival and disease-free survival results for the current treatment program at UT M. D. Anderson Hospital (see text for description of treatment program).

CONCLUSIONS

Currently, management programs for stages I and II Hodgkin's disease vary significantly among major institutions regardless of constitutional symptoms. The most common approach for patients with no constitutional symptoms continues to be sequential staging including laparotomy and followed by EF radiotherapy. However, at least one major institution, which does not use laparotomy, advocates treating all patients with chemotherapy and radiotherapy (Andrieu and Julien 1983, Koziner et al. 1981).

We have described an approach for giving effective minimum treatment that is based on negative laparotomy findings and retrospective information on clinical behavior for patients with laparotomy-staged disease who were treated with IF or mantle radiotherapy. Results for these different approaches can be approximately the same in terms of 5- and 10-year survival rates and, possibly, ultimate survival. Although disease-free survival figures may vary somewhat, with careful follow-up and appropriate rescue treatment, the freedom from second relapse can also be approximately the same. However, the quality of life can be significantly different. While adjuvant chemotherapy is indicated for certain clinical presentations of even laparotomy-staged I and II disease, it is questionable whether any of the current programs can be justified for all patients. In our series, one patient with stage I disease who received IF radiotherapy to the neck and six MOPP developed acute myelogenous leukemia five years after treatment. We have had several instances of cardiac failure in older people after treatment with CHOP-Bleo (cyclophosphamide, doxorubicin, vincristine, prednisone, and bleomycin, Rodriguez et al. 1977) for non-Hodgkin's lymphomas.

The advantage of more extensive treatment with either EF radiotherapy alone or with EF and combination chemotherapy is that such treatment can compensate for deficiencies in expertise in those disciplines that are involved in the investigative procedures of sequential staging. The success of truly minimal treatment programs primarily depends on the expertise of the diagnostic radiologist, surgeon, and pathologist in detecting minimal or occult disease during the initial investigative procedures. Since each step in sequential staging is dependent on the interpretation of the preceding procedures, it is essential that the physicians that are involved in staging and treatment function as a team. Otherwise, a truly minimum treatment cannot be safely given.

We have found that a weekly planning clinic is invaluable for review and exchange of information. This clinic is attended by representative members of the various disciplines. Data for all new patients are presented for discussion relative to treatment decisions and assignment to the appropriate treatment program.

ACKNOWLEDGMENT

This investigation was supported by grants CA-06294 and CA-16672 awarded by the National Cancer Institute, United States Department of Health and Human Services.

REFERENCES

Andrieu JM, Julien C. 1983. MOPP plus irradiation for Hodgkin's disease (HD), clinical stages (CS) IA to IIIB, 10 years later. (Abstract) Proceedings of the American Society of Clinical Oncology 24:213.

da Cunha MF, Meistrich ML, Saad MF. 1983. Impact of treatment for Hodgkin's disease on the reproductive function of adult patients. Cancer Bulletin 35:233–238.

Hagemeister FB, Fuller LM, Sullivan JA, North L, Velasquez W, Conrad FG, McLaughlin P, Butler JJ, Shullenberger CC. 1981. Treatment of stage I and II mediastinal Hodgkin's disease. Radiology 141:783–789.

Hagemeister FB, Fuller LM, Sullivan JA, Johnston D, North L, Butler JJ, Velasquez WS, Shullenberger CC. 1982a. Treatment of patients with stages I and II nonmediastinal Hodgkin's disease. Cancer 50:2307–2313.

Hagemeister FB, Fuller LM, Velasquez WS, Sullivan JA, North L, Butler JJ, Johnston DA, Shullenberger CC. 1982b. Stage I and II Hodgkin's disease: Involved field radiotherapy versus extended field radiotherapy versus involved field radiotherapy followed by six cycles of MOPP. Cancer Treat Rep 66:789–798.

Hoppe RT. 1983. Stage I-II Hodgkin's disease: Current therapeutic options and recommendations. Blood 62:32–36.

Ibrahim E, Fuller LM, Gamble JF, Jing B, Butler JJ, Gehan E. 1972. Stage I Hodgkin's disease. Comparison of surgical staging with incidence of new manifestations in lymphogram and prelymphogram studied patients. Radiology 104:145–151.

Koziner MD, Braun D, Myers J, Nisce L, Poussin-Rosillo H, Straus DJ, Lee BJ, Clakson BS. 1981. Combined modality of MOPP chemotherapy and radiotherapy for the treatment of stages I and II Hodgkin's disease. *In* Salmon SE, Jones SE, eds., Adjuvant Therapy of Cancer III. Grune and Stratton, New York, pp. 77–84.

Lee CKK, Bloomfield CD, Levitt SH. 1982. Results of lung irradiation for Hodgkin's disease patients with large mediastinal masses and/or hilar disease. Cancer Treat Rep 66:819–826.

Rodgers RW, Fuller LM, Hagemeister FB, Johnston DA, Sullivan JA, North LB, Butler JJ, Velasquez WS, Conrad FG, Shullenberger CC. 1981. Reassessment of prognostic factors in stage IIIA and IIIB Hodgkin's disease treated with MOPP and radiotherapy. Cancer 47:2196–2203.

Rodriquez V, Cabanillas F, Burgess MA, McKelvey EM, Valdivieso M, Bodey GP, Freireich EJ. 1977. Combination chemotherapy ("CHOP-Bleo") in advanced (non-Hodgkin) malignant lymphoma. Blood 49:325–333.

Vlasak MC, Martin RG, Fuller LM, Hagemeister FB, da Cunha MF, Shullenberger CC. 1983. Clinical staging of Hodgkin's disease: Results of staging laparotomy. Cancer Bulletin 35:209–214.

UT M.D. Anderson Clinical Conference on Cancer,
Vol. 27, edited by R.J. Ford, L.M. Fuller, and
F.B. Hagemeister. Raven Press, New York © 1984.

Development of Management Policies for Patients with Clinical Stages I and II Hodgkin's Disease

Daniel E. Bergsagel, Mary Gospodarowicz,* Simon Sutcliffe,†
Thomas C. Brown,† Theresa Chua,‡ and Raymond S. Bush**

*Departments of Medicine, *Radiation Oncology, †Pathology, ‡Biostatistics, and
**Director, Princess Margaret Hospital, Toronto, Ontario M4X 1K9, Canada*

Radiation therapy is widely regarded as the treatment of choice for most patients with early-stage Hodgkin's disease (HD). Disease-free survival is improved by extending the radiation fields (Hellman et al. 1978, Kaplan 1980, Hoppe et al. 1982, Hodgkin's Disease Collaborative Trial 1976) and adding combination chemotherapy (Hoppe et al. 1982, Hagemeister et al. 1982, Nissen and Nordentoft 1982) but without any improvement in overall survival. We have been reluctant to treat all early-stage HD patients with total nodal irradiation and combination chemotherapy because of the acute and chronic toxicity associated with added treatment.

Staging laparotomy has been advocated as a useful method for identifying patients who require additional treatment because they have HD in the spleen, liver, or abdominal lymph nodes that cannot be detected by clinical staging (CS) methods. An estimate of the potential benefit of a staging laparotomy for patients with CS I and II HD can be derived from Table 1. Kaplan (1980) found that among 100 patients with CS I and II disease, staging laparotomy revealed 20 patients with pathologic stage (PS) IIIA disease and 10 with PS IIIB and IV disease. The relapse-free survival rate (RFS) and overall survival figures reported for these patients with PS disease following treatment with extended field irradiation alone (Hoppe et al. 1982) and added chemotherapy for stages IIIB and IV (Kaplan 1980) are shown in Table 1. The overall results for 100 patients with CS I and II disease following laparotomy, calculated from the results reported for each PS, are 72% relapse free and 79% alive at 10 years. From these figures, we estimated the numbers of patients apparently "cured" by the first treatment.

By comparison, at the Princess Margaret Hospital (PMH) the actual results observed for all patients with CS I and II disease showed a RFS of 61% and a 10-year survival rate of 84%. It will be noted that there is a difference of 11 percentage points in RFS for patients with laparotomy-staged disease over the patients with CS disease but no increase in overall survival. In the Stanford series (Kaplan 1980, Hoppe et al. 1982), as a result of laparotomy, the radiation fields may have been

Table 1. *Results of Laparotomy in Patients with Clinically and Pathologically Staged I and II Disease*

100 Patients with CS I & II Hodgkin's disease	% Alive at 10 yr	% Relapse free at 10 yr	Number "cured" by first treatment	
			XRT	CT ± XRT
Following laparotomy				
PS I and II: 70	84	77	54	—
PS IIIA: 20	70	62	12	—
PS IIIB and IV: 10	65	60	—	6
Summary	79	72	66	6
100 CS I and II at PMH	84	61	61	

Results reported for laparotomy-staged patients from Stanford University (Kaplan 1980, Hoppe et al. 1982), and for clinically staged patients from the Princess Margaret Hospital.

extended for the 20 patients with PS IIIA disease, and chemotherapy was introduced for 10 patients with PS IIIB and IV disease.

We have analyzed our results in the treatment of patients with CS I and II disease in an attempt to define the prognostic factors that identify groups of patients with increased risk of relapse following treatment with radiation alone. The purpose of this paper is to present this analysis and to describe the changes we have introduced in our treatment policies in an attempt to reduce the relapse rate in patients with early-stage HD.

PATIENTS AND METHODS

Patient Population

The medical records of all patients referred to the PMH with diagnoses of HD between January 1, 1968 and December 31, 1977 were reviewed (Bergsagel et al. 1982). All biopsy specimens were examined and classified by Dr. T. C. Brown. Clinical staging, using the Ann Arbor criteria (Carbone et al. 1971), was done on the basis of the initial history and physical examination, chest radiograph, mediastinal tomograms, lymphangiogram, inferior venacavogram or intravenous pyelogram, liver and spleen scans, blood cell counts, and liver function tests.

Laparotomies were required to obtain diagnostic biopsies from 30 patients; in addition, staging laparotomies were done for the 33 patients younger than 17 years. Prior to 1973, laparotomy was part of the standard staging procedure for that age group. Since then, all younger patients have been treated with combination chemotherapy except for a subgroup with favorable CS IA disease (Jenkin et al. 1982). An additional 97 patients underwent laparotomy as part of the evaluation of the clinical patterns of HD (Peters et al. 1973) or because the pathologic extent of disease was considered to be important for treatment planning.

Since we were interested in determining the risk factors that predict relapse for patients with clinically staged disease who were treated with irradiation alone, we selected a subgroup of patients who had initially received only irradiation. Of the 790 patients who were eligible for analysis, we found 466 who were classified as having CS I or II disease. Thus, 214 patients were eliminated from the study for the following reasons: 103 had undergone laparotomy, 90 had received chemotherapy as part of initial treatment, 18 were younger than 17 years and had undergone routine laparotomy, 2 had undergone surgical resections of extranodal pulmonary lesions, and 1 elderly patient received palliative irradiation.

The subgroup, therefore, consisted of 252 patients older than 17 years, who had CS I and II disease, and who were treated initially with x-ray therapy (XRT) alone. Clinical features examined in the 252 XRT-only patients included age, sex, stage, and disease pathology.

Treatment

Of the patients treated with radiation, the majority (72%) received a tumor dose of 3500 cGy in 20 fractions over a four-week period; 21% of patients received doses less than 3500 cGy, and 7% received doses greater than 3500 cGy.

The tumor dose was delivered to the midplane, and compensators were used to reduce the dose variation to $\pm 5\%$. Radiation was delivered on ^{60}Co equipment with extended source-to-surface distance (130 cm). Shielding, compensators, and verification films were used for all patients.

The extend of radiation varied during the ten years covered by the review. Seventy-one patients (28%) received treatment to fields smaller than the upper mantle field or the abdominal inverted-Y field. One hundred thirty patients (52%) received treatment to either the upper mantle or the inverted-Y fields, and 51 patients (20%) received extended field radiation, covering either the upper abdomen or the para-aortic nodes only.

Many of the patients treated during this period were randomized to receive either local or extended radiation in the Canadian-American cooperative study comparing these two types of treatment (Hodgkin's Disease Collaborative Trial 1976). For rescue therapy, irradiation was used for relapses in marginal or solitary sites; chemotherapy, usually CVPP (cyclophosphamide, vinblastine, procarbazine, and prednisone) or MOPP (mechlorethamine, vincristine, procarbazine, and prednisone) was used for patients who suffered recurrence with constitutional B symptoms within previously irradiated areas, or extranodal or multiple sites. Chemotherapy and irradiation were combined for patients with bulky nodal relapses or relapses in extranodal sites, such as bone.

Complete response (CR) was defined as the absence of unexplained fever, night sweats, weight loss, pruritus, and all other biochemical and radiographic evidence of disease on physical examination, for at least four weeks. Patients who showed marked regression of lymph nodes but persistence of small hard nodes or regression of pulmonary infiltrates with persistence of fibrotic scars were judged to be in CR, if these uncertain signs of residual disease remained stable for three months after treatment was discontinued. Responses that did not fulfill the criteria for CR were judged to be inadequate. Biopsy confirmation of recurrent disease was obtained whenever possible, especially if there was doubt about clinical findings.

Survival curves were calculated by the actuarial life-table method. Overall survival rate was measured from the start of treatment to death from any cause. Relapse-free rates (RFR) were measured in patients who achieved CR from the start of initial treatment to the confirmation of relapse of the HD or to death from HD.

The significance of potential prognostic factors was tested first with an unadjusted logrank test. The four important factors (disease pathology, age, clinical stage, and presence of B symptoms) were then analyzed in adjusted logrank tests in which other important factors were controlled (Peto et al. 1977).

RESULTS

The clinical features of the XRT-alone subgroup are shown in Table 2. It will be noted that 34.1% of patients were over the age of 40; the majority presented with CS IIA disease, and only 24 patients (9.5%) had B symptoms.

Treatment

The radiation fields used in treatment of the XRT-alone subgroup and the results of treatment are shown in Table 3. Not shown in Table 3 are 67 patients with

Table 2.. *XRT-Alone Subgroup—*
Clinical Features

	n	%
Age		
17 – 39	166	(65.9)
≥ 40	86	(34.1)
Sex		
Male/female	144/108	
Stage		
IA	86	(34.1)
IB	10	(3.9)
IIA	135	(53.6)
IIAE	7	(2.8)
IIB	14	(5.6)
Pathology		
LP	34	(13.5)
NS	143	(56.7)
MC	65	(25.8)
LD	4	(1.6)
U	6	(2.4)

LP–lymphocyte predominant; NS–nodular sclerosing; MC–mixed cellularity; LD–lymphocyte depletion; U–undifferentiated; XRT–radiation treatment.

Table 3. *Treatment of the XRT-Alone Subgroup of Clinical Stage I and II Hodgkin's Disease Patients*

Radiation fields	CR/Total	(%)	% Relapse-free or alive		
			5 yrs	8 yrs	10 yrs
Local	66/71	(92.9)	59.9*	53. 8*	53.8*
			77.3†	68.2†	62.2†
Regional	125/130	(96.2)	67.2*	62.2*	62.2*
			85.1†	85.1†	85.1†
Extended	46/51	(90.2)	68.3*	68.3*	68.3*
			88.2†	83.9†	83.9†

*RFR.
†Survival from start of therapy (includes all deaths).
CR–complete remission; RFR–relapse-free rate. (See Table 3 for other abbreviations).

Table 4. *Treatment of Clinical Stage I and II Hodgkin's Disease Patients > 17 Years, 1968—1977*

	n	IA %	IIA %	I + IIB %	Mediastinal adenopathy % ⩾ 10 cm
Local XRT	71	64.8	28.2	7.0	4.2
Local and regional XRT	130	28.5	64.6	6.9	6.2
Extended XRT	51	5.9	74.5	19.6	5.9
Combined chemotherapy and XRT	67	10.4	50.7	38.8	37.3

(See Table 3 for abbreviations.)

CS I and II disease treated initially with combined chemotherapy and XRT. The composition of this group is shown in Table 4. It is noteworthy that 25 of the patients treated with chemotherapy and XRT presented with marked mediastinal adenopathy measuring 10 cm or more in width. Of the patients treated with combination chemotherapy (MOPP or CVPP) and XRT, 57 of 67 (85.1%) achieved CR; the RFR was 70.9%, 68.9%, and 68.9% at 5, 8, and 10 years respectively, and the proportion of patients alive for the same years are 79.8%, 77.8%, and 77.8%. The results of these different forms of treatment cannot be compared because the patient groups are so different (Table 4). Extended field irradiation and combined chemotherapy were clearly prescribed more frequently for patients with CS II disease, especially for those with mediastinal adenopathy ⩾ 10 cm and B symptoms, whereas local irradiation was used mainly for patients with CS IA disease.

Prognostic Factors for Relapse

The effect of various prognostic factors on the occurrence of relapses in the XRT-alone subgroup was tested (Tables 5 and 6). The sex of the patient, the

Table 5. *Prognostic Factors for Relapse of Clinical Stage I and II Hodgkin's Disease Patients Following Radiotherapy*

	No. of patients	8 Yr RFR %	Unadjusted logrank	
			RFR Observed/expected	P for trend
Sex				
Male	144	60.7	1.02	} 0.93
Female	108	61.9	0.98	
Diaphragm				
Above	228	62.3	0.96	} 0.36
Below	24	51.5	1.37	
Mediastinum				
Not involved	152	62.1	1.01	} >0.99
Adenopathy <10 cm	86	61.6	0.96	} 0.68
Adenopathy ⩾10 cm	14	50.0	1.25	

RFR–relapse-free rate.

Table 6. *Significant Prognostic Factors for Relapse of Clinical Stage I and II Hodgkin's Disease Patients Following Radiotherapy*

	Adjusted logrank	
	RFR Observed/expected	P for trend
Pathology		
LP/NS	0.80	} 0.0007
MC/LD	1.62	
Age		
<50	0.87	} 0.006
⩾50	1.61	
Stage		
IA + B	0.74	} 0.02
IIA + B	1.21	
Symptoms		
A	0.94	} 0.04
B	1.83	

RFR–relapse-free rate. (See Table 3 for other abbreviations.)

occurrence of the disease above or below the diaphragm, and the involvement of the mediastinum were not found to affect the RFR (Table 5). Univariate analysis showed that the RFR for patients registered between 1973 and 1977 was lower than for those registered in the preceding five years. However, when the logrank analysis was adjusted for age, stage, and disease pathology, the year of registration was found to have no influence on either the RFR or survival.

For patients treated with XRT alone, the pathologic classification of the type of HD, age, stage, and the presence of B symptoms proved to be important prognostic factors (Table 6). The risk of relapse was significantly increased for patients with mixed cellularity and lymphocyte-depleted HD, for patients older than 50 years, for patients with CS II disease, and for those with B symptoms. The significance of these factors was maintained when the logrank tests were controlled for the other important prognostic factors.

Relapse Rates in Patient Subgroups

We next constructed a table to compare the relapse rates for subgroups of patients divided on the basis of disease pathology, age, clinical stage, and the presence of B symptoms (Table 7). From this table, we identified subgroups of patients with low, intermediate, and high risks of relapse. In the low-risk group, relapses occurred in 49 of 171 patients (28.7%), in 19 of 42 patients (45.2%) in the intermediate-risk group, and in 24 of the 33 patients (72.7%) in the high-risk group.

Discussion

The factors predictive of relapse in HD are determined by many influences such as the composition of the patient study group and the treatment policies employed. It is difficult, therefore, to generalize about relapse prognostic factors for early stage HD. There is general agreement that relapse rates are higher in patients with stage II disease than in those with stage I (Hoppe et al. 1982, Hagemeister et al. 1982, Fuller and Hutchison 1982, Nissen and Nordentoft 1982) and that the risk of relapse is increased in patients with gross mediastinal adenopathy who are treated with XRT alone (Hoppe et al. 1982, Hagemeister et al. 1982, Nissen and Nordentoft 1982, Fuller and Hutchison 1982, Mauch et al. 1978, Thar et al. 1979, Lee et al. 1982). Treatment of patients who have gross mediastinal adenopathy with combination chemotherapy and XRT lowers the risk of relapse (Hoppe et al. 1982, Hagemeister et al. 1982, Nissen and Nordentoft 1982, Lee et al. 1982) and reduces the significance of a widened mediastinal adenopathy as a predictor of relapse.

Table 7. *Relapse Rates for 246* Patients with Clinical Stage I and II Hodgkin's Disease Treated with XRT Alone*

| Age | Pathology | Relapses/total (%) | | |
		IA	IIA	I + IIB
<50	LP/NS	12/46 (26.1)**	29/88 (32.9)**	3/13 (23.1)**
	MC/LD	3/10 (30.0)**	13/30 (43.3)†	6/6 (100.0)‡
≥50	LP/NS	2/14 (14.3)**	6/12 (50.0)†	3/4 (75.0)‡
	MC/LD	7/12 (58.3)‡	8/11 (72.7)‡	—‡

*Six patients with unclassified HD not included.
**Low risk, 49/171 (28.7).
†Intermediate risk, 19/42 (45.2).
‡High risk, 24/33 (72.7).
(See Table 3 for abbreviations.)

In our series of 252 CS I and II patients treated with XRT alone, 7 of 14 patients with mediastinal adenopathy ≥ 10 cm have relapsed. Although this is a high relapse rate, this degree of mediastinal adenopathy did not prove to be a significant predictor of relapse because the number of patients treated with XRT alone was small. We treated most patients who had mediastinal adenopathy ≥ 10 cm with combination chemotherapy and XRT (Table 4).

FUTURE TREATMENT PLANS

Based on the subgroups that we have identified as having low, intermediate, and high risks of relapse, we have developed our policies for treatment of CS I and II HD. Treatment for patients with disease above the diaphragm are shown in Table 8 and for those with disease below the diaphragm are shown in Table 9.

Patients who present with solitary involvement of nodes in the upper neck (above the notch of the thyroid cartilage) have good prognoses. We will continue to treat these patients regardless of age or pathologic classification using involved field XRT at 3500 cGy in 20 fractions.

Table 8. *Treatment Policies for Supradiaphragmatic Clinical Stages I and II Hodgkin's Disease Patients*

		IA			
Age	Pathology	Upper neck only	All others	IIA	I and IIB
<50	LP/NS MC/LD	Involved Field	Exclude mediastinum ≥10 cm		
			Upper mantle and upper abdomen XRT		
≥50	LP/NS MC/LD	XRT			MOPP × 3
			+ Upper mantle + upper abdomen XRT		

MOPP to adequate control + 3500 cGy/20 to nodal areas + 1750 cGy/20 (corrected) to both lungs.
(See Table 3 for abbreviations.)

Table 9. *Treatment Policies for Infradiaphragmatic Clinical Stage I and II Hodgkin's Disease Patients*

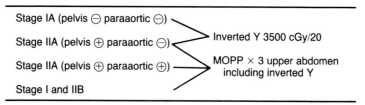

Stage IA (pelvis ⊖ paraaortic ⊖)
Stage IIA (pelvis ⊕ paraaortic ⊖) → Inverted Y 3500 cGy/20
Stage IIA (pelvis ⊕ paraaortic ⊕) → MOPP × 3 upper abdomen including inverted Y
Stage I and IIB

All patients with mediastinal adenopathy ≥ 10 cm will be treated with MOPP until adequate tumor regression is achieved; at least three courses of MOPP will be used. This will be followed by 3500 cGy in 20 fractions to the upper mantle plus 1750 cGy (correction for lung density as measured by computed tomographic lung scans) in 20 fractions to the lungs.

Other patients with low and intermediate risks of relapse will be treated with upper mantle (3500 cGy in 20 fractions) and upper abdominal radiation. The upper abdominal field will extend from the lower plate of the ninth dorsal vertebra (or a point matching the inferior border of the upper mantle field) to a line joining the superior border of the iliac crests and will cover the full width of the abdomen. The para-aortic region will receive 3500 cGy in 20 fractions midplane. The right and left lateral fields will be treated with 2000 cGy in 20 fractions. Individualized shielding of the left kidney will be used if doses of more than 2000 cGy are required for the treatment of the spleen and splenic pedicle.

The group at high risk to relapse will be treated initially with three courses of MOPP followed by irradiation to the upper mantle and upper abdomen, using the fields described above. The dose of irradiation will be reduced to 2000 cGy in 20 fractions to the upper mantle and the para-aortic region of the upper abdominal field.

The treatment policies for infradiaphragmatic presentations are shown in Table 9. Patients with CS IA disease with involvement of femoral or inguinal nodes and negative lymphangiogram will receive 3500 cGy in 20 fractions to an inverted-Y field extending from the lower plate of the ninth dorsal vertebra to include the inguinal and femoral nodes on both sides.

Patients with involved para-aortic nodes or B symptoms will be treated initially with three courses of MOPP, to be followed by irradiation to the upper abdomen and the para-aortic and pelvic nodes. A dose of about 3000 cGy will be delivered in 20 fractions to retroperitoneal and pelvic nodes with lateral attenuation of the upper abdominal field so that both lateral fields receive about 2000 cGy in 20 fractions.

Two treatment options are available for patients with CS IIA disease and involved pelvic nodes but with normal para-aortic nodes. These patients may be treated with either irradiation to an inverted-Y field or combined MOPP and irradiation, as described above.

We hope that these treatment policies will reduce the relapse rate for all patients. Careful adherence to these policies will allow us to identify patients with localized disease who require chemotherapy in addition to XRT and to define the effectiveness of abdominal irradiation in the control of upper abdominal disease.

REFERENCES

Bergsagel DE, Alison RE, Bean HA, Brown TC, Bush RS, Clark RM, Chua T, Dalley D, DeBoer G, Gospodarowicz M, Hasselback R, Perrault D, Rideout D. 1982. Results of treating Hodgkin's disease without a policy of laparotomy staging. Cancer Treat Rep 66:717–731.
Carbone PP, Kaplan HS, Musshoff H. 1971. Report of the Committee on Hodgkin's disease staging. Cancer Res 31:1860–1861.

Fuller LM, Hutchison GB. 1982. The collaborative clinical trial for Stage I and II Hodgkin's disease: significance of mediastinal and non-mediastinal disease in laparotomy and non-laparotomy-staged patients. Cancer Treat Rep 66:775–787.

Hagemeister FB, Fuller LM, Velasquez WS, Sullivan JA, North L, Butler JJ, Johnston DA, Shullenberger CC. 1982. Stage I and II Hodgkin's disease: Involved field radiotherapy versus extended field radiotherapy versus involved-field radiotherapy followed by six cycles of MOPP. Cancer Treat Rep 66:789–798.

Hellman S, Mauch P, Goodman RL, Rosenthal DS, Moloney WC. 1978. The place of radiation therapy in the treatment of Hodgkin's disease. Cancer 42:971–978.

Hodgkin's Disease Collaborative Trial. 1976. Survival and complications of radiotherapy following involved and extended field therapy of Hodgkin's disease, stages I & II. Cancer 38:288–305.

Hoppe RT, Coleman CN, Cox RS, Rosenberg SA, Kaplan HS. 1982. The management of Stage I-II Hodgkin's disease with irradiation alone or combined modality therapy: the Stanford experience. Blood 59:455–465.

Jenkin D, Chan H, Freedman M, Greenberg M, Gribbin M, McClure P, Saunders F, Sonley M. 1982. Hodgkin's disease in children: treatment results with MOPP and low-dose extended-field irradiation. Cancer Treat Rep 66:949–959.

Kaplan HS: 1980. Hodgkin's Disease, Ed. 2. Harvard University Press, Cambridge, MA, p. 689.

Lee CKK, Bloomfield CD, Levitt SH. 1982. Results of lung irradiation for Hodgkin's disease patients with large mediastinal masses and/or hilar disease. Cancer Treat Rep 66:819–825.

Mauch P, Goodman R, Hellman S. 1978. The significance of mediastinal involvement in early stage Hodgkin's disease. Cancer 42:1039–1045.

Nissen NI, Nordentoft AM. 1982. Radiotherapy versus combined modality treatment of Stage I and II Hodgkin's disease. Cancer Treat Rep 66:799–803.

Peters MV, Brown TC, Rideout DR. 1973. Prognostic influences and radiation therapy according to patterns of disease. JAMA, 223:53–59.

Peto R, Pike MC, Armitage P, Breslow N, Cox DR, Howard SV, Mantel N, McPherson K, Peto J, Smith PG. 1977. Design and analysis of randomized clinical trials requiring prolonged observation of each patient. II Analysis and examples. Br J Cancer 35:1–39.

Thar TL, Million RR, Housner RJ, McKetty MH. 1979. Hodgkin's disease, Stages I and II, relationship of recurrence to size, radiation dose and number of sites involved. Cancer 43:1101–1105.

Therapy for Advanced Hodgkin's Disease

UT M.D. Anderson Clinical Conference on Cancer,
Vol. 27, edited by R.J. Ford, L.M. Fuller, and
F.B. Hagemeister. Raven Press, New York © 1984.

The Use of Two MOPP and Radiotherapy for the Treatment of Stages IIIA and IIIB Hodgkin's Disease

Fredrick B. Hagemeister and Lillian M. Fuller*

*Departments of Hematology and *Radiotherapy, The University of Texas, M.D. Anderson
Hospital and Tumor Institute at Houston, Houston, Texas 77030*

The optimal treatment of stage III Hodgkin's disease continues to be controversial. Good results for patients without constitutional symptoms have been reported by various investigators who use a variety of programs ranging from total nodal irradiation, to chemotherapy only, to varying combinations of both. However, it has been difficult to compare results among institutions because of the use of different staging techniques and irradiation fields and the various types, amounts, and most important, the timing of chemotherapy used (Prosnitz et al. 1978, Rosenberg et al. 1978, Bergsagel et al. 1982, Hoppe et al. 1982, Stein et al. 1982, Mauch et al. 1983, O'Dwyer et al. 1983).

For patients with stage III disease and constitutional symptoms, the choices for therapy have been more restricted. Most investigators have continued to recommend primarily chemotherapy for patients with stage IIIB disease, because of the poor results reported using irradiation alone by the Stanford University group in the late 1960s (Rosenberg et al. 1978), and the encouraging results of 50% to 60% freedom from tumor mortality reported using MOPP (mechlorethamine, vincristine, procarbazine, and prednisone) alone (DeVita et al. 1980). More recently, some have returned to irradiation as a treatment modality in combination with chemotherapy in order to improve results (Prosnitz et al. 1982, Young et al. 1982, Santoro et al. 1983).

In 1965, our treatment plan for both stages IIIA and IIIB Hodgkin's disease was devised, using COP (cyclophosphamide, vincristine, prednisone) prior to irradiation (Gamble et al. 1971). In 1970, the protocol was changed to include two cycles of MOPP chemotherapy followed by sequential irradiation to the abdomen, pelvis, and mantle (Rodgers et al. 1981). From 1970 to February 1983, we treated 200 patients with this program. In the current analysis, we present our treatment results with an emphasis on prognostic factors, modifications of treatment technique, and resulting individualization of treatment.

MATERIALS AND METHODS

Staging

Two hundred patients underwent physical examinations, chemical and hemato-logic profiles, and chest radiographs. One hundred ninety-six patients underwent lymphangiography after giving informed consent; four others were allergic to iodine or had significant vascular disease, and abdominal involvement was diagnosed by means of computed tomographic (CT) scan, ultrasound, or laparotomy. Lung tom-ography, CT scan of the abdomen, gallium scanning, and laparoscopy were not routinely performed. One hundred seventeen patients with negative lymphangio-grams underwent staging laparotomy following informed consent. Patients with positive abdominal findings on lymphangiogram or during laparotomy were class-ified as having stages IIIA or IIIB disease, depending on the presence of consti-tutional symptoms. In patients with negative lymphangiograms, irradiation to the upper torso was performed prior to laparotomy because of the presence of signif-icant upper airway narrowing seen on chest radiographs, symptoms of dyspnea or cough, or painful nodal masses. After completion of planned irradiation in these patients, the laparotomy was performed.

TREATMENT PLAN

In the original study, all patients received two cycles of MOPP plus irradiation to the upper two-thirds of the abdomen, to the pelvis, and to the mantle. Treatment techniques have been previously reviewed (Rodgers et al. 1981). In brief, two cycles of MOPP chemotherapy were administered prior to irradiation to patients with positive lymphangiograms and to patients medically suited for laparotomy prior to any therapy. Doses of MOPP were as follows: intravenous mechlorethamine 6 mg/m^2 days 1 and 8, intravenous vincristine 2 mg/m^2 days 1 and 8, p.o. procarbazine 100 mg/m^2 days 1–10, and p.o. prednisone 40 mg/m^2 days 1–10. In these cases, irradiation was begun 28 days after the second cycle of MOPP. For patients with negative lymphangiograms who were unable to undergo laparotomy because of symptoms related to upper torso involvement, irradiation was first given to control disease in the upper torso, then laparotomy was performed. Ten to 14 days after laparotomy, MOPP chemotherapy was begun; after two cycles of MOPP, irradiation to the lower torso was begun.

Most patients in this study received two cycles of MOPP plus mantle, abdominal, and pelvic irradiation. However in 1981, results for the first 99 patients to be treated on this study were published (Rodgers et al. 1981). As a result of that analysis, treatment policy was modified; low-dose lung irradiation was added to the standard mantle field for patients presenting with hilar or large mediastinal involvement (Hagemeister et al. 1981, Lee et al. 1982), pelvic irradiation was omitted for those with celiac axis or splenic but no para-aortic or iliac involvement. Patients with mediastinal plus pelvic involvement (external iliac, femoral, or inguinal disease) were treated with CVPP (intravenous cyclophosphamide 300 mg/m^2 day 1, 8, and

15, intravenous vinblastine 6 mg/m^2 day 1, 8, and 15, P.O. procarbazine 100 mg/m^2 days 1–10, and P.O. prednisone 40 mg/m^2 days 1–10) (Bloomfield et al. 1976). The CVPP was alternated with ABDIC (intravenous doxorubicin 50 mg/m^2 day 1, intravenous bleomycin 5 μ/m^2 day 1 and 5, intravenous dacarbazine 200 mg/m^2 day 1–5, p.o. prednisone 100 mg/m^2 days 1–5, and p.o. chloroethyl cyclohexyl nitrosouria 40 mg/m^2 day 1) (Tannir et al. 1983) similar to our current treatment plan for stage IV disease. These drug combinations were repeated every 28 days. For this last group of patients, irradiation was given after completion of a minimum of eight cycles of chemotherapy. Irradiation was administered to sites of previous bulky disease, predominantly in the mediastinum. Finally, seven patients received six cycles of MOPP instead of abdominal irradiation for stage III$_s$ disease. In all, 139 patients were treated prior to modification of the protocol.

STATISTICAL EVALUATION

Standard patient pretreatment prognostic factors were chosen to determine their effect on complete remission rate, survival, and disease-free survival. The factors included sex, age, histopathologic subtype, lymphangiogram results, constitutional (B) symptoms, and presence of mediastinal involvement with disease. Extent of abdominal disease was also studied; patients with isolated splenic involvement were classified as having stage III$_s$ disease, and those with stage III$_1$ disease had celiac axis involvement but no para-aortic or iliac disease. Patients with para-aortic or common iliac involvement had stage III$_2$ disease, and those classified as having stage III$_3$ disease had external iliac, femoral, or inguinal involvement. This design has been described and was developed to detect differences in results for various subgroups treated with this modality of therapy (Rodgers et al. 1981). Differences in treatment were also analyzed for these subgroups. Features selected for study included elimination of pelvic irradiation for patients with stages III$_s$ or III$_1$, treatment with upper torso irradiation prior to laparotomy for patients with negative lymphangiograms, and the use of low-dose lung irradiation for patients with large mediastinal or hilar disease.

Overall survival and disease-free survival from the onset of therapy were calculated using the Kaplan-Meier method (1958), and differences among subgroups were analyzed according to Gehan's model (1965). Pretreatment factors were also analyzed using the logistic regression method, to detect relationships among these factors and identify the most important determinants of complete remission rate, overall survival, and disease-free survival (Prentice and Kalbefleisch 1979).

RESULTS

Patient Population

Of the 200 patients, 61% had nodular sclerosis, 75% were less than 40 years old, 60% had negative lymphangiograms, and 68% were male. The presence of constitutional symptoms (Table 1) was related to presence of mediastinal involve-

Table 1. *Stage III Hodgkin's Disease.*
Factors Related to Absence or Presence of
Constitutional Symptoms

	IIIA	IIIB	Total
Pathology			
Mixed cellularity	36	34	70
Nodular sclerosis	75	47	122
Other	5	3	8
Age			
< 40 yr	85	64	149
≥ 40 yr	31	20	51
Mediastinal disease			
Absent	53	34	87
Present	63	50	113
Sex			
Male	77	58	135
Female	39	26	65
Lymphangiogram			
Positive	31	48	79
Negative	84	33	117
Not performed	1	3	4
Total	116	84	200

ment with disease and to the positive lymphangiogram, whereas, sex, histology, and age had no bearing on the frequency of constitutional symptoms. When patients were segregated according to abdominal substage, different patterns for patients above and below the age of 40 emerged. The presence of constitutional symptoms for those over 40 was more indicative of stage III_3 disease than for those younger than 40, and the absence of these symptoms correlated strongly with substages III_s, or III_1. For the younger patients, constitutional symptoms were more evenly divided between those with stages III_2 or III_3 disease.

COMPLETE REMISSION

Complete remission was defined as having no evidence of disease after completing all proposed irradiation therapy to disease-involved areas. The complete remission rate for all 200 patients was 89%. This figure was not affected by any pretreatment patient characteristic, including age, sex, constitutional symptoms, presence of mediastinal disease, positive lymphangiogram, histopathology, or extent of disease in the abdomen, or any combination of these factors. By logistic regression, no factor could be detected that would indicate an inferior chance of attaining complete remission. In addition, patients receiving low-dose lung irradiation as a part of treatment for large mediastinal masses or hilar disease and those with stage III_s or III_1 who had pelvic irradiation had no improved response rate compared to patients not receiving adjuvant irradiation. Three of the four patients treated with CVPP/ABDIC entered complete remission. Five of the seven receiving six cycles of MOPP as adjuvant therapy for stage III$_s$ disease entered complete remission and completed all treatment.

Twenty-three patients did not achieve complete remission and nine of these were older than 40 years. Six failed to complete the proposed treatment plan; one developed irradiation hepatitis and two had significant thrombocytopenia, which precluded further therapy. One patient died in a motorcycle accident and two refused to complete upper abdominal irradiation or six cycles of MOPP for splenic disease that was discovered at laparotomy. Fourteen of the 23 patients who did not achieve complete remission had progressive disease and 3 others developed complications with progressive disease following therapy, including thrombocytopenia, pneumonia, and hepatitis. Only 4 of these 23 patients are alive without evidence of active disease and 10 are dead of Hodgkin's disease.

Survival and Disease-Free Survival

Results for all patients treated on this study are demonstrated in Figure 1. The five-year survival for all patients was 83%, and the disease-free survival was 77%. The five-year survival results for those with stage IIIA were 86% compared to 77% for those with stage IIIB, a difference that was not statistically significant (Figure 2). However, patients without constitutional symptoms had a significantly better disease-free survival, 84%, compared to 67% for those with symptoms ($P<.001$).

Patients with mediastinal and stage III$_3$ disease (Med III$_3$) had worse results than those patients with other substages of abdominal disease. The five-year survival for patients with Med III$_3$ was 57%, compared to 87% for other patients with mediastinal involvement ($P<.001$) (Table 2). Five-year disease-free survival figures

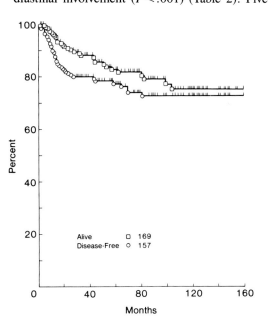

Figure 1. Overall survival and disease-free survival for 200 patients with stage III Hodgkin's disease.

Alive □ 169
Disease-Free ○ 157

Percent

Months

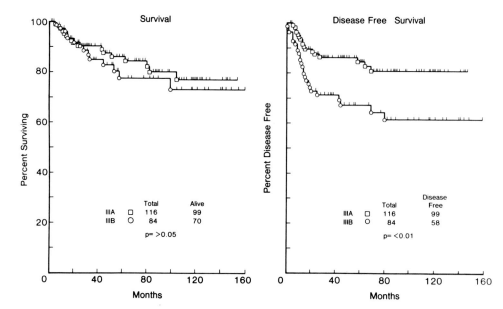

Figure 2. Survival and disease-free survival for patients with stages IIIA and IIIB Hodgkin's disease. There was no difference in curves for survival between these two groups; however, disease-free survival for those without constitutional symptoms was significantly better than for those with B symptoms.

Table 2. *Stage IIIA and IIIB Hodgkin's Disease.*
Survival and Disease-Free Survival Related to Presentation

Patient group	Mediastinal disease		Nonmediastinal disease	
	$III_{s,1,2}$	III_3	$III_{s,1,2}$	III_3
All patients				
Survival	87	57	86	83
Disease-free survival	80	40	89	76
Complete remission patients only				
Survival	92	56	94	85
Disease-free survival	86	41	95	85

were 40% for the Med III_3 group and 80% for the others ($P < .01$). There were no statistical differences in results for mediastinal patients with stages III_s, III_1, or III_2 disease. When we compared results for patients without mediastinal disease, with respect to presence of stage III_3 disease, no differences in abdominal substage could be demonstrated (Table 2). When we considered only the patients who entered complete remission, the same differences in patient subpopulations were observed. The five-year survival for Med III_3 patients entering complete remission was only 56%, compared to 92% for all other patients with mediastinal disease; corresponding values for disease-free survival were 41% and 86% ($P < .001$). For patients without mediastinal disease, results for substage III_3 were similar to those for stages III_s, III_1, or III_2.

Relationship of Patient Prognostic Features

When analyzed separately using Kaplan-Meier curves and Gehan's methods, age over 40, positive lymphangiogram, and mixed cellularity histology were unfavorable prognostic features for survival at five years. However, logistic regression analysis demonstrated that the positive lymphangiogram was the overwhelming adverse factor for survival and was positively correlated with mixed cellularity histology. Age over 40 remained an important factor. When Med III_3 disease was compared with the positive lymphangiogram, Med III_3 alone became the most important predictor of survival. Likewise, for disease-free survival results, presence of constitutional symptoms, the positive lymphangiogram, and Med III_3 disease were important prognostic factors when analyzed independently. When these factors were studied using logistic regression methods, however, Med III_3 disease was the most important prognostic feature, followed by the presence of constitutional symptoms. When only patients entering complete remission were studied, Med III_3 was the most important determinant of survival, and constitutional symptoms and age over 40 played no role for survival in the analysis. However, in the logistic regression analysis for disease-free survival, constitutional symptoms were also important, indicating a somewhat greater tendency for relapse for mediastinal patients with these symptoms and substages III_s, III_1, and III_2.

Because 11 of the 200 patients received chemotherapy other than two cycles of MOPP, we calculated results for the 189 patients treated with only two cycles of MOPP plus irradiation (Figure 3). In this analysis, the five-year survival rate for the 20 patients with Med III_3 disease was 56% compared to 86% for those with other substages ($P = .001$). Disease-free survival figures for the groups were 41% and 83%, respectively ($P < .001$). For patients entering complete remission, survival figures for Med III_3 and other substages were 56% and 92% ($P < .001$). Corresponding disease-free survival figures were 40% and 89% ($P < .001$). Using logistic regression methods, Med III_3 was the most important factor for survival and disease-free survival. Age was important for survival when all patients were considered, but for those entering complete remission, age was not a prognostic feature. Likewise, constitutional symptoms were important for disease-free survival but not for patients entering complete remission.

Treatment Related Factors

Effect of Eliminating Pelvic Irradiation

Ninety-nine patients in this study had either stage III_1 (celiac axis with or without splenic involvement) or stage III_s (splenic disease only) disease. No differences in results for complete remission, overall survival, or disease-free survival could be

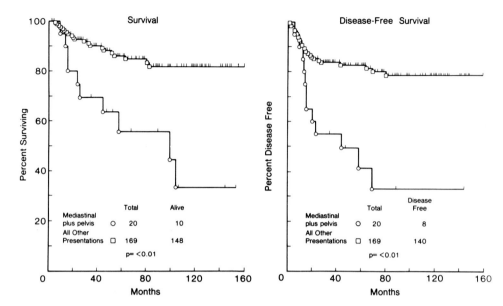

Figure 3. Results for patients with stage III Hodgkin's disease treated with two cycles of MOPP and irradiation. The groups of patients with mediastinal plus pelvic (III_3) disease had a significantly lower survival and disease-free survival than all other groups of patients treated. (See text for components of chemotherapeutic regimen.)

detected between these two groups. Ninety-two of these patients received irradiation to the lower torso as part of their primary treatment; 32 received upper abdominal irradiation alone, and 60 received upper abdominal followed by pelvic irradiation. The five-year survival and disease-free survival for those receiving irradiation to the upper abdomen alone were 96% and 84%. The results were not significantly different from the corresponding results of 87% and 83% for patients receiving upper abdominal and pelvic irradiation.

Effect of Laparotomy After Irradiation to the Upper Torso

In this study, 42 patients with negative lymphangiograms had laparotomies immediately following irradiation to the upper torso. Irradiation was performed because symptoms precluded laparotomy prior to therapy. These patients received MOPP after upper torso irradiation and prior to scheduled abdominal irradiation. Five-year survival for those undergoing irradiation first was 85% compared to 83% for those having staging laparotomy prior to therapy. Disease-free survival results were 87% and 83%.

Effect of Lung Irradiation

Seventy-two patients in this study presented with large mediastinal disease or hilar involvement and each received two cycles of MOPP plus irradiation. Sixty of these patients received irradiation to the mantle as therapy for upper torso involvement, and 12 received additional low-dose lung irradiation, similar to our treatment plan for stages I and II Hodgkin's disease. None of the patients treated with lung irradiation developed disease in the lung as the first site of relapse, whereas eight treated in the mantle field alone have developed pulmonary relapse.

Complications of Therapy

In general, the treatment plan was well tolerated, although complications were more frequent in the first 99 patients treated on this study. There was a tendency for patients to develop myelosuppression during irradiation, occasionally requiring dosage limitation and treatment delays. Thrombocytopenia caused three patients to be unable to complete proposed irradiation, and two of these are dead of progressive Hodgkin's disease. Another patient completed therapy but became pancytopenic and died of sepsis. Infection while on therapy was rare; only one patient developed and was successfully treated for neutropenic fever while on MOPP. Twelve patients developed localized herpes zoster during or within four months of completing all treatment and subsequently recovered.

Although mildly elevated serum hepatic enzymes were often seen during or following treatment, significant hepatitis was noted only in six patients early in the study. This occurred when doses of 2,000 to 2,500 rad were prophylactically used to treat the liver; one patient died of this complication. Following early recognition of this problem, the doses of hepatic irradiation were limited by shielding. Since 1973, there have been only three cases of treatment-related hepatitis and all three patients recovered without sequelae. Two patients developed irradiation pericarditis, and one died of this complication; three developed irradiation pneumonitis, which resolved, and one patient has had documented hypothyroidism.

Significant second malignancies were noted in eight patients; one patient died of adenocarcinoma of the lung and four developed large cell lymphoma. Only one of these patients is currently alive without disease. Three patients died of acute myelogenous leukemia at 44, 51, and 104 months, and one had evidence of Hodgkin's disease in the bone marrow, the only site of relapse. The other two patients were continuously free of disease after completing the original treatment for their Hodgkin's disease.

DISCUSSION

Treatment of Hodgkin's disease has become so successful that many investigators have turned their attention to decreasing toxicity of therapy. Attempts have included elimination of the staging laparotomy and its potential morbidity and expense (Bergsagel et al. 1982; Young et al. 1982; Andrieu and Julien 1983), limiting the use of lymphangiography by relying on gallium scans or CT scans of the abdomen (Castellino 1982), and reserving chemotherapy for those patients who demonstrate inferior survival rates after treatment with irradiation only (DeVita 1979, Stein et al. 1982). However, in our series of over 400 staging laparotomies for lymphan-

Table 3. *Current Treatment for Patients with Stages IIIA and IIIB Hodgkin's Disease*

A. Influence of extent of abdominal disease
   1. Celiac or splenic involvement only ($III_{s,1}$): two MOPP plus irradiation to mantle, upper two thirds of abdomen.
   2. Para-aortic or common iliac involvement (III_2): two MOPP plus irradiation to mantle, upper two thirds of abdomen, and pelvis.
   3. Pelvic but without mediastinal involvement ($NMIII_3$): two MOPP plus irradiation to mantle, upper two thirds of abdomen, and pelvis
   4. Patients with mediastinal and pelvic involvement ($MIII_3$): CVPP/ABDIC.
B. All patients with large mediastinal (≥ 7.5 cm in diameter) or hilar involvement receive low-dose XRT to lungs.

See text for components of chemotherapeutic regimens.

giogram-staged I and II Hodgkin's disease, only one patient died of a myocardial infarction in the immediate postoperative period, and serious morbidity, requiring hospitalization was less than 4%. More important, the laparotomies identified those patients needing irradiation only to the upper torso as primary management, and the resulting survival and disease-free survival rates were excellent (Hagemeister et al. 1982). This, combined with the preoperative lymphangiogram, has been a most effective staging system for our purposes.

The use of chemotherapy for treatment of patients with stage IIIA Hodgkin's disease and irradiation for stage IIIB has been debated. More evidence has recently been presented, demonstrating that most patients with stage IIIA disease require the addition of chemotherapy to irradiation in order to improve not only disease-free survival but also survival rates (Mauch et al. 1983). Most patients in this series who were treated with chemotherapy received six cycles; patients with stage III_1 disease had a 10-year survival rate of 96% and a disease-free survival rate of 91%. Those rates were significantly higher than 73% and 47% for similar patients treated with irradiation alone. Patients with lower abdominal disease had worse prognoses than those with stage III_1 disease, regardless of therapy. These conclusions are similar to those reported by Stein (1982).

In our current series, we demonstrate that two cycles of MOPP, if given prior to irradiation in the treatment of stage III Hodgkin's disease, offer an excellent chance of survival and disease-free survival for the majority of patients. However, with this form of treatment, the group of patients presenting with mediastinal and pelvic disease has an inferior survival and disease-free survival compared to the rest of the patients. This is the most important factor for survival and disease-free survival when this treatment is used. Age and constitutional symptoms are important for survival and disease-free survival, respectively, following adverse presentation, but these lose significance for patients entering complete remission.

Second, we have shown that patients with stage III Hodgkin's disease, limited to the celiac axis or spleen, can be treated without pelvic irradiation, as long as two cycles of MOPP are given prior to irradiation. Disease-free survival rates for these patients are excellent with or without the addition of pelvic irradiation. Finally, the majority of these patients tolerate treatment well. The risk of acute leukemia in patients treated for Hodgkin's disease has been previously presented in a large, well-analyzed series (Coltman and Dixon 1982). There was no risk following irradiation alone, but the risk following MOPP was approximately 7% at seven years, regardless of the addition of irradiation. The majority of patients in Coltman and Dixon's series received a minimum of six cycles of MOPP. In our series, only three patients have developed acute myelogenous leukemia.

Our recommendations for treatment of patients with stage III Hodgkin's disease are shown in Table 3. We currently stage disease by means of lymphangiography and chest radiographs. If the lymphangiogram is negative, a laparotomy is performed. For patients unable to undergo laparotomy because of threatening upper torso disease, irradiation to the mantle is given prior to laparotomy. Low-dose pulmonary irradiation is given for those with large mediastinal masses, 7.5 cm or greater in diameter on chest radiograph, and for those with hilar involvement. Patients with positive lymphangiograms and those with positive findings at laparotomy are treated with two cycles of MOPP plus irradiation to areas outlined in Table 3. Patients with the combination of mediastinal and pelvic disease are treated on our current stage IV protocol, CVPP/ABDIC. Longer follow-up is needed to determine whether any treatment modification can improve results for this group of patients.

REFERENCES

Andrieu JM, Julien C. 1983. MOPP plus irradiation for Hodgkin's disease (HD), Clinical stages (CS) IA to IIIB, 10 years later. (Abstract) Proceedings of the American Society of Clinical Oncology 24:213.

Bergsagel DE, Alison RF, Bean HA, Brown TC, Bush RS, Clark RM, Chua T, Dalley D, DeBoer G, Gospodarowicz M, Hasselback R, Perrault D, Rideout DF. 1982. Results of treating Hodgkin's disease without a policy of laparotomy staging. Cancer Treat Rep 66:717–732.

Bloomfield CD, Weiss RB, Fortuny I, Vosika G, Kennedy BJ. 1976. Combined chemotherapy with cyclophosphamide, vinblastine, procarbazine, and prednisone (CVPP) for patients with advanced Hodgkin's disease. Cancer 38:42–48.

Castellino RA. 1982. Imaging techniques for staging abdominal Hodgkin's disease. Cancer Treat Rep 66:697–700.

Coltman CA Jr., Dixon DO. 1982. Second malignancies complicating Hodgkin's disease: A Southwest Oncology Group 10-year followup. Cancer Treat Rep 66:1023–1034.

DeVita VT, Jr. 1979. The role of combined modality therapy in the treatment of stage IIIA Hodgkin's disease. Int J Radiat Oncol Biol Phys 5:913–914.

DeVita VT, Simon RM, Hubbard SM, Young RC, Berard CW, Moxley JH III, Frei E III, Carbone PP, Canellos GP. 1980. Curability of advanced Hodgkin's disease. Ann Intern Med 92:587–595.

Gamble JF, Fuller LM, Butler JJ, Shullenberger CC. 1971. Combined chemotherapy and radiotherapy for advanced Hodgkin's disease and reticulum cell sarcoma: A preliminary report. South Med J 64:775–783.

Gehan EA. 1965. A generalized Wilcoxon test for comparing arbitrarily singly-censored samples. Biometrika 52:203–223.

Hagemeister FB, Fuller LM, Sullivan JA, Johnston D, North L, Velasquez WS, Shullenberger CC. 1982. Treatment of patients with stages I and II non-mediastinal Hodgkin's disease. Cancer 50:2307–2313.

Hagemeister FB, Fuller LM, Sullivan JA, North L, Velasquez WS, Conrad FG, McLaughlin P, Butler JJ, Shullenberger CC. 1981. Treatment of stage I and II mediastinal Hodgkin's disease. Radiology 141:783–789.

Hoppe RT, Cox RS, Rosenberg SA, Kaplan HS. 1982. Prognostic factors in pathologic stage III Hodgkin's disease. Cancer Treat Rep 66:743–750.

Kaplan EL, Meier P. 1958. Nonparametric estimation from incomplete observations. Journal of the American Statistical Association 53:457–481.

Lee CKK, Bloomfield CD, Levitt SH. 1982. Results of lung irradiation for Hodgkin's disease patients with large mediastinal masses and/or hilar disease. Cancer Treat Rep 66:819–826.

Mauch PM, Rosenthal DS, Canellos GP, Hellman S. 1983. Improved survival for stage IIIA and IIIB Hodgkin's disease patients treated with combined radiation therapy (RT) and chemotherapy. (Abstract) Proceedings of the American Society of Clinical Oncology 24:213.

O'Dwyer PJ, Wiernik PH, Finlay R, Ungerleuder RS. 1983. A randomized trial of radiotherapy (RI) and MOPP (C) vs MOPP alone for stages IB-IIIA Hodgkin's disease. (Abstract) Proceedings of the American Society of Clinical Oncology 24:214.

Prentice RL, Kalbefleisch RD. 1979. Hazard rate models with covariates. Biometrics 35:25–29.

Proznitz LR, Farber LR, Kapp DS, Bertino JR, Nordlund M, Lawrence R. 1982. Combined modality therapy for advanced Hodgkin's disease: Long term follow-up data. Cancer Treat Rep 66:871–880.

Prosnitz LR, Rafael MD, Montalvo L, Fischer DB, Silberstein AB, Berger DS. 1978. Treatment of stage IIIA Hodgkin's disease: Is radiotherapy alone adequate. Int J Radiat Oncol Biol Phys 4:781–787.

Rodgers RW, Fuller LM, Hagemeister FB, Johnston DA, Sullivan JA, North L, Butler JJ, Velasquez WS, Conrad FG, Shullenberger CC. 1981. Reassessment of prognostic factors in stage IIIA and IIB Hodgkin's disease treated with MOPP and radiotherapy. Cancer 47:2196–2203.

Rosenberg SA, Kaplan HS, Glatstein EJ, Portlock CS. 1978. Combined modality therapy of Hodgkin's disease. Cancer 42:991–1000.

Santoro A, Viviani S, Zucali R, Ragni G, Confante V, Valagussa P, Banfi A, Bonadonna G. 1983. Comparative results and toxicity of MOPP vs ABVD combined with radiotherapy (RT) in PS IIB, III (A,B) Hodgkin's disease (HD). (Abstract) Proceedings of the American Society of Clinical Oncology 24:223.

Stein RS, Golomb HM, Wiernik PH, Mauch P, Hellman S, Ultmann JE, Rosenthal DA, Flexner JM. 1982. Anatomic substages of stage IIIA Hodgkin's disease: Followup of a collaborative study. Cancer Treat Rep 66:733–742.

Tannier N, Hagemeister FB, Velasquez WS, Cabanillas F. 1983. Long-term follow-up with ABDIC salvage chemotherapy of MOPP-resistant Hodgkin's disease. Journal of Clinical Oncology 1:432–439.

Young CW, Straus DJ, Myers J, Passe S, Nisce LZ, Lee BJ, Koziner B, Arlin Z, Kempin S, Gee T, Clarkson BD. 1982. Multidisciplinary treatment of advanced Hodgkin's disease by an alternating chemotherapeutic regimen of MOPP/ABVD and low-dose radiation therapy restricted to originally bulky disease. Cancer Treat Rep 66:907–914.

UT M.D. Anderson Clinical Conference on Cancer,
Vol. 27, edited by R. J. Ford, L. M. Fuller, and
F. B. Hagemeister. Raven Press, New York © 1984.

The Importance of Adjuvant Irradiation in the Management of Advanced Hodgkin's Disease

Leonard R. Prosnitz and Daniel S. Kapp*

*Division of Radiation Oncology, Duke University Medical Center, Durham, North Carolina 27710; and *Department of Therapeutic Radiology, Yale University School of Medicine, New Haven, Connecticut 06510*

The introduction of combination chemotherapy for the management of advanced Hodgkin's disease has resulted in a significant improvement in the outlook for patients with the disease (DeVita et al. 1980). Complete remissions are now accomplished with a variety of drug combinations in 55%–85% of advanced Hodgkin's disease patients (Cooper et al. 1980, Durant et al. 1978, Glick et al. 1982). Nevertheless, relapse remains a major problem; 35%–60% of those patients entering complete remission subsequently have reappearance of their Hodgkin's disease. A sustained second complete remission following relapse from the first complete remission is rare. Thus, the death rate resulting from Hodgkin's disease in patients treated with chemotherapy alone was 50%–65%, in the studies quoted above and in almost all other reports as well.

The effectiveness of combination chemotherapy varies inversely with the overall tumor cell burden; the chance of curing the patient is greatest when that burden is small. Therefore, chemotherapy is expected to be most effective against subclinical disease, and likely sites of relapse would be areas where clinically evident disease had been present initially (Fischer and Papac 1972). Since radiotherapy is an effective cytotoxic agent in Hodgkin's disease, its administration, following chemotherapy, to areas involved with Hodgkin's disease at the time of diagnosis might prevent relapse and increase the overall cure rate. Since some cell kill is achieved by the chemotherapy alone, only a low dose of radiation therapy is necessary (1500–2500 rad) rather than the dose necessary for local control when radiotherapy is the only treatment modality (3500–4000 rad).

Based on these concepts, a program of combined modality therapy was initiated at Yale University and affiliated institutions in 1969 for all patients with advanced Hodgkin's disease. These results have been reported (Prosnitz et al. 1976, Farber et al. 1980, Prosnitz et al. 1982). Additional 10-year follow-up data will be described in this chapter.

MATERIALS AND METHODS

All patients with newly diagnosed stages IIIB, IVA or IVB Hodgkin's disease seen at Yale University from 1969 to 1981 were included in this study. Patients who initially presented with early stage disease, received curative radiotherapy, and subsequently relapsed were also treated with the combined modality therapy program at the time of relapse. There were no exclusions because of age or general medical condition. Other selected categories of patients with Hodgkin's disease who were treated with combined modality therapy at the onset, including those with IIIA disease or large mediastinal masses or children, were not included but will be the subject of a separate report. Patients who received prior chemotherapy were excluded.

Disease in these patients was staged according to the Ann Arbor system. Disease was restaged and classified according to the Ann Arbor system in relapsing patients, and the letter R was added before the staging numerals. The staging evaluation was extensive in order to determine, as precisely as possible, the full anatomic extent of disease to facilitate subsequent planning of radiation therapy. The usual blood studies were obtained. Chest radiographs and tomographic studies, in the presence of a mediastinal mass, were done, lymphangiography with simultaneous intravenous pyelography, gallium and liver-spleen scans, bilateral iliac crest bone marrow aspiration and biopsy, needle biopsy of the liver and, more recently, computed tomographic (CT) scanning of the abdomen and chest were performed.

In the early years of the study, all patients underwent staging laparotomy, even if they appeared to have stage IV disease, because of our desire to document meticulously the full extent of disease. This policy was subsequently changed after it became apparent that treatment results were the same when the disease was staged with or without laparotomy, i.e., the decision of where to radiate the patient, when made on clinical staging grounds rather than following laparotomy, did not adversely effect the results (Newcomer et al. 1982). Thus, laparotomy is no longer done for patients with clinical stage IIIB disease, for example, those with unequivocally positive lymphangiogram, or those with obvious stage IV disease, for example, positive bone marrow or pulmonary parenchymal disease on chest radiograph. A full clinical evaluation of the abdomen, however, including lymphangiography and CT scan was carried out, even in those patients with obvious stage IV disease, for the purpose of determining subsequent radiation therapy portals. Almost all patients who entered the study after curative radiotherapy followed by relapse had undergone staging laparotomy at the time of diagnosis. Of the 76 relapsing patients who entered the study, only 5 had laparotomies at the time of entry. Fifty-three of the 84 patients with newly diagnosed disease had laparotomies at the time of diagnosis and entry into the treatment protocol.

Drug Therapy

Three different drug programs have been used in this study. At the onset in 1969, a five-drug combination MVVPP (mechlorethamine, vincristine, vinblastine, procarbazine, and prednisone) was used (Table 1). This program is very similar to the MOPP (mechlorethamine, vincristine, procarbazine, and prednisone) combination, but over six months, MVVPP delivers approximately 25% less mechlorethamine, 33% less procarbazine and vincristine but adds 50% more prednisone as well as vinblastine.

MVVPP was the drug combination used exclusively from 1969 to 1978. In 1978, a study directly comparing MVVPP with MOPP was undertaken. Patients were randomly assigned to either combination; both groups received involved-field low-dose radiation therapy. In addition, by 1978 it had been recognized that patients older than 40 years and those with multiple extranodal sites of involvement were considered "poor-risk" patients within the overall group of advanced stage disease patients. They had only a 50% chance of obtaining complete remission compared with 90% for "good-risk" patients with advanced stage disease. The poor-risk patients were started on a treatment program consisting of MOPP plus ABVD (doxorubicin, bleomycin, vinblastine, and dacarbazine) and low dose irradiation. The MOPP schedule followed was the same one described by DeVita et al. (1970). The ABVD schedule was outlined by Bonadonna et al. (1979) and consisted of 25 mg/m^2 of doxorubicin, 6 mg/m^2 of vinblastine, 10 mg/m^2 of bleomycin and 375 mg/m^2 of dacarbazine; all drugs were administered intravenously on days 1 and 15 of the cycle.

Patients were initially treated for six months with combination chemotherapy following which they underwent complete reevaluations of the disease status. This included appropriate radiographic and laboratory studies, and new biopsies of accessible sites of disease that had been involved at the time of diagnosis were also taken. Patients in complete remission then received low-dose radiation therapy. In some patients in partial remission, chemotherapy was continued for another three to four months. In others, in whom residual anatomic changes were thought to represent fibrosis rather than active disease (e.g., residual mediastinal widening), radiotherapy was instituted without additional chemotherapy. Patients who did not

Table 1. *MVVPP Program*

Drug	Days						
	1	8	15	22	29	36	43
Nitrogen mustard (0.4 mg/kg)	x						
Vincristine (1.4 mg/m^2)	x	x	x				
Vinblastine (6 mg/m^2)				x	x	x	
Procarbazine (100 mg/day)				xxxxxxxxxxxxxxxxxxxxxxxxxxxxxx			
Prednisone (40 mg/m^2)	xxxxxxxxxxxx and taper						

MVVPP–mechlorethamine, vincristine, vinblastine, procarbazine, and prednisone initially respond to chemotherapy or had regrowth of disease by the end of six months were treated with a variety of second-line chemotherapeutic programs.

Radiotherapy

Patients in complete remission were treated with radiotherapy directed to all sites of disease that had been clinically identified before chemotherapy was started. Prophylactic irradiation was not given to uninvolved areas; there were a few specific exceptions. If the para-aortic nodes were clinically determined to be involved and laparotomy had not been done, the spleen was irradiated, since splenic disease is very difficult to detect clinically and since the spleen is involved in greater than 75% of patients with disease in the para-aortic nodes. (Prosnitz et al. 1978). If even part of an organ was involved, the entire organ was usually treated, e.g. both lungs were treated even if parenchymal nodules were only demonstrated on one side.

Doses to parenchymal organs were limited to 1500 rad in 10 fractions. Nodal areas received approximately 2000 rad in 150–175 rad fractions; a few patients in partial remission received up to 3000 rad. The latter situation most commonly involved large mediastinal masses. Patients who had been previously irradiated and had relapsed within the treatment field were irradiated again with 1500 rad. In some instances, this raised the total dose to a given area over a period of several years to 4500–6000 rad. The spinal cord was protected using a variety of techniques, but otherwise, no special precautions were taken.

Following completion of radiation therapy, an additional three to four months of chemotherapy was given using the same treatment program that had been used for induction.

Statistical Methods

All patients treated between July 1969 and December of 1980 were evaluated as of July 1983. This comprised a minimum of 30 months of follow-up. All patients were considered evaluable. The data were entered into an IBM 370 computer, and the calculations were carried out by the biostatistics unit of the Yale Comprehensive Cancer Center. Survival and relapse-free survival were calculated from the start of therapy using the Berkson-Gage method (Berkson and Gage 1950). Patients who died of causes other than Hodgkin's disease were scored as alive but censored at the time of the last observation. Calculation of the relapse-free survival was based on the entire patient population at onset of treatment, not just those who achieved complete remission. Cox regression analysis (Cox 1972) was used to evaluate the impact of different prognostic variables. Differences between subgroups were analysed for statistical significance using the Gehan modification of the Wilcoxon method (Gehan 1965).

RESULTS

During the years of the study 160 patients were treated with the combined modality program. The chemotherapy used was MVVPP in 136 patients, MOPP in 12, and MOPP plus ABVD in 12. The treatment outcome is summarized in Table 2. A complete remission was achieved by 132 of 160 patients (82%). Twenty-eight patients were classified as induction failures, including those with no response to chemotherapy, those with disease regression but who had regrowth in subsequent cycles or prior to the onset of radiation, and those who died of drug toxicity during the induction phase (two patients). All of those classified as induction failures, except one patient, have died of their disease.

One hundred thirty-two patients achieved complete remission. One hundred seven remain in complete remission and are alive and well. Eighteen patients have relapsed, six of whom have died of disease, six are alive with disease, and six are alive and apparently free of disease following secondary treatment. Most of those who relapsed and then achieved a second complete remission with additional treatment had very limited disease at the time of relapse, usually confined to a few nodes or nodal areas.

Fatal second malignancies have occurred in six patients. Two patients have developed acute nonlymphocytic leukemia (ANLL), two non-Hodgkin's lymphoma (NHL), one carcinoma of the lung, and one carcinoma of the vulva. Both the lung and vulva tumors were outside of the radiation fields. The relationship of these two lesions to the treatment is unclear. The patient who developed lung carcinoma was a heavy cigarette smoker. One patient, 53 years, with a prior history of heart disease died of a myocardial infarction.

Actuarial survival and relapse-free survival curves are shown in Figure 1. The 10-year survival rate was 78%, and the relapse-free survival was 68%, including all patients started on the protocol, not just those who achieved CR. The follow-up is lengthy; 96 patients were at risk for five years or more and 32 patients were at risk for 10 years or more.

An analysis of the response to therapy by stage of disease, presence or absence of systemic symptoms, age of the patient, sites of involvement, and histology has been carried out. The survival of patients with newly diagnosed advanced stage disease and those who relapsed after failing initial radiation therapy for localized

Table 2. *Summary of Results*

Status	No. of patients
Total treated	160
Complete remission	132
Induction failures (includes 2 drug deaths)	28
Entered complete remission	132
Relapses	18
Acute leukemia	2
Non-Hodgkin's lymphoma	2
Carcinoma of lung	1
Carcinoma of vulva	1
Myocardiaı infarction	1
Remain in complete remission	107

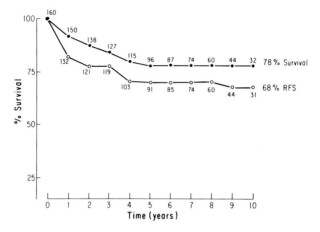

Figure 1. Actuarial survival and relapse-free survival (RFS) of all patients with advanced Hodgkin's disease treated with combined modality therapy.

disease and were then treated with the combined modality protocol is virtually identical, 77% and 78% 10-year survival rates, respectively. Eighty-eight patients had nodular sclerosing disease and 53 had mixed cellularity type, and the outlook was the same for both groups.

The presence of systemic symptoms conveyed a worse prognosis. One hundred one patients had B symptoms; their survival at 10 years was 70% versus 86% for the 59 patients without systemic symptoms ($P<.05$). The 33 patients older than 40 years did significantly worse than their younger counterparts, 52% versus 85% 10-year survival ($P<.01$). Finally, those patients with stage IV disease and multiple extranodal sites of involvement had a significantly worse prognosis than patients with stage IV disease with a single extranodal area involved, 55% versus 81% 10-year survival ($P<.01$).

The results of MOPP plus ABVD and radiation in the previously described poor-risk patients are shown in Figure 2 and compared with an earlier group of poor-risk patients who had been treated with MVVPP and radiotherapy. The survival rate in the former group was 73% at five years compared with 48% in the latter. This may also be contrasted with the good-risk advanced-disease patients (all others) who had an 89% survival at five years (Figure 3).

Complications

The drugs used in our treatment program are all standard agents with well-recognized side effects, both acute and chronic. Nevertheless, two patients died during the induction phase of chemotherapy, both with generalized sepsis, one from pneumococcal septicemia and the other from cryptococcal meningitis. Both patients had undergone splenectomies and were leukopenic at the time infection developed. The frequency of leukopenia, thrombocytopenia, gastrointestinal toxicity, and neurotoxicity with the drug combinations employed has been reported

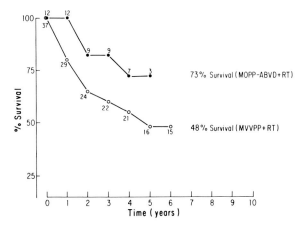

Figure 2. Actuarial survival of poor-risk patients with advanced Hodgkin's disease treated with MOPP plus ABVD and radiation (RT) versus MVVPP and radiation. (See text for components of chemotherapeutic regimens.)

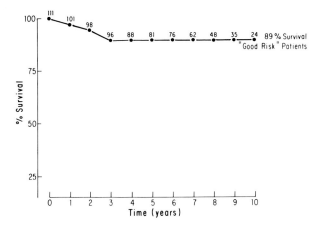

Figure 3. Actuarial survival of all good-risk patients with Hodgkin's disease treated with MVVPP or MOPP plus radiation. (See text for components of chemotherapeutic regimens.)

(Prosnitz et al. 1976) and does not differ significantly from the incidence reported with MOPP and other closely related combinations (DeVita et al. 1980). The addition of radiotherapy after six months of chemotherapy undoubtedly had an adverse effect on the ability to deliver full chemotherapeutic doses in subsequent cycles. The dose reductions necessary in the fourth and fifth cycles of MVVPP have also been described (Prosnitz et al. 1976).

Of more concern are the acute and chronic effects of organ irradiation following chemotherapy. The principal organs radiated were lungs and liver; 30 patients received whole lung irradiation and 10 received liver irradiation. Five of the 30 patients receiving whole lung radiation developed radiation pneumonitis as did two other patients who did not receive whole lung treatment but received mediastinal radiation. All patients recovered fully after receiving brief courses of corticosteroids. One patient developed radiation hepatitis but responded well to corticosteroids.

Serious long-term complications have included 6 fatal second malignancies, as described above, 1 case of thyroid carcinoma, apparently successfully treated with resection, and avascular necrosis of joints in 10 patients (Prosnitz et al. 1981). Sterility has presumably occurred in almost all men and about one half of the women, although we did not specifically assess the frequency of this event.

DISCUSSION

This chapter represents the continued accumulation of follow-up information on our series of advanced-stage Hodgkin's disease patients treated with combined modality therapy. The results have remained essentially the same as the numbers of patients in the series increased and the follow-up period lengthened. The actuarial survival of all patients treated is 78% at 10 years. For those patients who achieved complete remission, it is 95%. It must be emphasized that these are unselected advanced-disease patients thought to represent a cross section of patients seen in the average medical community.

These results appear to represent a significant advance over those achievable with chemotherapy alone. In the NCI series (DeVita et al. 1980), 52% of patients are alive and free of disease at 5 and 10 years corresponding to an 80% complete remission rate, with 35% of those achieving complete remission relapsing subsequently. The results of most other reported series were not as good. The major cooperative groups—Cancer and Leukemia Group B (CALGB), Southeastern Group (SEG), and the Eastern Cooperative Oncology Group (ECOG)—have generally obtained complete remissions ranging from 60%–80%, but relapse rates were from 40%–60%, resulting in five-year disease-free survivals of 30%–50% (Cooper et al. 1980, Durant et al. 1978, Glick et al. 1982). Similar results have been reported from Stanford University with a 74% complete remission rate in 81 MOPP-treated patients, a relapse rate of 45%, and a resulting five-year disease-free survival of 40% (Moore et al. 1973).

Results of treatment with the combined modality approach have now been reported from a number of other centers as well. Bonadonna et al. (1979) compared MOPP and radiation with ABVD and radiation for patients with newly diagnosed advanced-stage disease for those who had failed prior radiotherapy. Complete remission was achieved by 93 (96%) patients after chemotherapy and radiation; the overall relapse rate of those who achieved complete remission was 14% at five years. The authors specifically commented that the results were "almost superimposable" on the Yale University data (Prosnitz et al. 1976).

The Memorial Sloan-Kettering Hospital group reported a trial of MOPP plus ABVD and radiation therapy for patients with newly diagnosed advanced-stage disease (Young et al. 1982). The complete remission rate was 88%, the relapse rate was 16% at four years, and the actuarial survival was 80% at four years. It is of interest that patients who entered this study after failing radiation therapy did not receive the combined modality approach but were treated with chemotherapy only. These patients had a survival rate of 57%, compared to the patients with newly diagnosed disease who had an 80% survival rate. Almost all other studies have shown the prognosis of these two groups to be the same.

Additional support for the combined modality therapy concept comes from the results reported from a number of protocols of CALGB (Bloomfield et al. 1982). For example, in a study comparing patients with stage IIIA disease treated with chemotherapy alone or combined modality therapy, the patients who received BOPP [bis-chloroethyl nitrosouria (BCNU), vincristine, procarbazine, and prednisone] for stage IIIA disease had a 25% five-year disease-free survival rate compared to 80% for those who received total nodal irradiation followed by BOPP. Patients with stages IIIB and IV disease were randomized to receive COPP chemotherapy alone (cyclophosphamide, vinblastine, procarbazine, and prednisone) or chemotherapy plus radiation. The five-year survival rate was 78% in the irradiated patients versus 50% in those receiving chemotherapy alone (Rafla et al. 1982).

Two groups, on the other hand, have failed to demonstrate a clear advantage for combined modality therapy compared with chemotherapy alone. The Southwest Oncology Group (SWOG) compared 3 cycles of bleomycin and MOPP plus involved field radiotherapy to 10 cycles of bleomycin and MOPP for stages IIIA and IIIB disease and found no significant difference between the two. However, there was a suggestion of improved relapse-free survival in irradiated patients (Jones et al. 1982). The difference was significant in favor of irradiated patients with the nodular sclerosing Hodgkin's disease subtype.

A Stanford University trial compared MOPP plus full-dose total nodal irradiation to MOPP alone for stage IV disease (Rosenberg et al. 1978). No organ irradiation was given, so the treatment protocol differed significantly from our program. Fifteen patients received chemotherapy alone; 18 received combined approach. The relapse-free survival rate was approximately 55% at seven years in the combined modality group and 35% in the chemotherapy group, but the difference was not statistically significant.

Another approach to improving the results of combination chemotherapy in the management of advanced Hodgkin's disease has been the use of non–cross-resistant drug combinations. An alternating MOPP and ABVD program was introduced by the Milan group and compared in a randomized trial with MOPP alone (Santoro et al. 1982). The complete remission rate was 71% for the MOPP group and 92% for the MOPP–ABVD-treated patients. Actuarial survival was 36% for the former and 70% for the latter. These results are of considerable interest, but only small numbers of patients have been treated, four patients at risk at five years in one group and three in the other.

In contrast, the SEG compared the use of BCVPP (BCNU, cyclophosphamide vinblastine, procarbazine, and prednisone) plus ABD (doxorubicin, bleomycin and dacarbazine) versus BCVPP alone in a randomized trial. There were no apparent differences (Gams et al. 1979).

It is now well recognized that the treatment of advanced Hodgkin's disease is accompanied by serious long-term complications. Deaths resulting from sepsis during chemotherapy induction, secondary acute leukemias, and non-Hodgkin's lymphomas were all encountered in this series. Their frequencies were similar or less than those reported by other centers. The actuarial frequency of ANLL appears to be approximately 5% at five years (Coltman and Dixon 1982, Glicksman et al. 1982, Pedersen-Bjergaard and Larsen 1982). There is a similar risk of developing a non-Hodgkin's lymphoma (Krikorian et al. 1979). With reference to acute leukemia the three studies mentioned all failed to demonstrate any increased risk for patients receiving combined modality therapy compared to chemotherapy alone, despite earlier reports that suggested that the frequency of ANLL was greater in patients receiving radiation plus chemotherapy (Arseneau et al. 1977).

Other nonfatal long-term complications occurring in our patients were avascular necrosis of bone and sterility. The latter is due largely to chemotherapy; the former has been described in patients treated with chemotherapy alone but may be more frequent with combined modality therapy. It may also be possible to reduce its frequency by careful shielding of joints from radiation therapy fields.

In conclusion, we believe the data indicate a real advantage in adding radiation therapy, in the manner described, to combination chemotherapy for the treatment of advanced Hodgkin's disease. Furthermore, the risk to benefit ratio of using radiation along with chemotherapy seems heavily weighted in favor of this approach. Radiation therapy may be given at the conclusion of six months of chemotherapy, when the patient is in complete remission. Since additional chemotherapy as maintenance is probably unnecessary, one does not have to be concerned about compromising the ability to give more chemotherapy following the radiation. The frequency of second malignancies was not increased by the addition of radiation. Carefully shaping radiotherapy portals should reduce the risk of avascular necrosis. Finally, carefully monitoring the peripheral blood counts should prevent excessive bone marrow depression.

REFERENCES

Arseneau JC, Canellos GP, Johnson RR, DeVita VT Jr. 1977. Risk of new cancers in patients with Hodgkin's disease. Cancer 40:1912–1916.

Berkson J, Gage RP. 1950. Calculations of survival rates for cancer. Mayo Clin Proc 25:270–286.

Bloomfield CD, Pajak TF, Glicksman AS, Gottlieb AJ, Coleman M, Nissen NI, Rafla S, Vinciguerra V, Glidewell OJ, Holland JF. 1982. Chemotherapy and combined modality therapy for Hodgkin's disease: A progress report on cancer and leukemia Group B studies. Cancer Treat Rep 66:835–846.

Bonadonna G, Santoro A, Zucali R, Valagussa P. 1979. Improved five year survival in advanced Hodgkin's disease by combined modality approach. Cancer Clinical Trials 2:217–226.

Coltman CA, Dixon DO. 1982. Second malignancies complicating Hodgkin's disease: A Southwest Oncology Group 10 year follow-up. Cancer Treat Rep 66:1023–1034.

Cooper MR, Pajak TF, Nissen NI, Stutzman L, Brunner K, Cuttner J, Falkson G, Grunwald H, Bank A, Leone L, Seligman BR, Silver RT, Weiss RB, Haurani F, Blom J, Spurr CL, Glidewell OJ, Gottlieb AJ, Holland JF. 1980. A new effective four drug combination of CCNU, vinblastine, prednisone and procarbazine for the treatment of advanced Hodgkin's disease. Cancer 46:654–662.

Cox DR. 1972. Regression models and life tables. Journal of the Royal Statistical Society 34:187–220.

DeVita VT, Serpick AA, Zarbone PP. 1970. Combination chemotherapy in the treatment of advanced Hodgkin's disease. Ann Intern Med 73:881–895.

DeVita VT, Simon RM, Hubbard SM, Young RC, Berard CW, Moxley JH, Frei E, Carbone PP, Canellos GP. 1980. Curability of advanced Hodgkin's disease with chemotherapy. Ann Intern Med 92:587–595.

Durant JR, Gams RA, Velez-Garcia E, Bartolucci A, Wirtschafter D, Dorfman R. 1978. BCNU, velban, cyclophosphamide, procarbazine and prednisone (BVCPP) in advanced Hodgkin's disease. Cancer 42:2101–2110.

Farber LR, Prosnitz LR, Cadman EC, Lutes R, Bertino JR, Fischer DB. 1980. Curative potential of combined modality therapy for advanced Hodgkin's disease. Cancer 46:1509–1517.

Fischer JJ, Papac RJ. 1972. Theoretical considerations in combinations of localized and systemic therapy for neoplastic disease. J. Theor Biol 37:105–114.

Gams RA, Durant JR, Omura GA, Bartolucci AA. 1979. Remission duration and survival in advanced Hodgkin disease (HD): The influence of bleomycin and alternating non-cross resistant combination chemotherapy. (Abstract) Blood 54:187.

Gehan EA. 1965. A generalized Wilcoxon test for comparing arbitrarily singly-sensored samples. Biometrika 52:203–223.

Glick JH, Barnes JM, Bakemeier RR, Prosnitz LR, Bennett JM, Neiman RS, Costello W, Orlow EL. 1982. Treatment of advanced Hodgkin's disease: 10 Year experience in the Eastern Cooperative Oncology Group. Cancer Treat Rep 66:855–870.

Glicksman AS, Pajak TF, Gottlieb A, Nissen N, Stutzman L, Cooper MR. 1982. Second malignant neoplasms in patients successfully treated for Hodgkin's disease: A cancer and leukemia Group B study. Cancer Treat Rep 66:1035–1044.

Jones SE, Coltman CA, Grozea PN, DePersio EJ, Dixon DO. 1982. Conclusions from clinical trials of the Southwest Oncology Group. Cancer Treat Rep 66:847–854.

Krikorian JG, Burke JS, Rosenberg SA, Kaplan HS. 1979. Occurrence of non-Hodgkin's lymphoma after therapy for Hodgkin's disease. N Engl J Med 300:452–458.

Moore MR, Jones SE, Bull JM, William LA, Rosenberg SA. 1973. MOPP chemotherapy for advanced Hodgkin's disease. Cancer 32:52–60.

Newcomer LN, Cadman EC, Prosnitz LR, et al. 1982. Splenectomy in Hodgkin's disease: No therapeutic benefit. Am J Clin Oncol 5:393–398.

Pedersen-Bjergaard J, Larsen SO. 1982. Incidence of acute non-lymphocytic leukemia, preleukemia and acute myeloproliferative syndrome up to 10 years after treatment of Hodgkin's disease. N Engl J Med 307:965–971.

Prosnitz LR, Farber LR, Fischer JJ, Bertino JR, Fischer DB. 1976. Long term remissions with combined modality therapy for advanced Hodgkin's disease. Cancer 37:2826–2833.

Prosnitz LR, Farber LR, Kapp DS, Bertino JR, Nordlund M, Lawrence R. 1982. Combined modality therapy for advanced Hodgkin's disease: Long term follow-up data. Cancer Treat Rep 66:871–879.

Prosnitz LR, Montalvo RL, Fischer DB, Silverstein AB, Berger DS. 1978. Treatment of stage IIIA Hodgkin's disease: Is radiotherapy alone adequate? Int J Radiat Oncol Biol Phys 4:781–787.

Prosnitz LR, Lawson JP, Friedlaender GE, Farber LR, Pezzimenti JF. 1981. Avascular necrosis of bone in Hodgkin's disease patients treated with combined modality therapy. Cancer 47:2793–2797.

Rafla S, Coleman M, Pajak T, Vinciguerra V. 1982. The role of radiotherapy in the treatment of advanced Hodgkin's disease (a randomized study of cancer and leukemia Group B). Abstract. Int J Radiat Oncol Biol Phys 8:67–68.

Rosenberg SA, Kaplan HS, Glatstein EJ, Portlock CS. 1978. Combined modality therapy of Hodgkin's disease. Cancer 42:991–1000.

Santoro A, Bonadonna G, Bonfante V, Valagussa P. 1982. Alternating drug combinations in the treatment of advanced Hodgkin's disease. N Engl J Med 306:770–775.

Young CW, Straus DJ, Myers J, Passe S, Nisce LZ, Lee BJ, Koziner B, Arlin Z, Kempin S, Gee T, Clarkson BD. 1982. Multidisciplinary treatment of advanced Hodgkin's disease by an alternating chemotherapeutic regimen of MOPP/ABVD and low-dose radiation therapy restricted to originally bulky disease. Cancer Treat Rep 66:907–914.

UT M.D. Anderson Clinical Conference on Cancer,
Vol. 27, edited by R. J. Ford, L. M. Fuller, and
F. B. Hagemeister. Raven Press, New York © 1984.

The Treatment of Advanced Hodgkin's Disease with Alternating Potentially Non–Cross-Resistant Drug Combinations and Low-Dose Radiotherapy

David J. Straus, Jane Myers, Benjamin Koziner, Burton J. Lee,
Lourdes Nisce,† Beryl McCormick,† Charles W. Young,* and
Bayard D. Clarkson

The Hematology-Lymphoma and Developmental Chemotherapy Services,* Department of Medicine and the Department of Radiation Therapy†, Memorial Sloan-Kettering Cancer Center, New York, New York 10021

The introduction of the MOPP combination (mechlorethamine, vincristine, procarbazine, and prednisone) by De Vita and colleagues (1970) represented a dramatic advance in the treatment of patients with advanced Hodgkin's disease. They achieved an 80% complete remission (CR) rate, with approximately two-thirds of the complete responders remaining in unmaintained remission after a 10-year follow-up (De Vita et al. 1980). Others confirmed the dramatic improvement possible in the treatment of such patients, although CR rates were somewhat lower in other series (Frei et al. 1973, Huguley et al. 1975). The CR rate achieved at Memorial Sloan-Kettering Cancer Center with MOPP was at the lower end of those reported in the literature, perhaps reflecting the inclusion of patients with advanced Hodgkin's disease whose prognosis was worse than in those seen at other centers (Sahakian G, unpublished data).

In an attempt to improve upon these results, a new treatment program using two different strategies was started in January, 1975. The first was to add ABVD (doxorubicin, bleomycin, vinblastine, and dacarbazine), a drug combination potentially non–cross-resistant with MOPP (Santoro and Bonadonna 1979). The second was the use of adjunctive low-dose radiation therapy (RT) to areas initially involved with bulky nodal disease, which would be likely sites of relapse after chemotherapy alone (Frei et al. 1973).

In 1979, we made modifications of the MOPP/ABVD/RT protocol in an attempt to improve upon results and to decrease side effects. Dacarbazine was dropped from ABVD, and substitution of cyclophosphamide for mechlorethamine was allowed during the MOPP cycle in order to reduce nausea and vomiting. The size of the RT fields was enlarged to reduce the incidence of marginal recurrence (Young et al. 1982), although the dose was kept relatively low. In an attempt to improve upon overall results, a third potentially non–cross-resistant drug combination, CAD, which consists of lomustine (chloroethyl-cyclohexyl-nitrosourea) melphalan, and desacetyl vinblastine amide sulfate (DVA, vindesine), was added in alternation with MOPP and ABVD. Vindesine was active in a phase 2 trial in relapsed Hodgkin's disease patients following prior treatment with vincristine and vinblastine (Sklaroff et al. 1979). CAD alone and CAD/MOPP/ABV were as active as other "rescue" regimens for previously treated patients with Hodgkin's disease when the prognostic factors of the patients were considered (Straus et al. 1981). Patients on this 10-drug regimen, CAD/MOPP/ABV/RT, were then randomized against patients on the standard 8-drug regimen, MOPP/ABVD/RT, for previously untreated patients with advanced Hodgkin's disease.

In this chapter we will bring up to date the results of the original MOPP/ABVD/RT trial for which follow-up now extends to nine years (median of 6½ years) and report on more recent results with our current randomized trial of MOPP/ABVD/RT versus CAD/MOPP/ABV/RT.

MATERIALS AND METHODS

Between January, 1975 and December, 1978, a total of 118 patients with advanced Hodgkin's disease were entered into the MOPP/ABVD/RT program. Fifty-seven evaluable patients were previously untreated; 12 patients had stage IIB; 9, IIIA "unfavorable" (age >35 years or mixed cellularity histology); 23, IIIB; and 13, IV Hodgkin's disease. Fifty-one relapsed patients were also treated. Twenty-three of these had received irradiation or small amounts of single agent chemotherapy or both (minimally pretreated), while 28 others had been heavily pretreated with chemotherapeutic agents in combination and, in many cases, irradiation as well. Clinical staging conformed to the guidelines of the Ann Arbor Conference (Carbone et al. 1971), and pathologic staging by laparotomy was performed in 11 patients. Histologic classification was made according to the Rye modification of the Lukes and Butler scheme (Lukes et al. 1966).

Ninety-one of the 118 patients started on treatment were evaluable for response, 57 were previously untreated, 16 had relapsed after radiation therapy or small amounts of single agent chemotherapy (minimally pretreated), or both, and 18 had been heavily pretreated. Of the 27 patients who were unevaluable for response, 13 had received less than three cycles of treatment because of severe nausea and vomiting, 6 had no measurable prior disease, and there were major protocol violations in the treatment of 8 others. Nodular sclerosis was the histologic subtype in 63% of the patients, and 69% had stages IIIB or IV disease. Detailed descriptions of this regimen have also been reported (Case et al. 1976, Straus et al. 1980). To recapitulate briefly, the first regimen was the standard MOPP of De Vita and colleagues (1970): mechlorethamine 6 mg/m^2 i.v. (maximum $= 10$ mg) days 1 and 8; vincristine 1.4 mg/m^2 i.v. (maximum $= 2$ mg) days 1 and 8; procarbazine 100 mg/m^2 p.o. (maximum $= 150$ mg), days 1–14; and prednisone 40 mg/m^2 p.o., days

1–14 in cycles 1 and 8. The second regimen was ABVD: doxorubicin 25 mg/m^2 i.v. days 1 and 14; vinblastine 6 mg/m^2 i.v. days 1 and 14; dacarbazine 250 mg/m^2 i.v., days 1 and 14; and bleomycin 2 mg c.c. daily, days 4–12 and 8–26. MOPP and ABVD were alternated monthly during months one through four, six through nine and then every two months for an additional seven cycles of maintenance chemotherapy. Radiation consisting of 2,000 rad tumor dose in two weeks was administered to areas of initial bulky (>5 cm) nodal disease in month five. Relapsed patients who had received prior radiation therapy were not reirradiated. Patients were randomized to receive either levamisole 150 mg p.o. daily on days 1–6 and 15–20 or no treatment in the intervening periods between their bimonthly maintenance chemotherapy in months 10 through 24.

Starting in December, 1978, 15 patients with Hodgkin's disease who were in relapse were treated with the CAD regimen. This consisted of lomustine 100 mg/m^2 p.o. on day one; melphalan 6 mg/m^2 p.o. on days one through four; and DVA 3 mg/m^2 i.v. on days one and eight. Cycles were repeated every five to six weeks for up to six cycles of treatment, depending upon the response. We then began to treat relapsed Hodgkin's disease patients with CAD in alternation with two other drug combinations. One was the MOPP or (C)MOPP (cyclophosphamide instead of mechlorethamine) regimen. The other was the same as ABVD with the omission of dacarbazine. CAD was administered first followed by (C)MOPP on day 36 or 43. ABV was administered on day 29 following (C)MOPP, and CAD was then recycled on day 29 following ABV. A total of nine cycles, three of each regimen, were administered. Twenty-five patients experiencing relapse of Hodgkin's disease were entered onto this protocol. Twenty-three received no RT as part of the program. Two patients each received approximately 2,000 rad to nodal areas involved with disease over two weeks, between cycles six and seven.

From January, 1979 to June, 1983, 102 consecutive previously untreated patients with advanced Hodgkin's disease were entered into a randomized trial of CAD/MOPP/ABV/RT versus MOPP/ABVD/RT (Figure 1). Seventy-one patients completed treatment with chemotherapy and RT. Thirty-four were randomized to CAD/MOPP/ABV/RT and 37 to MOPP/ABVD/RT. Thirty-one have not completed treatment. Patients on the CAD/MOPP/ABV/RT arm received nine cycles of chemotherapy, three of each combination (Figure 2). Patients on MOPP/ABVD/RT also received nine alternating cycles of chemotherapy; five of MOPP and four of ABVD (Figure 2). Attenuation of doses of the drugs was made when patients were leukopenic or thrombocytopenic and in cycle seven immediately following the RT, even if the white blood cell (WBC) and platelet counts were normal.

An interruption in chemotherapy was made between the sixth and seventh cycles for radiotherapy to the nodal regions that were initially involved with disease. The three regions were the mantle port, the para-aortic nodes and spleen, and the iliac nodes. The dose was 2,000 rad in approximately 2½ weeks (250 rad per treatment, four treatments per week). A booster dose of 1,000 rad was permissible to areas of bulky disease. Areas of direct extension into extranodal sites were included in the portals, and adequate margins were allowed.

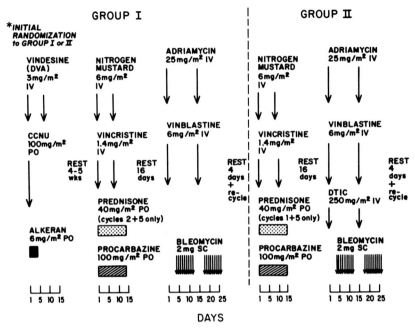

Figure 1. Schedule of the two treatment arms in the randomized trial of two (MOPP/ABVD) versus three (MOPP/ABV/CAD) alternating potentially non–cross-resistant drug combinations and low-dose radiotherapy for patients with advanced Hodgkin's disease (1979–1983). (See text for components of chemotherapeutic regimens.)

Group I		Group II	
Cycle 1	CAD	Cycle 1	MOPP
2	MOPP	2	ABVD
3	ABV	3	MOP
4	CAD	4	ABVD
5	MOPP	5	MOPP
6	ABV	6	ABVD
R.T. - 2 wks rest		R.T. - 2 wks rest	
7	CAD	7	MOP
8	MOP	8	ABVD
9	ABV	9	MOP

2nd Randomization

Levamisole (5 cycles) every other mo. x10	Observation

Figure 2. Drug combinations used in the randomized trial of two versus three alternating potentially non–cross-resistant drug combinations and low-dose radiotherapy for patients with advanced Hodgkin's disease (1979–1983). (See text for components of chemotherapeutic regimens.)

Patients who achieved CR were randomized to the immunotherapy with levamisole group or the observation group following completion of chemotherapy and RT. Levamisole was administered in a dose of 150 mg per day for 6 days every 14 days every other month for 10 cycles (Figure 2).

CR was defined as disappearance of all symptoms attributable to Hodgkin's disease as determined by physical examination, radiographic films, scans, bone marrow biopsy, and blood biochemical studies. Partial remission (PR) was defined as disappearance of constitutional symptoms and reduction by greater than 50% in the sum of the products of the largest perpendicular diameters of all measurable disease. Response duration had to be greater than one month to be counted as a remission. Clinical restaging employing the appropriate studies was performed for each patient at the completion of treatment. Contingency tables were analyzed using the chi-square statistic. Survival and remission duration curves were obtained by the product limit method (Kaplan and Meier, 1958) and differences in the curves were determined by the logrank method (Peto and Pike, 1973).

RESULTS

MOPP/ABVD/RT (1975–1978)

There were 67 patients entered in the study who were previously untreated, 10 of whom were not evaluable for response. Seven of the 10 discontinued treatment before receiving three cycles, 1 had no measurable initial disease, and there were major protocol violations in the treatment of 2 patients. Among 57 evaluable previously untreated patients, 50 (88%) achieved CR, 7 (12%) PR, and no patient failed to respond. Four of those patients initially categorized as achieving PR (Straus et al. 1980) were upgraded to CR status because of further normalization and stabilization seen on follow-up radiographs. Results were similar for patients who had relapsed after radiation therapy or small amounts of single agent chemotherapy or both, with the exception of two who failed to respond to treatment. Among the 18 heavily pretreated patients, 9 (50%) achieved CR, 4 (22%) PR, and 5 (28%) failed to respond to treatment (Table 1).

Overall, there were 19 relapses among the patients achieving CR, 10 among previously untreated, 3 among minimally pretreated, and 6 among heavily pretreated patients (Figure 3). Twenty percent of the patients in the previously untreated group had relapsed at a median follow-up time of 78 months. There were only two relapses later than 36 months. Among previously untreated patients achieving CR, one suffered relapse in an irradiated field and two other patients suffered relapses at the margins of the irradiated fields. There was no difference in remission duration or survival between patients randomized to receive levamisole during maintenance and those who did not receive levamisole.

Table 1. *MOPP/ABVD/RT in Advanced Hodgkin's Disease: Response by Prior Therapy*

	Total	CR (%)	PR (%)	Disease progression (%)
No prior treatment	57	50 (88)	7 (12)	0
Minimal prior treatment	16	11 (69)	3 (19)	2 (12)
Heavy prior treatment	18	9 (50)	4 (22)	5 (28)
Totals	91	70 (77)	14 (15)	7 (8)

CR–complete remission; PR–partial remission.

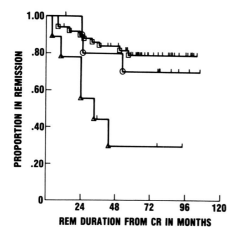

Figure 3. Duration of remission by amount of prior therapy for all patients achieving complete remission in the original MOPP/ABVD/RT trial (1975–1983). □–No prior treatment (50 patients, 40 in remission); ○–Minimal pretreatment = prior radiation therapy or minimal chemotherapy or both (11 patients, 8 in remission); △–Heavy pretreatment (9 patients, 3 in remission); Tick mark (′)–Last follow-up; REM–Remission. (See text for components of chemotherapeutic regimens.)

REM DURATION FROM CR IN MONTHS

Table 2. *MOPP/ABVD/RT in Advanced Hodgkin's Disease (1975–1978)*

Toxicity	Patients/total (%)
Hematologic	
WBC $< 2,000/mm^3$	18/118 (15)
Platelet count $< 50,000/mm^3$	7/118 (6)
Sideroblastic anemia	4/118 (3)
Acute leukemia	4/118 (3)
Total previously untreated	2/67 (3)
Pulmonary	
Bleomycin related	6/118 (5)
Lung fibrosis: RT related	4/118 (3)
Pneumocystis	3/118 (2)
Severe neuropathy	2/118 (2)
Cardiomyopathy	1/118 (1)
Pericarditis	1/118 (1)
Aseptic bone necrosis	2/118 (2)
Graft-vs-host disease	2/118 (2)

The major toxicities are summarized in Table 2. There have been four cases of acute leukemia among the total of 118 patients, two among prior-treated and two among previously untreated patients. In two instances, this was preceded by sideroblastic anemia. The ages of the patients were 41, 52, 54 and 64 years, and three of the four received RT below the diaphragm.

There were six bleomycin-related pulmonary toxic events. Three patients had acute bronchospasm that resolved with discontinuation of bleomycin, one had acute pneumonitis and two had pulmonary fibrosis on chest radiographic examination. None of the six had permanent pulmonary symptoms, and all six completed treatment without bleomycin successfully. One patient, the oldest to receive low-dose mediastinal RT, developed symptomatic congestive heart failure during a relapse and died of progressive Hodgkin's disease. She was found to have a cardiomyopathy at autopsy. No other patients developed cardiac symptoms, and resting and exercise radionuclide cardiac angiography and echocardiography in 19 asymptomatic patients studied at a median time of two years after completion of treatment showed cardiac function to be well preserved (Straus et al. 1982). There were two instances of graft-versus-host disease (GVHD) resulting from blood transfusions, one of which was proven by HLA typing (Dinsmore et al. 1980) and another was suspected. A major problem for the patients receiving MOPP/ABVD/RT was severe nausea and vomiting, particularly related to dacarbazine. Thirteen patients (11%) stopped treatment before receiving three cycles and 24 patients (28%) failed to complete maintenance treatment. Among the entire group of previously untreated patients, 67 evaluable and 10 unevaluable for response, there have been 18 deaths, 16 due to Hodgkin's disease and 2 to secondary acute leukemia (Figure 4).

CAD and CAD/MOPP/ABV for Relapsed Hodgkin's Disease Patients

A total of 15 Hodgkin's disease relapsed patients were treated with CAD. The median age was 28 years, with a range between 18 and 59 years. Two thirds of the patients had the nodular sclerosis histology. Four patients had mixed cellularity histology and the fifth was not subclassified because the diagnosis was obtained by mediastinoscopy from a small fragment of tissue. Two thirds of the patients had extranodal sites of relapse prior to the initiation of CAD. Thirteen of the 15 patients (87%) had B symptoms when they were started on CAD. Most of the patients were failing treatment before they were started on CAD, and the longest disease-free interval was 17 months. Thirteen of the 15 patients had been previously treated with extended field RT and chemotherapy. Nine had received MOPP/ABVD or MOPP/ABV, and four received MOPP alone. These patients were treated relatively late in the course of the disease. The median time from initial diagnosis to initiation of CAD was 49 months.

The results are shown in Table 3. Only two patients achieved CR (13%). One of these occurred in the patient who had received RT only and no chemotherapy.

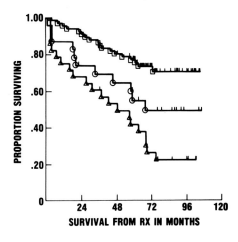

Figure 4. Survival by amount of prior therapy for all patients in the original MOPP/ABVD/RT trial (1975–1983). □–No prior treatment (67 patients, 49 alive); ○–Minimal pretreatment = prior radiation therapy or minimal chemotherapy or both (23 patients, 12 alive); △–Heavy pretreatment (28 patients, 7 alive); Tick mark (')–Last follow-up. (See text for components of chemotherapeutic regimens.)

Table 3. *Results of Rescue Treatment*

	CAD group	CAD/MOPP/ABV group
No. of patients	15	25
CR	2 (13.3%)	11 (44%)
PR	5 (33.3%)	7 (28%)
Minor or no response	5 (33.3%)	0
Disease progression	3 (20.0%)	7 (28%)
Relapses from CR	1 (4 mo.)	5 (3,6,9,13,21 mo.)

CR–complete remission; PR–partial remission.

The toxicity was acceptable. One patient developed sepsis during a period of neutropenia. CAD had to be discontinued in four of the early patients because of prolonged thrombocytopenia. All four had received extensive prior chemotherapy and RT, and this problem was subsequently eliminated by an attenuation of the initial doses of lomustine and melphalan. Ten of the 15 patients treated with CAD have died, and the median survival was 14 months from the start of CAD treatment.

Twenty-five patients were treated with CAD/MOPP/ABV. The median age was 23 years with a range between 17 and 53 years. Twenty of the 25 patients (80%) had nodular sclerosing histology. The histology was not subclassified in one patient because of the poor quality of the original biopsy material. Thirteen of the 25 patients (52%) had only nodal sites of relapse. Twenty of the 25 patients had B symptoms when they were started on CAD/MOPP/ABV. In contrast with most of the patients treated with CAD, the majority of patients were treated while in relapse with CAD/MOPP/ABV rather than during progression of disease. The median disease-free interval was five months (range 0–51 months). Seventeen patients (68%) had previously received combination chemotherapy, usually with MOPP or a variant of MOPP, and extended field RT. The patients were treated with CAD/MOPP/ABV earlier in the course of their disease than with CAD. The median time from initial diagnosis to rescue treatment was 19 months (range 3–107 months).

The response rate is shown on Table 3. Eleven of 25 patients (44%) achieved CR, and 5 of these patients have relapsed. Eight of the 11 patients in CR had B symptoms. The CR rate was slightly higher for patients with disease-free intervals ≥ 11 months than for those with disease-free intervals <11 months ($P = .09$, Fisher Exact Test). Three of five patients who had received prior RT achieved CR.

The toxicity of CAD/MOPP/ABV was acceptable and was comparable to that of CAD. There were no instances of prolonged pancytopenia. There were three episodes of sepsis related to neutropenia, and one patient developed epistaxis with thrombocytopenia. The incidence of vinca alkaloid-related neuropathy was slightly higher for CAD/MOPP/ABV than for CAD alone. It was reversible in all cases except for the patient with orthostatic hypotension. One patient developed a mild paralytic ileus while on MOPP. Drug rashes, probably related to procarbazine, occurred in two patients. Severe nausea and vomiting, as reported by the patients and documented in their records, were relatively infrequent with CAD/MOPP/ABV and occurred less often than with ABVD or MOPP/ABVD (Straus et al. 1980, 1981). Thirteen of the 25 patients have died, and the median survival was 22 months from initiation of treatment.

CAD/MOPP/ABV/RT Versus MOPP/ABVD/RT for Previously Untreated Patients with Hodgkin's Disease (1979–1983)

The patients' characteristics are described in Table 4. There was a slight preponderance of females in the CAD/MOPP/ABV/RT arm. The median age was approximately 30 years in both arms. Nodular sclerosis was the predominant histologic type; approximately 60% of the patients had stage IIIB or IV disease and most of the rest had stage IIB. Median follow-up time was 27 months for the CAD/MOPP/ABV/RT patients and 25 months for the MOPP/ABVD/RT patients. Total follow-up extends to 50 months.

The response rates for patients on the two arms of the trials are shown in Table 5. Twenty-eight of 34 patients (82%) achieved CR, 4 (12%) PR, and 2 patients' (6%) disease progressed with CAD/MOPP/ABV/RT. Twenty-nine of 37 patients (78%) achieved CR, 6 (16%) PR, and 2 (6%) experienced disease progression on MOPP/ABVD/RT. The difference in response rates lacked statistical significance ($P = .864$). Nineteen of the 28 patients who achieved CR on CAD/MOPP/ABV/RT achieved their CR before RT, and 5 achieved CR without RT. On MOPP/ABVD/RT, 24 of the 29 CR occurred before RT, and 4 occurred without the RT.

Table 4. *CAD/MOPP/ABVD/RT versus MOPP/ABVD/RT (1979–1983): Advanced Hodgkin's Disease Previously Untreated, Randomized Patients, and Patient Characteristics*

	CAD/MOPP/ABV/RT	MOPP/ABVD/RT
Total patients	50	52
Unevaluable (lost to follow-up)	3	1
Too early for evaluation	13	14
Evaluable patients	34	37
Male	13	23
Female	21	14
Median age in yr (range)	29 (16–57)	30 (17–61)
Histology		
Nodular sclerosis	27	25
Mixed cellularity	4	10
Lymphocyte predominance	1	0
Lymphocyte depletion	1	1
Not subclassified	1	1
Stage		
IIAE	0	1
IIB	14 (4 IIBE)	11 (2 IIBE)
IIIA	1	0
IIIB	11 (1 IIIBE)	16
IVA and B	8	9

Table 5. *CAD/MOPP/ABV/RT Versus MOPP/ABVD/RT (1979–1983): Advanced Hodgkin's Disease Previously Untreated, Randomized Patients, Results*

	Total	CR (%)	PR (%)	Progression	(%)	Relapses	Death
CAD/MOPP/ABV/RT	34	28 (82)	4 (12)	2	(6)	5 (2 CR) (3 PR)	3 (1 PR) (2 Prog)
MOPP/ABVD/RT	37	29 (78)	6 (16)	2	(6)	6 (3 CR) (3 PR)	5 (1 PR) (1 Prog) (3 CR) P = .864

CR–complete remission; PR–partial remission; Prog–disease progression.
(See text for components of chemotherapeutic regimens.)

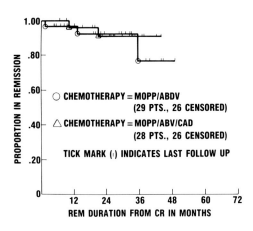

Figure 5. Remission duration (relapse-free survival) for patients treated with CAD/MOPP/ABV/RT and MOPP/ABVD/RT from date of complete remission. REM–Remission. (See text for components of chemotherapeutic regimens.)

Six patients have relapsed on the MOPP/ABVD/RT arm, three from CR and three from PR. Two patients who achieved CR and three who achieved PR relapsed on CAD/MOPP/ABV/RT. The differences in remission duration between CAD/MOPP/ABV/RT and MOPP/ABVD/RT were not statistically significant (Figure 5, $P = .652$). There have been eight deaths, seven of which were due to Hodgkin's disease and one to diffuse histiocytic lymphoma. The difference in survival between CAD/MOPP/ABV/RT patients and MOPP/ABVD/RT was not statistically significant (Figure 6, $P = .465$). The differences between the response rates for the patients divided according to initial stage were not statistically significant ($P = .065$). Ten of 17 patients (59%) with stage IV disease achieved CR, 5 of 8 on CAD/MOPP/ABV/RT and 5 of 9 on MOPP/ABVD/RT. PR and progressive disease were seen among patients with initial bulky nodal disease in stages IIB, IIIB, and IVB.

The toxicity of the two regimens is shown in Table 6. Over twice as many patients on the CAD/MOPP/ABV/RT arm experienced platelet count drop below 80,0000/mm³ and WBC count below 2,000/mm³ as on MOPP/ABVD/RT arm. This was most frequent after CAD. Prolonged pancytopenia was seen in three patients, two on CAD/MOPP/ABV/RT and one on MOPP/ABVD/RT. All three

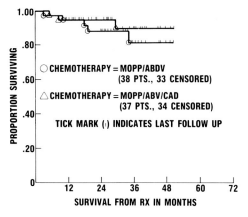

Figure 6. Survival for patients treated with CAD/MOPP/ABV/RT and MOPP/ABVD/RT from date of initiation of treatment. (See text for components of chemotherapeutic regimens.)

Table 6. *CAD/MOPP/ABV/RT Versus MOPP/ABVD/RT (1979–1983): Advanced Hodgkin's Disease, Toxicity*

	CAD/MOPP/ABV/RT Total = 34 No. Pts. (%)	MOPP/ABVD/RT Total = 37 No. Pts. (%)
Hematologic		
WBC <2,000 mm³	19 (56)	11 (30)
Platelet count <80,000 mm³	20 (59)	5 (14)
Prolonged pancytopenia	2 (6)	1 (3)
Sepsis	2 (6)	1 (3)
Hemorrhage	2 (6)	1 (3)
Neurologic		
Paresthesias	6 (18)	8 (22)
Jaw pain	1 (3)	1 (3)
Myalgias	2 (6)	2 (6)
Orthostatic hypotension	2 (6)	0
Constipation	7 (21)	6 (16)
Alopecia	5 (15)	3 (8)
Mouth sores	4 (12)	3 (8)
Second malignancy	0	1 (3) (DHL)
Severe nausea and vomiting	9 (26)	37 (100)

patients received RT below the diaphragm. None of the three patients was able to complete the last three cycles of chemotherapy following the RT. Three patients developed sepsis with neutropenia, and there were three episodes of bleeding due to thrombocytopenia. The incidence of neurologic complications was comparable in both arms and was usually due to one of the vinca alkaloids. One patient developed a diffuse histiocytic lymphoma one year following completion of MOPP/ABVD/RT.

An important difference between the two regimens, which greatly influenced their acceptability to patients, was the incidence of severe nausea and vomiting. All patients on MOPP/ABVD/RT complained of this side effect while it was seen in only 26% of patients treated with CAD/MOPP/ABV/RT.

DISCUSSION

Combination chemotherapy has dramatically improved the outlook for patients with advanced Hodgkin's disease. Complete remission rates with MOPP and variants of MOPP have ranged between 47.5% and 80% (De Vita et al. 1970, Huguley et al. 1975). The latter result was achieved only by De Vita and co-workers (1970, 1980). The long-term follow-up from the National Institutes of Health (NIH) group has shown that 68% of the complete responders have remained in unmaintained remission beyond 10 years from the end of treatment (De Vita et al. 1980). We suspect, although we cannot absolutely prove, that our own low CR rate with MOPP and variants of MOPP might have been due to an accrual of difficult cases. This may be because our institution is a cancer referral center in a large metropolitan area where patients also have access to other sources of cancer treatment.

Since we wished to improve upon our own results with MOPP alone in the treatment of our patients with advanced Hodgkin's disease, we made two major modifications of the classic MOPP combination chemotherapeutic scheme. The first was to add a potentially non–cross-resistant combination of drugs, ABVD. Bonadonna and colleauges (Santoro et al. 1979) achieved a comparable CR rate to MOPP with this combination in untreated patients, and they also were able to rescue a number of "MOPP-resistant" patients. Although patient characteristics are also extremely important in the outcome of rescue chemotherapy in patients either relapsing after or failing to respond to combination chemotherapy (Straus et al. 1981), others have confirmed the concept of non–cross-resistant drug combinations in Hodgkin's disease. Hodgkin's disease resistant to MOPP might be sensitive to ABVD. For this reason, we decided to use both drug combinations.

The second modification was the use of adjuvant low-dose irradiation to areas of frequent relapses in patients treated with chemotherapeutic agents alone (Frei et al. 1973). We postulated that a low dose of radiation therapy might be sufficient to eradicate any remaining nodal disease in patients on combination chemotherapy. Our decision to keep the radiation dosage low was also influenced by a concern that doxorubicin and mediastinal irradiation together might have a synergistic potential for inducing cardiac toxicity.

Our 100% response rate in 57 untreated patients who could be evaluated has been particularly gratifying in view of the 13%-35% primary failure rate reported for MOPP (De Vita et al. 1970, Frei et al. 1973, Huguley et al. 1975). However, 7 of the 10 previously untreated patients who were unevaluable for response were dropped before completing three cycles of treatment because of intolerable nausea and vomiting. The patients who could not tolerate the treatment have to be considered in the overall assessment of its effectiveness.

Our 20% relapse rate among CR patients at a median of 78 months of follow up compares very favorably with the 32%–65% relapse rates reported for MOPP alone (De Vita et al. 1970, Frei et al. 1973, Huguley et al. 1975). A similar superiority of MOPP/ABVD to MOPP for stage IV Hodgkin's disease without RT has recently been reported by Santoro et al. (1982). Low-dose irradiation combined with chemotherapy seemed to be effective in achieving local disease control, since only one patient from the previously untreated group suffered relapse in an irradiated field. A similar success in local control was reported by the Yale group who observed only 3 of 10 patients suffering relapses in areas treated with low-dose irradiation in addition to a five-drug combination that added vinblastine to the drugs used in MOPP (Farber et al. 1980).

Encouraged by these results, it seemed possible that the addition of a third potentially non–cross-resistant drug combination might eradicate any tumor remaining after MOPP/ABVD/RT and thus further increase the disease-free survival. The third potentially non–cross-resistant drug combination employed in this trial included two conventional agents with proven activity against Hodgkin's disease, lomustine (Wasserman et al. 1974) and melphalan (Wolin et al. 1979). The third drug, vindesine, we found to be active in Hodgkin's disease patients who had been previously treated with both vincristine and vinblastine (Sklaroff et al. 1979). The lomustine, melphalan, vindesine combination was active in patients who had been extensively treated with MOPP with or without RT. The CAD/MOPP/ABV regimen achieved a 44% CR rate in the group of relapsed Hodgkin's disease patients with more favorable prognoses. When the prognostic factors of these relapsed Hodgkin's disease patients were considered, both CAD alone and CAD/MOPP/ABV were found to be comparable to other rescue chemotherapeutic regimens (Straus et al. 1981).

The response rate for previously untreated patients in the randomized trial was slightly higher in CAD/MOPP/ABV/RT than for MOPP/ABVD/RT, although the difference was not statistically significant. The CR rate for MOPP/ABVD/RT in the current randomized trial was somewhat lower than in the original MOPP/ABVD/RT trial. Also, there were four primary treatment failures in the present trial, in contrast with the original MOPP/ABVD/RT trial, in which all patients responded to treatment. We believe that we are currently seeing more patients with bulky stage B disease who have worse prognoses, and we plan to analyze the prognostic factors in both trials to see if this impression is correct.

Low-dose RT was retained in the current randomized protocols, since there were no relapses from CR in the original MOPP/ABVD/RT trial within the RT treatment portals. The toxicity of such low-dose RT seems to be minimal. Cardiac function in patients receiving mediastinal RT was well preserved with the exception of one patient. The size of the RT portals was increased in the current trial, since two patients had recurrences in the margins of the RT portals in the original MOPP/ABVD/RT trial.

Levamisole did not affect either remission duration or survival in the original MOPP/ABVD/RT trial. Chemotherapy maintenance has been dropped from the current trial, since there is now no evidence that it prolongs either relapse-free or total survival (Coltman et al. 1976). It is too early to assess the true rates of remission duration and survival and the effect of levamisole maintenance in the current trial. We are optimistic, however, that the relapse rate will be low in both arms.

The toxicities of the CAD/MOPP/ABV/RT and MOPP/ABVD/RT regimens were comparable with the exception of myelosuppression. The incidence of severe leukopenia and thrombocytopenia was greater with the CAD/MOPP/ABV/RT than MOPP/ABVD/RT regimen. The myelosuppression was usually transient with both regimens, which may be due to the long rest period following CAD and the routine use of a drug attenuation schedule according to the levels of the WBC and platelet counts. The use of such an attenuation schedule has not adversely affected the results in the present trial or in our original MOPP/ABVD/RT trial. There were three episodes of hemorrhage associated with thrombocytopenia and three episodes of sepsis with neutropenia. The three instances of prolonged pancytopenia occurred following RT below the diaphragm. It seems desirable to limit such RT as much as possible in combined modality treatment programs. There were two cases of graft-versus-host disease in the original MOPP/ABVD/RT trial. We now irradiate to 2,000 rad all blood products administered in all Hodgkin's disease patients on combined modality protocols to eliminate donor lymphocytes that might engraft in the recipient.

The incidence of secondary acute leukemia among our previously untreated patients in our original MOPP/ABVD/RT protocol was approximately 3% at a median follow-up time of 6½ years, which is at the lower end of the range reported by others for combined modality treatment (Coleman et al. 1977). It is too early to assess the secondary leukemia rate for the current randomized trial. There has been only one second malignancy so far in the current trial, a diffuse histiocytic lymphoma that occurred one year after the completion of treatment in a patient on MOPP/ABVD/RT.

The use of alternating potentially non–cross-resistant drug regimens combined with RT has improved the outlook for our patients with advanced Hodgkin's disease. The response rate with CAD/MOPP/ABV/RT has been at least as high as that for MOPP/ABVD/RT. The omission of dacarbazine has greatly reduced the incidence of severe nausea and vomiting and has made CAD/MOPP/ABV/RT more acceptable to our patients than MOPP/ABVD/RT. If the relapse-free and total survival rates for CAD/MOPP/ABV/RT are as high and the long-term side effects as low as anticipated, the CAD/MOPP/ABV/RT regimen may be preferable to MOPP/ABVD/RT.

ACKNOWLEDGMENT

We would like to acknowledge Ms. Constance Cirrincione for her help with the biostatistics and Ms. Dorothy Hemphill for typing the manuscript.

REFERENCES

Carbone PP, Kaplan HS, Musshoff K, Smithers DW, Tubiana M. 1971. Report of the committee on Hodgkin's disease classification. Cancer Res 31:1860–1861.
Case DC, Young CW, Nisce L, Lee BJ, Clarkson BD. 1976. Eight drug combination chemotherapy (MOPP and ABVD) and local radiotherapy for advanced Hodgkin's disease. Cancer Treat Rep 60:1217–1223.

Coleman CN, Williams CJ, Flint A, Glatstein EJ, Rosenberg SA, Kaplan HJ. 1977. Hematologic neoplasia in patients treated for Hodgkin's disease. N Engl J Med 297:1249–1252.

Coltman CA. 1976. MOPP maintenance (MM) vs unmaintained remission (UMR) for MOPP induced complete remission (CR) of advanced Hodgkin's disease (HD). 7.2 year follow-up. (Abstract) Proceedings of the American Society of Clinical Oncology 1:269.

De Vita VT, Serpick AA, Carbone PP. 1970. Combination chemotherapy in the treatment of advanced Hodgkin's disease. Ann Intern Med 73:881–895.

De Vita VT, Simon RM, Hubbard SM, Young RC, Berard CW, Moxley JH, Frei E, Carbone PP, Canellos GP. 1980. Curability of advanced Hodgkin's disease with chemotherapy. Long term follow-up of MOPP-treated patients at the National Cancer Institute. Ann Intern Med 92:587–595.

Dinsmore RE, Straus DJ, Pollack MS, Woodruff JM, Garrett TJ, Young CW, Clarkson BD, Dupont B. 1980. Fatal graft-versus-host disease following blood transfusion in Hodgkin's disease documented by HLA typing. Blood 55:831–834.

Farber LR, Prosnitz LR, Cadman EC, Lutes R, Bertino JR, Fischer DB. 1980. Curative potential of combined modality therapy for advanced Hodgkin's disease. Cancer 46:1509–1517.

Frei E, Luce JK, Gamble JF, Coltman CA, Constanzi JJ, Talley RW, Monto RW, Wilson HE, Hewlet JS, Delaney FC, Gehan E. 1973. Combination chemotherapy in advanced Hodgkin's disease. Induction and maintenance of remission. Ann Intern Med 79:376–382.

Huguley CM, Durant JR, Morres RR, Chan YK, Dorfman RF, Johnson L. 1975. A comparison of nitrogen mustard, vincristine, procarbazine and prednisone (MOPP) vs nitrogen mustard in advanced Hodgkin's disease. Cancer 37:1227–1240.

Kaplan EL, Meier P. 1958. Non-parametric estimation from incomplete observations. Journal of the American Statistical Association 53:457–481.

Lukes RJ, Craver LF, Hall TL, Rappaport H, Rubin P. 1966. Report of the nomenclature committee. Cancer Res 26:1311.

Peto R, Pike MC. 1973. Conservation of the approximation $(O-E)^2/E$ in the logrank test for survival data or tumor incidence data. Biometrics, 29:579–584.

Santoro A, Bonadonna G. 1979. Prolonged disease-free survival in MOPP-resistant Hodgkin's disease after treatment with adriamycin, bleomycin, vinblastine and dacarbazine (ABVD). Cancer Chemother Pharmacol 2:101–105.

Santoro A, Bonadonna G, Bonfante V, Valagussa P. 1982. Alternating drug combinations in the treatment of advanced Hodgkin's disease. N Engl J Med 306:770–775.

Sklaroff RB, Straus D, Young C. 1979. Phase II trial of vindesine in patients with malignant lymphoma. Cancer Treat Rep 63:793–794.

Straus DJ, Myers J, Passe S, Young CW, Nisce LZ, Lee BJ, Koziner B, Arlin Z, Kempin S, Gee TS, Clarkson BD. 1980. The eight-drug/radiation therapy program (MOPP/ABVD/RT) for advanced Hodgkin's disease. A follow-up report. Cancer 46:233–240.

Straus DJ, Passe S, Koziner B, Lee BJ, Young CW, Clarkson BD. 1981. Combination chemotherapy salvage of heavily-pretreated patients with Hodgkin's disease: An analysis of prognostic factors in two chemotherapy trials and the literature. Cancer Treat Rep 65:207–211.

Straus DJ, Yeh S, La Monte CS, Myers J, Clarkson BD. 1982. Effect of low-dose adriamycin-containing chemotherapy (MOPP/ABVD) and low-dose mediastinal radiotherapy (RT) on cardiac function in untreated advanced Hodgkin's disease (HD). (Abstract) Proceedings of the American Association for Cancer Research 23:113.

Wasserman TH, Slavik M, Carter SK. 1974. Review of CCNU in clinical cancer therapy. Cancer Treat Rev 1:131–151.

Wolin EM, Rosenberg SA, Kaplan HS. 1979. A randomized comparison of PAVe and MOP(P) as adjuvant chemotherapy for Hodgkin's disease. In Salmon SE and Jones SE, eds., Adjuvant Therapy of Cancer II. Grune and Stratton, New York, pp. 119–127.

Young CW, Straus DJ, Myers J, Passe S, Nisce LZ, Lee BJ, Koziner B, Arlin Z, Kempin S, Gee TS, Clarkson BD. 1982. Multidisciplinary treatment of advanced Hodgkin's disease by an alternating chemotherapeutic regimen MOPP/ABVD and low-dosage radiation therapy restricted to originally bulky disease. Cancer Treat Rep 66:907–914.

NON-HODGKIN'S LYMPHOMA

Etiology and Immunology

UT M.D. Anderson Clinical Conference on Cancer,
Vol. 27, edited by R. J. Ford, L. M. Fuller, and
F. B. Hagemeister. Raven Press, New York © 1984.

Lymphotropic Viruses—Epstein-Barr Virus (EBV) and Human T-Cell Leukemia Virus (HTLV)—As Etiologic Agents in Non-Hodgkin's Lymphoma (NHL)

David T. Purtilo, *† Shinji Harada, *
George Manolov, * Eiji Tatsumi, *
Helen Lipscomb, * and Yanka Manolova *

The Department of Pathology and Laboratory Medicine and †The Eppley Institute for Research in Cancer and Allied Diseases and The Department of Pediatrics, University of Nebraska Medical Center, Omaha, Nebraska 68105

Environmental and genetic factors interact in the development of non-Hodgkin's lymphoma (NHL). Development of NHL usually includes a phase of increased lymphoproliferation that is polyclonal. This may be followed by specific cytogenetic alterations, which seem to endow a cell with the ability to escape the host regulatory mechanism. Subsequently, a monoclonal malignancy emerges (Klein 1979). Cofactors in the induction and promotion of NHL may include radiation, nutrition, chemicals, immunosuppressive drugs, parasites, and plant products. Two viruses have been etiologically linked to NHL: Epstein-Barr virus (EBV) and human (adult) T-cell leukemia virus (HTLV or ATLV). This chapter focuses on the roles of EBV and HTLV in the induction of non-Hodgkin's lymphoma and related disorders.

We discuss EBV and the spectrum of diseases resulting from several groups of patients with defective immune responses to the virus: (1) Primary immune deficiency disorders. Males with X-linked lymphoproliferative (XLP) syndrome serve as a model. (2) Organ allograft recipients. Renal and cardiac allograft recipients serve as examples of secondary immune deficiency. (3) Acquired immune deficiency syndrome (AIDS). AIDS will be presented regarding induction of benign and malignant lymphoproliferative diseases by EBV. Male homosexuals will serve as a model.

HTLV is a retrovirus that has been incriminated in the induction of T-cell lymphoproliferative malignancies. The evidence supporting the association of HTLV with adult T-cell leukemia and T-cell lymphomas will be summarized. The controversial role of HTLV in the induction of AIDS will be discussed.

We consider the possibility that pathogenetic mechanisms of acquisition and progression of immune deficiency allow the above lymphotropic viruses to induce benign and malignant lymphoproliferative disorders. The evidence suggesting that thymic epithelium is damaged by viral infection and then immune regulation further declines is discussed and illustrated. The supporting evidence for the hypothesis that multiple steps occur in the conversion of polyclonal B- and T-cell proliferation to monoclonal malignancy results from rearrangements of chromosomal segments and immunoglobulin gene loci. In this context, oncogenes c-*myc* and b-*lym* may be key participants in B-cell lymphomagenesis. We conclude the chapter by comparing biological features of EBV and HTLV.

EPSTEIN-BARR VIRUS–INDUCED
LYMPHOPROLIFERATIVE DISEASES

EBV was associated first with Burkitt's lymphoma, then infectious mononucleosis (IM), and then nasopharyngeal carcinoma (NPC) (Klein 1975). Acquisition of knowledge in immunopathology and virology permitted the recognition of a wider spectrum of diseases associated with EBV (Figure 1) in families with XLP (Purtilo et al. 1975) and also renal allograft recipients (Hanto et al. 1981). We hypothesize that the outcome of EBV infections is determined by socioeconomic status, age at occurrence of primary infection, concurrent viral infection, and immunocompetence at the time of infection (Purtilo and Sakamoto 1982). Discussed below are patients with primary immune deficiency, allografts and AIDS and their diseases associated with EBV.

Primary Immune Deficiency and EBV-Induced Non-Hodgkin's Lymphoma

The XLP syndrome serves as an excellent model for uncovering the role of EBV in the induction of a variety of lymphoproliferative and aproliferative diseases (Figure 2). Recognition of the variability of expression of EBV-induced diseases was possible through study of the Duncan kindred with X-linked recessive progressive combined variable immunodeficiency disease (Purtilo et al. 1975). In 1978, a registry of XLP syndrome was established (Hamilton et al. 1980) to develop criteria for diagnosis, explore mechanisms in the pathogenesis of the various phenotypes, and provide consultation. To date, 35 kindreds are being investigated for the XLP syndrome (Purtilo et al. 1982).

Among the initial 100 cases of XLP syndrome, approximately two-thirds of the individuals had developed IM. Most of these patients died from massive hepatic necrosis or aplastic anemia (Purtilo et al. 1982). In addition, 35 individuals developed NHL of the B-cell type. IM preceded NHL in approximately one-third of the cases. In the other cases, NHL arose de novo. Several patients have developed life-threatening IM. Nineteen percent of the individuals developed hypogammaglobulinemia, and IM often was its antecedent. The mortality rate has been approximately 85% in patients with the XLP syndrome.

Assessment of individuals prior to EBV infection and after EBV infection in survivors has revealed preexisting defects in immunity to the virus. In our initial report (Purtilo et al. 1975) we proposed that immune defects to EBV were respon-

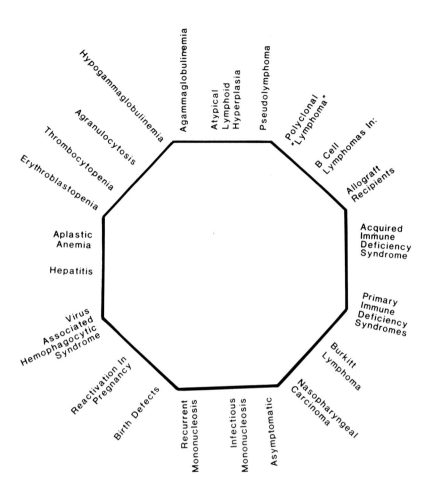

Figure 1. A spectrum of EBV-associated diseases. Depending on the type and degree of immune deficiency, we propose that a variety of diseases can be associated with this virus.

sible for the various phenotypes. In 1976, we (Purtilo 1976) proposed that immunoregulatory defects were responsible for the phenotypes of the XLP syndrome. This hypothesis has been borne out by our studies.

Salient diagnostic features of the XLP syndrome include the occurrence of phenotypes of XLP (agammaglobulinemia, aplastic anemia, agranulocytosis, red-cell aplasia, chronic or acute IM, pseudolymphoma, or malignant B-cell lymphoma) in maternally related males.

Cardiovascular birth defects are excessive in males and females in the families. Invariably, the EBV genome is present in tissues at times of acute infection. Variable antibody responses to viral capsid antigen (VCA) and early antigen (EA) are found. However, boys do not possess the T-cell competence necessary to mount anti-EB

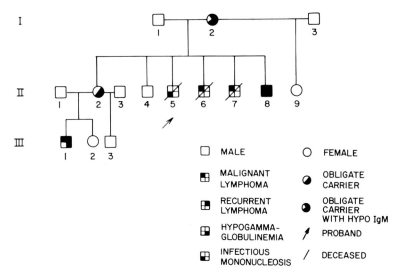

Figure 2. Pedigree of family with the X-linked lymphoproliferative (XLP) syndrome. This family, originally reported from Chicago (Mauer et al. 1976), was thought to have only malignant lymphoma. Reevaluation of the family has revealed multiple phenotypes of the XLP syndrome.

nuclear-associated antigen (EBNA). Often the mothers will show elevated anti-VCA of IgG (80% of cases), IgA, and IgM, and EA antibodies are often present (Sakamoto et al. 1980).

Immune studies in the survivors with XLP syndrome reveal normal numbers of T cells by rosetting with sheep erythrocytes, and immunoglobulin levels vary from normal to agammaglobulinemia. Enumeration of subsets of T cells using monoclonal antibodies reveals inversion of the helper T-cell subpopulations (Seeley et al. 1982). Natural killer (NK) cell activity is impaired by EBV infection in the majority of the individuals (Seeley et al. 1982). In addition, following EBV infection, defective helper T-cell activity with reduced secretion of immunoglobulin in vitro is found when lymphoid cells are stimulated by pokeweed mitogen (Lindsten et al. 1982). The patients fail to mount IgG antibodies to bacteriophage ØX174 owing to defects in switching from IgM to IgG anti-ØX174 antibodies.

Prospective studies of males at risk for XLP syndrome have focused on males whose mothers showed paradoxically elevated antibodies to EBV or whose brothers or maternally related male cousins or uncles developed phenotypes of the XLP syndrome. These studies revealed, prior to EBV infection, only subtle immune deficiency. NK cell activity, for instance, is normal in these individuals (Seeley et al. 1984). Subsets of suppressor and helper T cells show normal ratios prior to EBV infection. However, following EBV infection, inversion of the ratio occurs. Hypogammaglobulinemia often ensues after the viral infection.

We have learned from studying individuals with the XLP syndrome that immunoregulatory defects predispose specifically to EBV (Figure 3). Normally, immu-

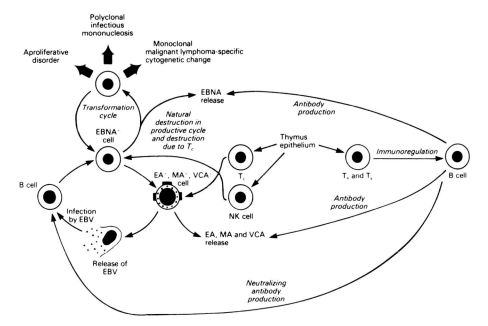

Figure 3. In patients with XLP, infection by EBV of B cells is not recognized by the immune surveillance apparatus because of the inherited lymphoproliferative control locus on the X chromosome (defective immune responses are outlined in the right side of the diagram). The defective cytotoxic responses by T, and natural killer (NK) cells permit proliferation of EBV-transformed B cells, through monoclonal or polyclonal pathways. Aproliferative diseases (i.e., agammaglobulinemia and aplastic anemia) occur owing to unregulated and excessive T-cell responses to infected B cells. Immunoregulation becomes progressively defective due to destruction of thymic epithelium following EBV infection. EBNA–EBV nuclear antigen; EA–early antigen; MA–membrane antigen; VCA–viral capsid antigen; T_c, T_h, T_s, cytotoxic, helper, and suppressor T cells, respectively. (From Purtilo DT, 1983 with permission of Immunology Today.)

noregulatory T-cell populations, especially T-suppressor/lytic cells, subdue EBV-infected B cells. Owing to the infection of the immune system itself and the reliance on immune surveillance by immunoregulatory T cells to thwart B-cell proliferation, individuals with immune deficiency are vulnerable to life-threatening EBV infections. However, patients with the XLP syndrome have effective immune surveillance against most viruses that infect target cells outside the immune system. The immune systems of males with the XLP syndrome cannot recognize viruses in the infected immune system; EBV thereby escapes immunological recognition.

Other primary immune deficiency disorders that have been documented to show defective responses to EBV and lymphoproliferative diseases include Steinbrinck-Chédiak-Higashi syndrome, ataxia-telangiectasia, common variable immunodeficiency, Wiskott-Aldrich syndrome, severe combined immune deficiency following thymic epithelial transplant, and many ill-defined disorders characterized by dysgammaglobulinemia (summarized in Purtilo, 1984).

Organ Allograft Recipients and EBV-Induced
Lymphoproliferative Disorders

In 1970, investigators had noted an increased frequency of NHL in children with primary immune deficiency disorders (Gatti and Good 1971) and a similar situation in renal transplant recipients (Starzl and Penn 1971). More than a decade passed before EBV was recognized as being responsible for these B-cell neoplasms. Perhaps the reason for the delay in identifying EBV as a primary cause of lymphoproliferative malignancies in immune deficient individuals was a lack of close association between the basic scientist and the clinician seeing the patients.

Approximately 1 in 100 renal allograft recipients develop fatal lymphoproliferative disease. Seronegative, young individuals are apt to develop a disseminated fatal IM-like clinical picture, whereas older patients show reactivation patterns of EBV serology and tend to acquire localized tumor masses. Many of these tumors are polyclonal, and virtually all contain the EBV genome (Hanto et al. 1984). Later, we discuss the cytogenetic aberrations that may be pivotal in conversion to a monoclonal malignancy.

Cardiac allograft recipients are also at increased risk for developing EBV-induced lymphoproliferative diseases (Anderson et al. 1978). Penn (1984) has estimated that approximately 20–30% of cardiac allograft recipients surviving five years after transplantation will develop NHL. Bieber et al. (1984) has summarized clinical and pathologic features of NHL in these patients. Nine of 10 B-cell lymphomas in cardiac allograft recipients at Stanford University have shown EBV DNA in their tumors (Cleary et al. 1984). Cyclosporin A impairs T-cell surveillance against EBV in vitro (Bird 1981). This and other immunosuppressive agents may be responsible for ablating cytotoxic T cells, which provide immune surveillance against the virus.

Vulnerability to EBV-induced lymphoproliferative diseases in immune-deficient individuals who are immunologically reconstituted by either thymic epithelium or bone marrow transplant differs. Approximately 10% of patients receiving thymic epithelial transplant have developed EBV-associated polyclonal B-cell lymphoproliferative diseases (Borzy et al. 1979). A Montreal group has demonstrated the EBV genome in such a patient (Reece et al. 1981). In contrast, patients immunologically reconstituted by bone marrow allografting do not develop NHL (Neudorf et al. 1984). Their resistance to EBV may be due to destruction of target B cells for transformation, the brevity of the immune suppression, and the activation of suppressor cells. Rapid immunologic reconstitution occurs in the patients who receive bone marrow transplants (Meuwissen and Purtilo, 1984).

Acquired Immune Deficiency and Non-Hodgkin's Lymphoma

Male homosexuals with AIDS develop cellular immune defect and often manifest opportunistic infections and three malignancies also common in renal allograft recipients—Kaposi's sarcoma, NHL, and squamous cell carcinoma (Sonnabend et al. 1983, Purtilo and Linder 1983). Moreover, during a prodromal phase of AIDS, chronic lymphadenomegaly is often found (Lipscomb et al. 1983). An outbreak of a Burkitt's-like lymphoma in homosexual men was recognized in 1982 (Ziegler et al. 1982). One-hundred percent of the 250 male homosexuals we have studied from Greenwich Village have been seropositive for EBV as opposed to 90% of normal adult controls (Lipscomb et al. 1983). Furthermore, we have noted that the EBV genome may be present in the lymph nodes of patients without serological evidence of reactivation of the virus. They lack the immunocompetence to mount antibody responses. EBNA has been demonstrated in Burkitt's-like lymphomas (Ziegler et al. 1982). We have demonstrated EBV DNA in such a tumor (Petersen et al. 1984).

We have proposed that chronic exposure to multiple infectious agents and to sperm may induce immunoregulatory disturbances in a subset of homosexual men (Sonnabend et al. 1983). Should the immunoregulatory disturbances persist, then the destruction of thymic epithelium, which we have observed at autopsy, may further impair immune regulation. Ubiquitous, opportunistic infections may become very active because of loss of immune surveillance. In our view, immune response genes develop to cope with one infectious agent at a time. Multiple, simultaneous infections may result when multiple sexual partners transmit infectious agents that probably overload the immune system.

The favorite hypothesis to explain AIDS is that a unique viral agent is responsible for the induction of AIDS in male homosexuals, hemophiliacs, Haitians, and children (Fauci 1983). In our view, this is a reductionist approach to complex and different acquired immune deficiency syndromes. The controversy regarding HTLV and AIDS will be dealt with in the next section.

A retrovirus, HTLV, was identified in long-term T-cell cultures derived from a patient with Sézary syndrome (Poiesz et al. 1980). A recent editorial describes the history of the discovery of this virus (Groopman 1983). Gallo's group cultured the cells from the patient with Sézary syndrome by adding T-cell growth factor or interleukin-2. They thereby identified HTLV. The virus associated with adult T-cell leukemia was first described by Hinuma and co-workers in Japan as ATLV (Hinuma et al. 1981). The investigations by groups in the United States and Japan both strongly suggest that HTLV or ATLV cause adult T-cell leukemia. Hinuma thinks that ATLV is a different retrovirus from HTLV (Yorio Hinuma, personal communication, 1983), whereas others considered them synonymous.

Human T-Cell Leukemia Virus and Induction of Adult T-Cell Leukemia

Adult T-cell leukemia usually occurs in elderly individuals, producing skin lesions, hepatosplenomegaly, lymphadenomegaly, and high white blood cell counts (Uchiyama et al. 1972). A rapid course occurs in these patients, who live predominantly in southern Japan. In addition, cases of adult T-cell lymphoma associated with HTLV have been described in the West Indies (reviewed in Bunn et al. 1983). Diagnosis is often made by observing multilobular leukemic cells, which possess helper T-cell phenotype markers in the peripheral blood. In addition, skin biopsies often show epidermal tropism and form Pautrier's microabscesses.

Seroepidemiologic studies in Japan strongly suggest that HTLV is the etiologic agent of ATL. High titer of antibodies against HTLV-infected T-cell lines and also structural proteins of the virus are found in the serum of the majority of patients from Japan and the Caribbean region who have T-cell leukemia or lymphoma. In Japan, approximately 25% of the individuals living in the southern region show antibodies (Yorio Hinuma, personal communication, 1983). Only rarely does ATL occur in seropositive individuals. Hence, one might presume that immune surveillance against the virus is effective in most instances. The seroepidemiology is unique for viruses in that seroconversion occurs usually after the third or fourth decade. In contrast, for EBV and most ubiquitous viruses, seroconversion occurs in the initial years of life. Intrafamily transmission of HTLV may occur.

Human T-Cell Leukemia Virus and Adult T-Cell Lymphoma

The retrovirus HTLV is associated with some ATL in the southeastern United States (Bunn et al. 1983). Bunn and his group described 11 patients with ATL associated with HTLV. Predominantly, they were young and black and were born in the southeastern United States. An aggressive course characterized by disseminated skin lesions or hypercalcemia was noted. Rapidly enlarging peripheral, hilar, and retroperitoneal lymph nodes with sparing of the mediastinum was found. The lymphomatous cells often had invaded the central nervous system, lungs, or gastrointestinal tract. Opportunistic infections including *Pneumocystis carinii* often developed owing to the T-cell immunologic defects. Similar clinical features have been described in patients in Japan and the West Indies.

To date, no benign (nonmalignant) expression of HTLV has been described. This contrasts with EBV. For example, IM is regarded as the benign counterpart to BL (Klein 1975).

Human T-Cell Leukemia Virus as Possible Etiologic Agent of AIDS

Claims have been made that HTLV-I is linked etiologically to AIDS (Essex et al. 1983a). Essex, using serological techniques, found approximately 25% seropositivity of patients with AIDS. Gallo's group (Gallo et al. 1983) found the HTLV genome in 2 of 29 peripheral blood samples. A French group found a retrovirus in a lymph node of one AIDS patient (Barre-Sinoussi et al. 1983). Moreover, Essex's group has demonstrated HTLV-I antibodies in approximately one-third of patients with hemophilia and AIDS (Essex et al. 1983b).

These groups have proposed that HTLV-I infects promiscuous homosexual males. They have speculated that the virus has been carried from African and Caribbean, to North American regions. They draw an analogy with the feline leukemia virus (Essex 1982). The feline leukemia virus induces an acquired immune deficiency in the majority of cats and leukemia in a minority. They have proposed that this is a model for the induction of AIDS.

In 1983 we began HTLV serology testing in our laboratory. Given that we were studying patients with AIDS, we began to investigate whether they were seropositive for this virus. Our studies of more than 100 male homosexuals, including many individuals with AIDS, have failed to demonstrate antibodies to HTLV-I. Furthermore, using a monoclonal antibody (GIN-14), we find no viral structural proteins (p2 and p14) in the patients' sera.

The induction of AIDS by HTLV-I does not make biological sense in our opinion for the following reasons:

1. No T-cell leukemias have been reported in AIDS patients.
2. No AIDS is found in Japan, yet more than 500,000 Japanese are seropositive.
3. HTLV has low virulence and acts slowly; AIDS has a fulminating course.
4. B-cell lymphomas carrying EBV are found in AIDS patients.
5. Our ATLV antibody studies were negative (HTLV different virus?).
6. No obvious immunodeficiency is found in the 25% normal HTLV seropositive persons in Kyushu, Japan.
7. HTLV titers tested by Essex's group were very low (1:4) in AIDS patients. Humoral immunity is very reactive in AIDS patients and hence possibly false seropositivity was detected by Essex.
8. HTLV proviral sequences were isolated in only 2 of 29 patients with AIDS (Gallo et al. 1983).
9. The AIDS patients we have studied have shown cytomegalovirus (CMV) and EBV antibodies in 100% of cases (Lipscomb et al. 1983).
10. ATLV is not necessarily a human T-cell leukemia virus as the antibody is also found in most monkeys from Japan. B cells can be infected with HTLV-I as can rabbit lymphocytes.
11. No antibodies reactive to viral structural polypeptides of ATLV were found by Hinuma's group in the sera of patients with AIDS.
12. Hinuma has not been able to identify anti-ATLV in the sera of 15 AIDS patients from Chicago (personal communication, 1983) and Karpas, in England, cannot reproduce the results (Abraham Karpas, personal communication, 1983).
13. Recently, Gallo et al. (1984) have identified a different retrovirus, HTLV-II, in AIDS patients.

The history of research on viruses in cancer is replete with examples of failure to appreciate the potential value of following empirical leads from patients to find a viral etiology in immune deficient patients (i.e., B-cell lymphoma, Kaposi's sarcoma, and squamous cell carcinoma). Failure to recognize that the very restricted forms of cancer are probably due to ubiquitous viruses has delayed control of virus-induced cancers. The recognition that EBV was responsible for many lymphoproliferative malignancies in children with primary immune deficiency disorders and allograft patients required more than 10 years from recognition of the cancer (Purtilo and Linder 1983). The induction of AIDS is a very complex phenomenon resulting from multifactorial etiological agents and requires multiple steps.

MECHANISMS OF INDUCTION OF VIRALLY INDUCED
IMMUNODEFICIENCY AND NEOPLASIA

Thymic Epithelial Destruction and Progressive Immune Deficiency

The pathogenesis of EBV-induced lymphomas is a multistep process. In inherited and acquired immune deficiency disorders, the pathogenesis of the immune defects may include thymic epithelial destruction. A group in Montreal has demonstrated that thymic epithelial destruction occurs in cases of severe combined immune deficiency syndrome (Seemayer and Bolande 1980) and AIDS (Seemayer et al. 1984). Either introduction of immunocompetent lymphoid cells or virus can initiate lesions (Figure 4). Graft-versus-host response in F_1 mouse hybrids, maternal fetal transfusion leading to severe combined immune deficiency, fatal infectious mononucleosis in XLP, Steinbrinck-Chédiak-Higashi syndrome, fatal IM, and AIDS manifest thymic epithelial destruction. A spectrum of malignant lymphomas or pseudolymphomas occurs in patients with EBV (Purtilo 1984).

Reasons for the destruction of thymic epithelium in EBV patients are unknown. Hypotheses to be investigated might include alteration of HLA antigens by EBV in the virally infected thymus gland with consequent misdirection of cytotoxic T cells, which destroy epithelium. The epithelium could be an innocent bystander to cytotoxic T cells or NK cells, which may be activated anomalously and thereby might destroy epithelium. A third possibility would be fusion of infected B cells with thymic epithelium. The productive cycle of the virus could be unleashed in the heterokaryon cell. Thus, lysis and death of the epithelial cells might occur.

In individuals with XLP syndrome, defective NK function and inverted helper to suppressor T-cell ratios develop after infection by EBV. We have speculated that destruction of thymic epithelium may account for the progression of the immune defect. Persistent polyclonal B-cell lymphoproliferation, driven by transforming EBV, may be converted to monoclonal malignancy due to specific molecular or cytogenetic rearrangements in a cell (Figure 3).

Conversion from Polyclonality to Monoclonality by Rearrangement
of Genes and Chromosomes

When polyclonal B-cell proliferation initiated by EBV persists, fatal IM or other related diseases develop. NHL can occur if the proliferation is sustained for a period sufficient to allow a cytogenetically altered cell to grow and clone into a monoclonal malignancy. George Klein suggested that the final step in the development of Burkitt's lymphoma is a specific translocation involving chromosomes 8 and 14 (Klein 1979). In 1971, Manolov and Manolova described the 14q+ alteration in BL. During the 1980s, molecular cytogenetic studies revealed that gene loci located at the sites of breakpoints in the chromosomes 14, 2, and 22, involved in the translocations of Burkitt's lymphoma, code for immunoglobulin. For example, chromosome 14 contains the heavy-chain genetic locus, #2 kappa and #22 lambda genes (Klein 1983). Chromosome 8 contains the oncogene c-*myc*

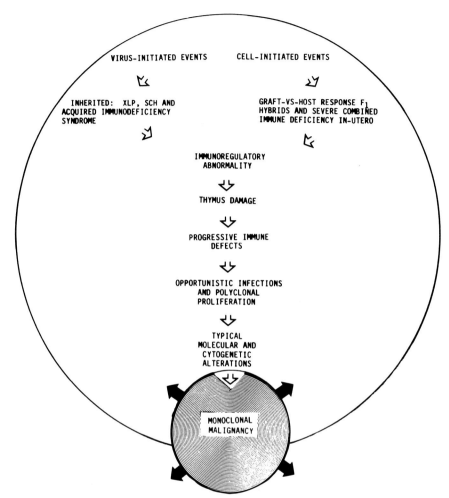

Figure 4. Hypothesis of induction of acquired immune deficiency and malignancy by virus or cells. This process can be initiated by virus or immunocompetent lymphoid cells in thymic epithelium. Thereafter a decline in immunity occurs. Viral burden thus increases. If target cells proliferate, a specific cytogenetic transposition in a cell may convert a polyclonal cellular proliferation to a monoclonal malignancy. In other patients, fatal opportunistic infections occur before evolution of malignancy. XLP–X-linked lymphoproliferative syndrome; SCH–Steinbrinck-Chédiak-Higashi syndrome.

at the breakpoint. The juxtaposition of an immunoglobulin locus with the c-*myc* oncogene appears to enhance lymphoproliferation and thereby allows escape of the altered cell from host immune surveillance. The following cases support the hypothesis. Typical BL translocations are present NHL in AIDS patients.

We (Petersen et al. 1984), as well as investigators at Memorial Sloan-Kettering Cancer Center (Chaganti et al. 1983), have described Burkitt's-like lymphoma monoclonal malignancies in male homosexuals with AIDS. Often these patients manifest lymphadenomegaly as prodromal phase, as described above (Lipscomb et al. 1983), and these lymph nodes often contain the EBV genome. We have observed the typical BL translocation with breakpoints in 8 at c-*myc* and at the heavy chain locus on 14 in a Burkitt's-like lymphoma of a patient with AIDS.

Molecular Events in B-Cell Lymphomagenesis

Employing NIH 3T3 mouse cells, investigators have transinfected cells with transforming genes from a wide variety of neoplasms including carcinomas, sarcomas, lymphomas, and leukemias (Cooper 1983). DNA extracted from six Burkitt's lymphomas with the chromosome 8;14 translocation and three EBV-immortalized diploid lymphoblastoid cell lines were assayed for transforming activity by transinfection of NIH 3T3 cells (Diamond et al. 1983). DNA from all six Burkitt's lymphoma induced transformation with high efficiency. In contrast, DNA from the lymphoblastoid cell line lacked transforming activity. Molecular cloning studies have revealed that the transforming gene in Burkitt's lymphoma is identical to that found in chicken B-cell lymphomas. The chicken B-cell lymphoma-transforming gene is designated ChBlym-1. The transforming gene activated in Burkitt's lymphoma is designated Blym-1. The investigators have suggested that in both chickens and man a multistep process, including preneoplastic and neoplastic stages, evolves. They propose that c-*myc* and Blym-1 may be involved in different stages of progression to the neoplastic phenotype. Moreover, the group from Boston (Diamond et al. 1983) propose that the same two transforming genes are involved in B-cell lymphomas. Land et al. (1983) have supplied evidence that conversion to malignancy requires at least two cooperating oncogenes. David Volsky (personal communication, 1983) has termed this an oncogene cascade.

A second provocative molecular finding in EBV-induced malignant lymphomas is rearrangement of immunoglobulin genes. This phenomenon was identified by molecular hybridization studies in malignant lymphomas carrying EBV in cardiac transplantation recipients (Cleary et al. 1983). Nine of ten of the malignant lymphomas in cardiac allograft patients recently studied at Stanford University have carried the EBV genome. These lymphomas lack detectable surface or cytoplasmic immunoglobulin; however, heavy- and light-chain immunoglobulin gene rearrangements were found, and this revealed their B-cell origin. Importantly, the gene rearrangements were monoclonal. This highly sensitive technique offers the advantage that the immunoglobulin gene in DNA can be extracted from frozen tissue biopsy specimens. This provides a major advantage over cytogenetic evaluation.

SUMMARY AND COMPARISON OF EPSTEIN-BARR AND HUMAN T-CELL VIRUSES

In this chapter we have described the role of two lymphotropic viruses in the induction of NHL. Marked differences in biological and molecular characteristics of these viruses are summarized in Table 1. The existence of EBV has been known for 20 years, and it has been studied extensively, whereas HTLV has been inves-

Table 1. *Comparison of Epstein-Barr Virus and Human T-Cell Virus*

Characteristic	EBV	HTLV
Age at infection	<30 years	>30 years antibodies appear, but infection in childhood
Distribution	Ubiquitous	Southern Japan, Caribbean, Southeastern United States
Detection	Serology, genome	Serology, genome
Viral type	DNA (Herpesvirus)	RNA (retrovirus)
Target cells	B cells, oropharyngeal epithelium, marmoset B cells	T cells, and B lymphoblastoid cells, rabbit and monkey lymphocytes
Paraneoplastic syndrome	Extremely rare	Hypercalcemia Common with T-cell lymphoma
Karyotype	BL reciprocal translocation 8, 14, 22 and 2	Information incomplete 14q+
Predominant location of neoplasm	Blood, head, and visceral organs	Blood, skin, lymph nodes, and visceral organs
NHL	BL, IBS, pseudolymphoma	High grade (chiefly diffuse histiocyte)
Clonality	Polyclonal benign, monoclonal malignant	Monoclonal
Immune Deficiency	Variable, subtle to profound	Variable, T-cell defects chiefly
Chemotherapy	Cyclophosphamide, good response	Combination drugs, poor response
Antiviral therapy	Acyclovir, interferon	Unknown
Diseases	IM, BL, NPC, and atypical lymphoproliferative and aproliferative diseases in immune deficient individuals	Adult T-cell leukemia, smoldering ATL, and lymphoma

EBV–Epstein-Barr virus; HTLV–human T-cell leukemia virus; NHL–non-Hodgkin's lymphoma; IM–infectious mononucleosis; BL–Burkitt's lymphoma; NPC–nasopharyngeal carcinoma; IBS–immunoblastic sarcoma.

tigated for only 3 years. It appears, however, that the virus of Epstein and Barr is more important in the induction of lymphoma and other diseases overall than is HTLV. HTLV-I has been implicated (Essex et al. 1983a) etiologically with AIDS, yet we have summarized our evidence to the contrary. More likely EBV, CMV, and other agents that infect simultaneously induce AIDS (Sonnabend et al. 1983). HTLV-III is a new candidate for causing AIDS. Ubiquitous viruses common in a subset of male homosexuals very likely overwhelm the immune system. The lymphomas in the male homosexuals, to date, have carried the EBV genome, and the HTLV-I genome has not been identified.

ACKNOWLEDGMENT

This study was supported in part by PHS grant 30196, awarded by the National Cancer Institute, DHHS, the American Cancer Society RD161, the Nebraska Department of Health LB506, and the Lymphoproliferative Research Fund.

REFERENCES

Anderson, JL, Fowles, RE, Bieber CP, Stinson EB. 1978. Idiopathic cardiomyopathy, age, and suppressor-cell dysfunction as risk determinants of lymphoma after cardiac transplantation. Lancet ii:1174–1177.

Barre-Sinoussi F, Chermann JC, Rey F, Nugeyre MT, Chamaret S, Gruest J, Dauguet C, Zxler-Blin C, Vezinet-Brun F, Rouzioux C, Rozenbaum W, Motagnier L. 1983. Isolation of T-lymphotropic retrovirus from a patient at risk for acquired immune deficiency syndrome (AIDS). Science 220:868–871.

Bieber CP, Heberling RL, Jamieson SW, Oyer PE, Cleary M, Warnke R, Saemundsen AK, Klein G, Henle W, Stinson E. 1984. Lymphoma in cardiac transplant recipients associated with cyclosporine A, prednisone, and anti-thymocyte globulin (ATG). *In* Purtilo DT, ed., Immune Deficiency and Cancer: Epstein-Barr Virus and Lymphoproliferative Malignancies. Plenum Press, New York, pp. 309–320.

Bird AG. 1981. Cyclosporine A promotes spontaneous outgrowth in vitro of Epstein-Barr virus-induced B-cell lines. Nature 289:300–301.

Borszy M, Hong R, Horowitz S, Gilbert E, Kaufman D, DeMendonca W, Oxelius V-A, Dictor M, Pachman L. 1979. Fatal lymphoma after transplantation of cultured thymus in children with combined immunodeficient diseases. N Engl J Med 301:565–568.

Bunn PA, Schechter GP, Jaffey E, Glayney D, Young RC, Matthews MJ, Blattner W, Broder S, Robert-Guroff M, Gallo RC. 1983. Clinical course of retrovirus associated adult T cell lymphoma in the United States. N Engl J Med 309:257–264.

Chaganti RSK. 1983. Significance of chromosome change to hematopoietic neoplasms. Blood 61:1269–1272.

Cleary ML, Chao J, Warnke R, Sklar J. 1984. Immunoglobulin gene rearrangements as aid to the diagnosis of B cell lymphoma. Proc Natl Acad Sci USA 81:593–597.

Cooper GM. 1983. Cellular transforming genes. Science 218:801–806.

Diamond A, Cooper GM, Ritz J, Lan MS. 1983. Identification and molecular cloning of human Blym transforming gene activated in Burkitt's lymphoma. Nature 305:112–116.

Essex ME. 1982. Feline leukemias: a naturally occurring cancer of infectious origin. Epidemiol Rev 4:189–203.

Essex ME, McLane MF, Lee TH, Falk L, Howe CWS, Mullins JI, Cabradilla C, Francis DP. 1983a. Antibodies to cell membrane antigens associated with human T-cell leukemia virus in patients with AIDS. Science 220:859–864.

Essex M, McLane MF, Lee TH, Tachibana N, Mullins JI, Kreiss J, Kaspar CK, Poon M-C, Landay A, Stein SF, Francis DP, Cabradilla C, Lawrence DN, Evatt BL. 1983b. Antibodies to human T cell leukemia virus membrane antigens (HTLV-MA) in hemophiliacs. Science 23:1061–1063.

Fauci AS. 1983. The acquired immune deficiency syndrome. The ever-broadening clinical spectrum. JAMA 249:2375–2376.

Gallo RC, Salahuddin SZ, Popovic M, et al. 1984. Frequent detection and isolation of cytopathic retroviruses (HTLV-III) from patients with AIDS and at risk for AIDS. Science 224:500–502.

Gallo RC, Sarin PS, Gelmann EP, Robert-Guroff M, Richardson E, Kalyanaraman VS, Mann D, Sidhu GD, Stahl RE, Zolla-Pazner S, Leibowitch J, Popovic M. 1983. Isolation of human T cell leukemia virus in acquired immune deficiency syndrome (AIDS). Science 220:865–868.

Gatti RA, Good RA. 1971. Occurrence of malignancy and immunodeficiency diseases. Cancer 28:89–98.

Groopman JE. 1983. Viruses and human neoplasia approaching etiology. Am J Med 79:377–380.

Hamilton JK, Paquin LA, Sullivan JL, Maurer HS, Cruzi PG, Provisor AJ, Steuber CP, Hawkins E, Yawn D, Cornet J, Clausen K, Finkelstein GZ, Landing B, Grunnet M, Purtilo DT. 1980. X-linked lymphoproliferative syndrome registry report. J Pediatr 96:669–673.

Hanto D, Sakamoto K, Purtilo DT, Simmons RL, Najarian JS. 1981. The Epstein-Barr virus in the pathogenesis of posttransplant lymphoproliferative disorders. Surgery 90:204–213.

Hanto DW, Frizzera G, Gajl-Peczalska KJ, Simmons RL, Najarian JS, Balfour HH. 1982. Epstein-Barr virus-induced B-cell lymphoma after renal transplantation. N Engl J Med 307:896–897.

Hanto DW, Frizzera G, Gajl-Peczalska KJ, Purtilo DT, Simmons RL. 1984. Lymphoproliferative diseases in renal allograft recipients. *In* Purtilo DT, ed., Immune Deficiency and Cancer: Epstein-Barr Virus and Lymphoproliferative Malignancies. Plenum Press, New York, pp. 321–348.

Hinuma Y, Nagata K, Hanaoka M, Nakai M, Matsumoto T, Kinoshita K-I, Shirakawa S, Miyoshi I. 1981. Adult T cell leukemia: antigen in an ATL cell line and detection of antibodies to the antigen in human sera. Proc Natl Acad Sci USA 78:6476–6480.

Klein G. 1975. The Epstein-Barr virus and neoplasia. N Engl J Med 293:1353–1357.

Klein G. 1979. Lymphoma development in mice and humans: diversity of initiation is followed by convergent cytogenetic evolution. Proc Natl Acad Sci USA 76:2442–2446.

Klein G. 1983. Specific chromosomal translocation and the genesis of B cell derived tumors in mice and men. Cell 32:311–315.

Land H, Parada LF, Weinberg RA. 1983. Tumorigenic conversion of primary embryofibroblasts requires at least two cooperating oncogenes. Nature 304:596–602.

Lindsten T, Seeley JK, Sakamoto K, Yetz J, Harada S, Bechtold T, Rogers G, Purtilo DT. 1982. Immune deficiency in the X-linked lymphoproliferative syndrome. II. Immunoregulatory T cell defects. J Immunol 129:2536–2540.

Lipscomb HL, Tatsumi E, Harada S, Sonnabend J, Wallace J, Yetz J, Davis J, McClain K, Metroka C, Tubbs R, Purtilo DT. 1983. Epstein-Barr virus, chronic lymphadenomegaly, and lymphoma in male homosexuals with acquired immunodeficiency syndrome (AIDS). AIDS Research 1:59–83.

Manolov G, Manolova Y. 1971. A marker band in one chromosome No. 14 in Burkitt Lymphomas. Hereditas 69:300–303.

Mauer HS, Gotoff SP, Allen L, Bolan J. 1976. Malignant lymphoma of the small intestine in multiple family members. Association with an immunologic deficiency. Cancer 37:2224–2231.

Meuwissen H, Purtilo DT. 1984. Epstein-Barr virus and marrow transplantation. *In* Purtilo DT, ed., Immune Deficiency and Cancer: Epstein-Barr Virus and Lymphoproliferative Malignancies. Plenum Press, New York (In press).

Neudorf SL, Filipovich AH, Kersey JH. 1984. Immunoreconstitution by bone marrow transplantation decreases lymphoproliferative malignancies in Wiskott-Aldrich and severe combined immune deficiency syndromes. *In* Purtilo DT, ed. Immune Deficiency and Cancer: Epstein-Barr Virus and Lymphoproliferative Malignancies. Plenum Press, New York, pp. 471–480 .

Penn I. 1984. Allograft Transplant Cancer Registry. *In* Purtilo DT, ed., Immune Deficiency and Cancer: Epstein-Barr Virus and Lymphoproliferative Malignancies. Plenum Press, New York (In press).

Petersen JM, Tubbs RR, Savage RA, Calabrese LC, Proffitt MR, Manolova Y, Manolov G, Schumaker A, Tatsumi E, McClain K, Purtilo DT. 1984. Small noncleaved B cell Burkitt-type lymphoma with chromosome t(8;14) translocation and carrying Epstein-Barr virus in a male homosexual with the acquired immune deficiency syndrome. Am J Med (In press).

Poiesz BJ, Ruscetti FW, Gazdar AF, Bunn PA, Minna JD, Gallo RC. 1980. Detection and isolation of type C retrovirus particles from fresh and cultured lymphocytes of a patient with cutaneous T cell leukemia. Proc Natl Acad Sci USA 77:7415–7419.

Purtilo DT, Yang JPS, Cassel CK, Harper P, Stephenson SR, Landing BH, Vawter GF. 1975. X-linked recessive progression combined variable immunodeficiency (Duncan's disease). Lancet i:935–950.

Purtilo DT. 1976. Hypothesis: Pathogenesis and phenotypes of an X-linked recessive lymphoproliferative syndrome. Lancet ii:882–885.

Purtilo DT. 1983. Immunopathology of X-linked lymphoproliferative syndrome. Immunology Today 4:291–297.

Purtilo DT, ed. 1984. Immune Deficiency and Cancer: Epstein-Barr Virus and Lymphoproliferative Malignancies. Plenum Press, New York (In press).

Purtilo DT, Linder J. 1983. Oncological consequences of impaired immune surveillance against ubiquitous virus. J Clin Immunol 3:197–206.

Purtilo DT, Sakamoto K. 1982. Reactivation of Epstein-Barr virus in pregnant women, social factors, and immune competence as determinants of lymphoproliferative disease. Med Hypothesis 8:401–408.

Purtilo DT, Sakamoto K, Barnabei V, Seeley J, Bechtold T, Rogers G, Yetz J, Harada S. 1982. Epstein-Barr virus-induced diseases in males with the X-linked lymphoproliferative syndrome (XLP). Am J Med 73:49–56.

Reece ER, Gartner JG, Seemayer TA, Joncas JH, Pagano JS. 1981. Epstein-Barr virus in a malignant lymphoproliferative disorder of B-cells occurring after thymic epithelial transplantation for combined immunodeficiency. Cancer Res 41:4243–4247.

Sakamoto K, Freed H, Purtilo DT. 1980. Antibody responses to Epstein-Barr virus in families with the X-linked lymphoproliferative syndrome. J Immunol 125:921–925.

Seeley JK, Sakamoto K, Ip S, Hansen P, Purtilo DT. 1981. Abnormal subsets in the X-linked lympho-proliferative syndrome. J Immunol 127:2618–2620.

Seeley JK, Bechtold T, Lindsten T, Purtilo DT. 1982. NK deficiency in X-linked lymphoproliferative syndrome. *In* Herberman RB, ed., NK Cells and Other Natural Effector Cells. Academic Press, New York, pp. 1211–1218.

Seeley J, Lindsten T, Ballow M, Sakamoto K, Purtilo DT. 1982. Defective lymphocyte function in x-linked lymphoproliferative syndrome. *In* Yohn D, ed., Comparative Leukemia and Related Diseases. Elsevier North Holland, New York, pp. 571–572.

Seemayer TA, Bolande RP. 1980. Thymic involution mimicking thymic dysplasia, a consequence of transfusion-induced graft-versus-host disease in a premature infant. Arch Pathol Lab Med 104:141–144.

Seemayer TA, Laroch AC, Russo P, Malebrance R, Arnoux E, Guerin J-M, Pierre G, Dupuy J-M, Gartner JG, Lapp WS, Spira TJ, Elie R. 1984. Precocious thymic involution manifest by epithelial injury in the acquired immune deficiency syndrome. Human Pathol (In press).

Sonnabend J, Witkin SS, Purtilo DT. 1983. Acquired immunodeficiency syndrome, opportunistic infections, and malignancies in male homosexuals. A hypothesis of etiologic factors in pathogenesis. J Am Med Assoc 249:2370–2374.

Starzl TE, Penn I, Putnam CW, Groth CG, Halgrimson CG. 1971. Iatrogenic alterations of immunologic surveillance in man and their influence on malignancy. Transplant Rev 7:112–145.

Uchiyama T, Yodoi J, Sagawa T, Takatsuki K, Uchino H. 1972. Adult T cell leukemia: clinical and hematologic features of 16 cases. Blood 50:481–492.

Ziegler J, Drew WL, Miner RC, Mintz L, Rosenbaum E, Gershow J, Casavant C, Yamamoto K, Lennette ET, Greenspan J, Shillitoe E, Beckstead J. 1982. The outbreak of Burkitt's-like lymphoma in homosexual men. Lancet ii:631–633.

UT M.D. Anderson Clinical Conference on Cancer,
Vol. 27, edited by R. J. Ford, L. M. Fuller, and
F. B. Hagemeister. Raven Press, New York © 1984.

Transforming Genes of Lymphoid Neoplasms

Alan Diamond, Joan Devine, Mary-Ann Lane,* and Geoffrey Cooper

Laboratory of Molecular Carcinogenesis and Laboratory of Molecular Immunobiology,
Dana-Farber Cancer Institute and Department of Pathology, Harvard Medical School,
Boston, Massachusetts 02115*

TRANSFORMING GENES DETECTABLE BY TRANSFECTION

Recent advances in molecular biology have provided new insight into the genetic events that occur during neoplastic development. It was discovered in 1971 that cellular DNA containing the genomes of Rous sarcoma virus (RSV) could induce the morphological transformation of chicken embryo fibroblasts (Hill and Hillova 1971). The transfer of either total genomic DNA or specific fragments of DNA that confer some biological alteration on recipient cells is termed transfection. This procedure is often performed using NIH 3T3 mouse fibroblasts as recipient cells because they efficiently take up and integrate exogenous DNA.

Acutely transforming DNA tumor viruses or retroviruses are viruses that can induce tumors in susceptible hosts after a relatively short latent period. These viruses contain specific DNA sequences within which the transforming function of the virus is contained. These transforming genes have nontransforming homologs in normal DNA, and it is generally believed that the viral transforming genes have been acquired from host DNA during the evolution of the highly oncogenic retroviruses (Bishop 1981).

The DNA of approximately 50% of the neoplasms examined also contain sequences that can transform mouse cells by transfection (for review, see Cooper 1982). These neoplasms include carcinomas, sarcomas, and lymphoid neoplasms and represent both primary (1°) isolates and established cell lines. In the case of a number of lung, colon, and bladder carcinomas, it has been determined that the activated transforming genes of these neoplasms are homologous to the *ras*-transforming genes of the Harvey and Kirsten murine sarcoma viruses (Der et al. 1982, Parada et al. 1982, Shimizu et al. 1983). This work has also revealed that there exists a family of *ras*-related genes in normal DNA, and these genes show strong sequence conservation throughout vertebral evolution. Activated members of the *ras* family capable of transforming mouse cells by transfection have also been detected as the transforming gene in a variety of neoplasms including pancreatic, gall bladder and ovarian carcinomas, a rhabdomyosarcoma, fibrosarcoma, and neuroblastoma, promyelocytic leukemia, acute myelogenous leukemia, and a Burkitt's lymphoma

(Murray et al. 1983, Balmain and Pragnell 1983, Yuasa et al. 1983, Hall et al. 1983, Feig et al. 1984). Thus, although members of the *ras* family of transforming genes appear to be activated in a wide variety of neoplasms, they are only found in approximately 20% of any particular type of neoplasm.

TRANSFORMING GENES OF LYMPHOID NEOPLASMS

Approximately 90% of those lymphoid neoplasms investigated contain activated transforming genes detectable by transfection (Cooper and Neiman 1980, Lane et al. 1982a, 1982b). It is not yet understood why the percentage of lymphoid neoplasms containing detectable transforming genes is higher than that of other types of neoplasm. In contrast to these results observed for those tumors containing an activated *ras* gene, the activated transforming genes observed in lymphoid neoplasms show strong cell type specificity (Lane et al. 1982a). Using the sensitivity to restriction enzyme digestion of the transforming activity observed in the DNA of a variety of neoplasms, the same gene was detected by transfection in multiple isolates of neoplasms representing either early, intermediate, or late stages of B- and T-cell differentiation. These genes were different for each of the neoplasms and represented different stages of the B- and T-cell lineages. For example, 19 different isolates of pre-B neoplasms from both mice and man exhibit the same pattern of restriction enzyme sensitivity and thus is distinguishable from that observed for lymphoid neoplasms representing different stages of differentiation (Lane et al. 1982a). The reproducibility with which these genes are activated in any neoplasm of a particular type implies that the genes are involved in carcinogenesis and further suggests that they may be involved in the normal differentiation of these cells.

THE Blym-1 TRANSFORMING GENE OF CHICKEN B-CELL LYMPHOMAS

Chicken bursal lymphomas arise after a long latency period following infection of susceptible birds with avian lymphoid leukosis virus (LLV). LLV are retroviruses that do not contain oncogenic sequences of their own but induce tumors as a result of integration of the LLV genome next to a cellular gene (Hayward et al. 1981). This cellular gene, c-*myc*, is the chicken gene homologous to the transforming gene of the MC-29 retrovirus. C-*myc* becomes activated as a result of coming under the influence of LLV regulator sequences and increased levels of c-*myc* mRNA are evidence of this activation (Hayward et al. 1981). However, using the Southern blot analysis of the DNA of mouse cells transformed by bursal lymphoma DNA, it was shown that c-*myc* is not the transforming gene whose biological activity is detectable by transfection (Cooper and Neiman 1981). This indicated that in addition to c-*myc*, a second gene that is detectable by transfection is involved in lymphomagenesis.

In order to isolate the activated transforming gene of bursal lymphoma DNA, a recombinant phage library was constructed from the DNA of NIH 3T3 cells transformed by the DNA of the bursal lymphoma cell line RP9 (Goubin et al. 1983). This library was screened by sib selection, using the biological assay of transfection to determine which phage contained the transforming sequences. In this manner, a single recombinant phage with transforming activity ($1-5 \times 10^3$ transformants per μg of DNA) was isolated. Initial experiments indicated that this clone had an insert of 4.5 kb of chicken DNA and the cloned transforming gene was designated ChBlym-1.

Analyzing the gene by means of Southern blot hybridization revealed that ChBlym-1 was not homologous to any of the known retroviral transforming genes (Goubin et al. 1983). Thus, ChBlym-1 represents the first cloned active transforming gene that does not have a known retroviral homolog. Further analysis of ChBlym-1 indicated this gene codes for a small protein of only 65 amino acids in length and that the coding sequence was interrupted once by a noncoding intervening sequence. The deduced amino acid sequence of ChBlym-1 was shown to be rich in arginine and lysine (9.2% and 12.3% respectively) and hydrophilic at the termini, while containing a central 14 amino acid sequence that is hydrophobic. In addition, a computer assisted homologic search revealed that the predicted amino acid sequence of ChBlym-1 showed 36% homology to the amino-terminal portions of the transferrin family of proteins. The segment of transferrins that show homology to ChBlym-1 is the same region that is strongly homologous among the different members of the family, suggesting that the observed homology may be biologically significant. Transferrins are a family of high molecular weight, iron-binding proteins that are essential growth factors for lymphocytes grown in culture. Expression of transferrin-related molecules (Brown et al. 1982) and transferrin receptors (Omary et al. 1980, Reinherz et al. 1980, Judd et al. 1980, Goding et al. 1981, Haynes et al. 1981, Sutherland et al. 1981) has been correlated with cell proliferation. Furthermore, transferrin may act as a lymphocyte mitogen (Dillner-Centerlind 1979). Recently, the product of the simian sarcoma virus transforming gene, v-*sis*, has been shown to be homologous to platelet-derived growth factor (Waterfield et al. 1983, Doolittle et al. 1983). It is intriguing that transforming genes are homologous to growth factors, and it remains to be seen if this will be a general phenomenon.

ChBlym-1 hybridizes to multiple bands when the DNA of either normal chicken or lymphoma cells is digested with a variety of restriction endonucleases and is analyzed by means of Southern blot hybridization (Goubin et al. 1983). This provides evidence that there are multiple fragments (6-7) within the chicken genome that are homologous to ChBlym-1. This observation was extended to show that multiple sites homologous to ChBlym-1 are also present in human DNA, which indicates these sequences are well conserved between chicken and man (Goubin et al. 1983). This observation led to the hypothesis that sequences homologous to ChBlym-1 are activated in human neoplasms. Burkitt's lymphoma represents a human B-cell lymphoma at the intermediate stage of B-cell development, as are chicken bursal lymphomas, and for this reason, the transforming activity of Burkitt's lymphoma DNA was investigated.

TRANSFORMING ACTIVITY OF BURKITT'S LYMPHOMA DNA

The DNA of six Burkitt's lymphoma cell lines were examined for transforming activity (Diamond et al. 1983). The Raji and Namalwa Burkitt's lymphoma cell lines represent Epstein-Barr virus (EBV)-associated African cell lines. BJAB is an African Burkitt's cell line with no EBV-associated sequences, and the American cell lines CW678, EW36, and MC116 are also non-EBV associated. The DNA of all six of these cell lines transformed mouse cells with an efficiency of 0.1 to 1.0 transformants per μg of DNA. In contrast, the DNA of either peripheral or cord blood lymphocytes, immortalized by EBV infection, failed to transform cells by transfection. This indicates that the observed transforming activity of Burkitt's lymphoma DNA is specific for the lymphomas.

In order to characterize further the observed transforming activities, the DNA from the above described cell lines were investigated by restriction enzyme sensitivity studies (Diamond et al. 1983). The DNA of these six Burkitt's lymphoma cell lines were inactivated by digestion with BamH1; digestion with Hind III, EcoRl, and XhoI did not alter transforming activity. The observation that the DNA of all six Burkitt's lymphoma cell lines had the same pattern of restriction enzyme sensitivity indicates that in each case the transforming activity observed was due to activation of the same gene.

THE ISOLATION OF THE HuBlym-1 TRANSFORMING GENE

The observation that ChBlym-1 was homologous to a small gene family in human DNA (Goubin et al. 1983) prompted speculation that a gene homologous to Ch-Blym-1 was the activated transforming gene detected in the DNA of Burkitt's lymphomas. To test this hypothesis, a recombinant phage library was constructed from the DNA of the CW678 American Burkitt's lymphoma cell line (Diamond et al. 1983), a cell line with a transforming activity of 1.0 foci per μg of DNA. The library was then screened by means of plaque hybridization using ^{32}P-labelled ChBlym-1 sequences as a hybridization probe. In this manner, 14 positively hybridizing clones were detected. Each of these was isolated and tested in the transfection assay for transforming activity. Only 1 of these 14 clones efficiently transformed mouse cells and was designated λHuBlym-1. The other 13 clones represented either the normal, nontransforming allele of HyBlym-1 (J. Devine unpublished observations) or other members of the family of sequences showing homology to ChBlym-1.

CHARACTERIZATION OF HuBlym-1

A restriction map of those sequences hybridizing to ChBlym-1 was obtained by blot hybridization techniques (Diamond et al. 1983). In order to determine if those sequences that hybridized to ChBlym-1 are the same sequences with transforming activity, a 2.2 kb Hind III fragment of λHuBlym-1 that contained ChBlym-1 homologous sequences was tested by transfection. This fragment had the same transforming activity as did the entire clone, indicating that the ChBlym-1 homologous sequences and the transforming sequences are the same. The same fragment was examined with a number of restriction enzymes for sensitivity to digestion. The transforming activity of the fragment was abolished by prior digestion with BamH1 and was not affected by digestion with Hind III, EcoR1, or XhoI. This pattern of enzyme sensitivity exactly matches the pattern observed for total Burkitt's lymphoma DNA, indicating that the gene cloned from a recombinant phage library was the same gene detected by transfection of genomic DNA.

Using HuBlym-1 as a hybridization probe, it was determined that HuBlym-1 is not homologous to any of the retroviral transforming genes *myc*, *ras*^{H}, *ras*^{K}, *fms*, *erb*, *abl*, *src*, *sis*, *fes*, *mos*, and *rel* (Diamond et al. 1983). HyBlym-1 is not homologous to Tlym-1 a transforming gene isolated from a T-cell lymphoma (Lane et al. 1984). In addition, HuBlym-1 is not homologous to another member of the *ras* family of transforming genes, *ras*^{N}. *Ras*^{N} has been observed to be the activated transforming gene in the AW Ramos Burkitt's lymphoma cell line (Murray et al. 1983).

HuBlym-1 hybridizes to a single 5.0 kb Hind III fragment in the DNA of normal human fibroblasts, six Burkitt's lymphoma cell lines, and the DNA of NIH 3T3 cells transformed by Burkitt's lymphoma DNA but not in the DNA of untransformed mouse cells (Diamond et al. 1983). These results provide direct evidence that the mouse cells have indeed become transformed due to the acquisition of HuBlym-1. These hybridization data also indicate that activation of HuBlym-1 is not accompanied by gross gene rearrangements or gene amplification. Furthermore, activation does not appear to be associated with increased levels of HuBlym-1 transcription (J. Devine unpublished observations). Single base mutations are responsible for the activation of members of the *ras* family of transforming genes (Reddy et al. 1982, Tabin et al. 1982, Taparowsky et al. 1982, Capon et al. 1983, Shimizu et al. 1983, Yuasa et al. 1983) and it seems possible that similar point mutations are associated with activation of HuBlym-1.

The chromosomal location of HuBlym-1 has been determined by in situ hybridization to human metaphase chromosomes (Morton et al. 1984). HuBlym-1 has, in this manner, been mapped to chromosome 1 at position 1P32. Burkitt's lymphoma cells typically exhibit a reciprocal translocation between chromosome 8 either chromosome 14, 2, or 22 (Klein 1981, Rowly 1982). Thus, the activated transforming gene of Burkitt's lymphoma DNA, HuBlym-1, does not map to any of those chromosomes involved in the characteristic translocations.

SUMMARY AND CONCLUSIONS

The majority of lymphoid neoplasms tested contain DNA capable of efficiently transforming mouse NIH 3T3 cells. To date, only two transforming genes that show specificity for lymphoid neoplasms have been isolated, although the presence of others is indicated by restriction endonuclease sensitivity studies (Lane et al. 1982). Tlym-1 has been isolated from a T-cell lymphoma (Lane et al. 1984) and

Blym-1 from B-cell lymphomas (Goubin et al. 1983, Diamond et al. 1983). ChBlym-1 has been isolated from a chicken B-cell lymphoma cell line (Goubin et al. 1983). Chicken B-cell lymphomas arise after a long latency period following infection with LLV; this period is thought to be a necessary consequence in order for a number of events to occur before tumor progression begins (Neiman et al. 1980). Activation of both the chicken c-*myc* and Blym genes appear to be necessary for lymphomagenesis. In Burkitt's lymphoma, there also appears to be evidence indicating the requirement for activated c-*myc* and Blym genes. The characteristic translocations between chromosome 8 and 14, and 2 or 22 occur in all Burkitt's lymphoma cell lines and the human c-*myc* gene has been mapped to the breakpoint on chromosome 8 and translocates to the recipient chromosome (Dalla-Favera et al. 1982, Taub et al. 1982, Neel et al. 1982, Marcu et al. 1983). These results implicate c-*myc* in the disease process, although HuBlym-1 is the transforming gene detected by transfection (Diamond et al. 1983). The localization of HuBlym-1 to chromosome 1 implies that this gene is not activated as a direct result of chromosomal translocations, although it is possible that small aberrations of chromosomes have not yet been detected. Thus, the consistent observation of c-*myc* and Blym involvement in these lymphomas provides evidence that these events are significant, and neoplastic development occurs by a process involving at least two steps. Tumor development by a multistep process has also been suggested for pre–B-cell neoplasms induced by Abelson murine leukemia virus (AbMuLV). Although the expression of the viral transforming gene, v-*abl*, is required to induce neoplastic growth, a second gene, distinct from and not linked to viral sequences, transforms mouse cells by transfection (Lane et al. 1982b). Carcinogenesis is generally considered a multistep process, and it seems likely that lymphoid neoplasms may provide useful model systems for the examination of the molecular and cellular events involved in neoplastic development.

ACKNOWLEDGMENT

These studies were supported by a fellowship to Dr. Diamond from the Damon Runyon-Walter Winchell Cancer Fund, a Travel Fellowship to Dr. Devine from the Imperial Cancer Research Fund, London, and a faculty research award to Dr. Cooper from the American Cancer Society.

REFERENCES

Balmain A, Pragnell IB. 1983. Mouse skin carcinomas induced in vivo by chemical carcinogens have a transforming Harvey-ras oncogene. Nature 303:72–74.

Bishop JM. 1981. Enemies within: The genesis of retrovirus oncogenes. Cell 23:5–6.

Brown JP, Hewick RM, Hellstrom I, Hellstrom KE, Doolittle RM, Dreyer WJ. 1982. Human melanoma-associated antigen is structurally and functionally related to transferrin. Nature 296:171–173.

Capon DJ, Chen EY, Levinson AD, Seeburg PH, Goeddel DV, 1983. Complete nucleotide sequence of the T24 human bladder carcinoma oncogene and its normal homologue. Nature 302:33–37.

Cooper GM. 1982. Cellular transforming genes. Science 217:801–806.

Cooper GM, Neiman PE. 1980. Transforming genes of neoplasms induced by avian lymphoid leukosis viruses. Nature 287:656–659.

Cooper GM, Neiman PE. 1981. Two distinct candidate transforming genes of lymphoid leukosis virus induced neoplasms. Nature 292:857–858.

Dalla-Favera R, Gregni M, Erikson J, Patterson D, Gallo RC, Croce CM. 1982. Human c-myc onc gene is located on the region of chromosome 8 that is translocated in Burkitt lymphoma cells. Proc Natl Acad Sci USA 79:7824–7827.

Der CJ, Krontiris TG, Cooper GM. 1982. Transforming genes of human bladder and lung carcinoma cell lines are homologous to the *ras* genes of Harvey and Kirsten sarcoma viruses. Proc Natl Acad Sci USA 79:3637–3640.

Diamond A, Cooper GM, Ritz J, Lane M-A. 1983. Identification and molecular cloning of the human Blym transforming gene activated in Burkitt's lymphomas. Nature 305:112–116.

Dillner-Centerlind ML, Hammarstrom S, Perlman P. 1979. Transferrin can replace serum for in vitro growth of mitogen-stimulated T lymphocytes. Eur J Immunol 9:942–948.

Doolittle RF, Hunkapillar MW, Hood LE, Devare SG, Robbins KC, Aaronson SA, Antoniades HN. 1983. Simian sarcoma virus onc gene, v-sis, is derived from the gene (or genes) encoding a platelet-derived growth factor. Science 221:275–277.

Feig LA, Bast RC, Knapp RC, Cooper GM. 1984. Somatic activation of ras^K gene in a human ovarian carcinoma. Science 223:698–701.

Goding JW, Burns GF. 1981. Monoclonal antibody OKT-9 recognizes the receptor for transferrin on human acute lymphocytic leukemia cells. J Immunol 127:1256–1258.

Goubin G, Goldman DS, Luce J, Neiman PE, Cooper GM. 1983. Molecular cloning and nucleotide sequence of a transforming gene detected by transfection of chicken B-cell lymphoma DNA. Nature 302:114–119.

Hall A, Marshall CJ, Spurr NK, Weiss RA. 1983. Identification of transforming gene in two human sarcoma cell lines as a new member of the *ras* gene family located on chromosome 1. Nature 303:396–400.

Haynes BF, Hemler M, Cotner T, Mann DL, Eisenbarth GS, Strominger J, Fauci AS. 1981. Characterization of a monoclonal antibody (5E9) that defines a human cell surface antigen of cell activation. J Immunol 127:347–351.

Hayward, WS, Neel BG, Astrin SM. 1981. Activation of a cellular onc gene by promotor insertion in ALV-induced lymphoid leukosis. Nature 290:475–480.

Hill M, Hillova J. 1971. Production virale dans les fibrobastes de poules traites par l'acide desoxyri-bonucleique de cellules XC de rat transforme' es par lo virus de Rous. C R Seances Acad Sci [III] 272:3094–3097.

Judd W, Poodry CA, Strominger JL. 1980. Novel surface antigens expressed on dividing cells but absent from non-dividing cells. J Exp Med 152:1430–1435.

Klein G. 1981. The role of gene dosage and genetic transpositions in carcinogenesis. Nature 294:313–318.

Lane M-A, Sainten A, Cooper GM. 1982a. Stage-specific transforming genes of human and mouse B- and T-lymphocyte neoplasms. Cell 28:873–880.

Lane M-A, Sainten A, Doherty KM, Cooper GM. 1984. Isolation and characterization of a stage-specific transforming gene, Tlym-1, from T cell lymphomas. Proc Natl Acad Sci USA 81:2227–2231.

Lane M-A, Neary D, Cooper GM. 1982b. Activation of a cellular transforming gene in tumors induced by Abelson murine leukemia virus. Nature 300:659–661.

Marcu KB, Harris LJ, Stanton LW, Erikson J, Watt R, Croce CM. 1983. Transcriptionally active c-myc oncogene is contained within NIARD, a DNA sequence with chromosome translocations in B-cell neoplasia. Proc Natl Acad Sci USA 80:519–523.

Morton CC, Taub R, Diamond A, Lane M-A, Cooper GM, Leder P. 1984. Mapping of the human Blym-1 transforming gene activated in Burkitt's lymphomas to chromosome 1. Science 223:173–175.

Murray MJ, Cunningham JM, Parada LF, Dautry F, Lebowitz P, Weinberg RA. 1983. The HL-60 transforming sequence: A ras oncogene coexisting with altered myc genes in hematopoietic tumors. Cell 33:749–757.

Neel BG, Jhanwar SC, Changant RSK, Hayward WS. 1982. Two human c-onc genes are located on the long arm of chromosome 8. Proc Natl Acad Sci USA 79:7842–7846.

Neiman PE, Payne LN, Jordan L, Weiss R. 1980. Malignant lymphoma of the bursa of fabricius: Analysis of early transformation. Cold Spring Harbor Symp Quant Biol 7:519–528.

Omary MB, Trowbridge IS, Minowada J. 1980. Human cell-surface glycoprotein with unusual properties. Nature 286:888–891.

Parada LF, Tabin CJ, Shih C, Weinberg RA. 1982. Human EJ bladder carcinoma oncogene is a homolog of Harvey sarcoma virus *ras* gene. Nature 297:474–478.

Reddy EP, Reynolds RK, Santos E, Barbacid M. 1982. A point mutation is responsible for the acquisition of transforming properties by the T24 human bladder carcinoma oncogene. Nature 300:149–153.

Reinherz EL, Kung PC, Goldstein G, Levey RH, Schlossman SF. 1980. Discrete stages of human intrathymic differentiation: Analysis of normal thymocytes and leukemic lymphoblasts of T-cell lineage. Proc Natl Acad Sci USA 77:1588–1592.

Rowley J. 1982. Identification of constant chromosome regions involved in human hematologic malignant disease. Science 216:749–751.

Shimizu K, Goldfarb M, Suard Y, Perucho M, Li Y, Kamata T, Feramisco J, Staunezer E, Togh J, Wigler MH. 1983. Three human transforming genes are related to the viral *ras* oncogenes. Proc Natl Acad Sci USA 80:2112–2116.

Sutherland R, Delia D, Schneider C, Newman R, Kemshead J, Greaves M. 1981. Ubiquitous cell-surface glycoprotein on tumor cells is proliferation-associated receptor for transferrin. Proc Natl Acad Sci USA 78:4515–4519.

Tabin CJ, Bradley SM, Bargmann CI, Weinberg RA, Papageorge AG, Scolnick EM, Dhar R, Lowy DR, Chang EH. 1982. Mechanism of activation of a human oncogene. Nature 300:143–149.

Taparowsky E, Suard Y, Fasano O, Shimizu K, Goldfarb M, Wigler M. 1982. Activation of the T24 bladder carcinoma transforming gene is linked to a single amino acid change. Nature 300:762–765.

Taub R, Kirsch I, Morton C, Lenoir G, Swan D, Tronick S, Aaronson S, Leder P. 1982. Translocation of the c-myc gene into the immunoglobulin heavy chain locus in human Burkitt lymphoma and murine plasmacytoma cells. Proc Natl Acad Sci USA 79:7837–7841.

Waterfield MD, Scrace GT, Whittle N, Strvobant P, Johnssan A, Wasteson A, Westermark B, Heldin C-H, Huang JS, Deuel T. 1983. Platelet derived growth factor is structurally related to the putative transforming protein p28[sis] of simian sarcoma virus. Nature 204:305–307.

Yuasa Y, Srivatava SK, Dunn CY, Rhim JS, Reddy EP, Aaronson SA. 1983. Acquisition of transforming properties by alternative point mutations with c-bas/has human proto-oncogene. Nature 303:775–779.

UT M.D. Anderson Clinical Conference on Cancer,
Vol. 27, edited by R. J. Ford, L. M. Fuller, and
F. B. Hagemeister. Raven Press, New York © 1984.

Burkitt's Lymphoma: Chromosome Translocations and Oncogene Activation

Peter C. Nowell, Janet Finan, Jan Erikson,* and Carlo M. Croce*

*Department of Pathology and Laboratory Medicine, University of Pennsylvania School of Medicine, and *The Wistar Institute of Anatomy and Biology, Philadelphia, PA 19104*

Recent studies of the cytogenetics and molecular genetics of various forms of human lymphoma and leukemia have demonstrated a number of chromosomal translocations that occur with nonrandom frequency, have indicated that these cytogenetic changes confer a selective growth advantage on the neoplastic cell, and have led to the suggestion that these translocations indicate sites in the human genome where genes that are important in neoplastic development are located (Klein 1981, Nowell 1983, Yunis 1983). Among the non-Hodgkin's lymphomas, the most common translocations typically involve the terminal portion of the long arm of chromosome 14 (band q34); the other chromosomes very frequently involved in the translocation are numbers 8, 11, or 18 (Fukuhara et al. 1978, Yunis et al. 1982).

The cytogenetic rearrangements in the Burkitt's lymphoma have been of particular interest and most extensively studied. In 1972, Manolov and Manolova observed an abnormally long chromosome 14 in the Burkitt's tumor, which was later shown to be the result of a reciprocal translocation between chromosomes 8 and 14 (Zech et al. 1976). Subsequently, two variant translocations have been described in 10% of Burkitt's lymphomas (Van Den Berghe et al. 1979, Lenoir et al. 1982), one involving a reciprocal translocation between chromosomes 8 and 22 and the other, a reciprocal translocation between chromosomes 2 and 8. Interestingly, the breakpoint in chromosome 8 in all instances is consistently at band q24 (Van Den Berghe 1979, Lenoir et al. 1982).

The use of somatic cell genetic techniques allowed the mapping of the genes for human immunoglobulin heavy chains to chromosome 14 (Croce et al. 1979), of λ light-chain genes to chromosome 22 (Erikson et al. 1981), and of κ light-chain genes to chromosome 2 (McBride et al. 1982, Malcolm et al. 1982). These findings suggested that the immunoglobulin chain genes might be involved in the various chromosomal translocations observed in Burkitt's lymphoma (Erikson et al. 1981).

Furthermore, recent analysis of rodent-human hybrids for the presence of the human homologues of known retroviral oncogenes has allowed the chromosomal localization of several human "oncogenes" (Dalla Favera et al. 1982a,b,c). One of these, the so-called c-*myc* oncogene, that is homologous to the avian virus oncogene v-*myc*, which can induce B-cell lymphoma in chickens, was located on the terminal portion of the long arm of chromosome 8 (band q24). This observation suggested that the c-*myc* oncogene might also have a role in the development of the Burkitt's tumor, since this is the segment of chromosome 8 that translocates to chromosome 14 in the typical t(8;14) translocation (Neel et al. 1982).

Using a combination of cytogenetic and somatic genetic techniques, we have examined various aspects of the structure and function of the immunoglobulin genes and the c-*myc* oncogene in Burkitt's tumor cell lines with the usual t(8;14) translocation and also with the variant t(8;22) and t(2;8) rearrangements. Some of our findings and conclusions to date are summarized below.

INVOLVEMENT OF IMMUNOGLOBULIN GENES AND THE c-*myc* ONCOGENE IN THE t(8;14) TRANSLOCATION IN BURKITT'S TUMORS

The involvement of the immunoglobulin heavy-chain locus in Burkitt's lymphomas with the t(8;14) chromosome translocation was shown using somatic cell hybrids between mouse myeloma cells and the Daudi Burkitt's tumor cell line (Erikson et al. 1982). Analysis of the hybrids indicated that genes for the variable regions of heavy chains translocated to the involved chromosome 8, and genes for the constant regions, remained on chromosome 14 (Erikson et al. 1982). Thus, the heavy-chain locus in these cells was split by the chromosomal break occurring in chromosome 14 in the generation of the t(8;14) translocation (Erikson et al. 1982).

Subsequently, similar techniques were used to demonstrate that the segment of chromosome 8 translocated to the long arm of chromosome 14 contained the c-*myc* oncogene (Dalla Favera et al. 1982a). By using restriction enzyme analysis and probes for the *myc* oncogene and for human immunoglobulin genes, several laboratories have now found rearrangements of the c-*myc* oncogene and head-to-head rearrangements between the c-*myc* and the C-μ gene in a number of Burkitt's lymphomas with the t(8;14) translocation (Dalla Favera et al. 1982a, Taub et al. 1982, Dalla Favera et al. 1983). These findings have been further confirmed by analysis of recombinant DNA clones containing the chromosomal breakpoint (Hamlin and Rabbits 1983). Diagrammatic representation of the involvement of the immunoglobulin and c-*myc* genes in the t(8;14) translocation, as we have observed it in the P3HR1 Burkitt's tumor cell line, is given in Figure 1.

ACTIVATION OF THE TRANSLOCATED c-*myc* ONCOGENE IN BURKITT'S LYMPHOMAS

High levels of c-*myc* transcripts have been observed in a number of Burkitt's lymphoma cell lines (Erikson et al. 1983a). These findings have now been extended to additional Burkitt's lymphomas, not only with the t(8;14) translocation but also with the t(8;22) and t(2;8) chromosome rearrangements, which have either a normal

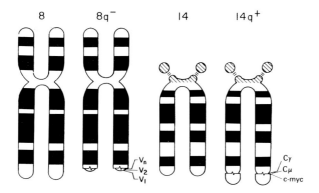

Figure 1. The t(8;14) chromosome translocation in Burkitt's lymphoma. The V$_H$ genes translocate from chromosome 14 to the involved 8 (8q⁻), while the c-*myc* oncogene translocates to the heavy-chain locus. (Reproduced from Erikson et al. 1983a, with permission of Proc Natl Acad Sci USA)

or a rearranged c-*myc* oncogene (Nishikura et al. 1983). In all circumstances, the levels of c-*myc* transcripts were consistently high, regardless of whether the gene appeared to be rearranged. In Burkitt's lymphoma cell lines with the t(8;14) translocation, the levels of *myc* transcripts were similar to or higher than those expressed in the HL-60 cell line derived from human promyelocytic leukemia that contains an amplified c-*myc* gene and expresses levels of c-*myc* transcripts 20- to 40-fold higher than normal cells (Dalla Favera et al. 1982d).

In our studies of somatic cell hybrids derived from Burkitt's cell lines with the t(8;14) translocation, only the hybrids containing the 14q⁺ chromosome expressed high levels of human c-*myc* transcripts. Hybrids containing the untranslocated c-*myc* gene on the normal chromosome 8 did not express such transcripts. Thus, we concluded that the translocated c-*myc* gene and the untranslocated c-*myc* gene are under different transcriptional control and that the c-*myc* gene that is close to the heavy-chain locus on the 14q⁺ chromosome is activated, whereas the normal c-*myc* gene, remaining on chromosome 8, is repressed (Nishikura et al. 1983). This finding, in conjunction with similar studies of hybrids derived from mouse plasmacytoma cells (Nishikura et al. 1983) and Epstein-Barr virus (EBV)–transformed human lymphoblastoid cells, indicates that the normal human c-*myc* oncogene is not active in a mouse plasmacytoma background, while the translocated oncogene in the same circumstances is expressed at high levels.

We have also investigated the levels of human c-*myc* transcripts in hybrid cells between mouse fibroblasts and Burkitt's lymphoma cells, and in this instance, we found a dramatic reduction of the levels of human *myc* transcripts in the hybrids (Nishikura et al. 1983). Thus, although the translocated c-*myc* oncogene appears to be expressed at abnormally high levels in a lymphoid cell background, it also appears clear that in cells of another differentiation lineage (e.g., fibroblasts), expression of the gene can be repressed.

INVOLVEMENT OF THE c-*myc* ONCOGENE IN BURKITT'S LYMPHOMAS WITH THE t(8;22) TRANSLOCATION

A Burkitt's cell line with the variant t(8;22) chromosome translocation has also been studied using the somatic cell genetics approach to explore the involvement of the c-*myc* oncogene and mechanisms of its activation in these circumstances. Somatic cell hybrids between mouse plasmacytoma cells and the BL2 Burkitt's lymphoma cell line, carrying a t(8;22) translocation, were examined for the presence and expression of human λ chains and the c-*myc* oncogene. Our data indicate that in these cells the c-*myc* oncogene remains on the 8q$^+$ chromosome, and the excluded and rearranged immunoglobulin C-λ allele translocates from chromosome 22 to this chromosome 8 (Croce et al. 1983). As a result of the translocation, transcriptional activation of the c-*myc* oncogene on the rearranged chromosome 8 (8q$^+$) occurs, while the c-*myc* oncogene on the normal chromosome 8 is transcriptionally silent.

These findings suggest that activation of a c-*myc* oncogene can occur through translocation of a rearranged immunoglobulin gene to the site of an unrearranged c-*myc* oncogene, as well as the reverse situation observed in the t(8;14) translocation. These results, coupled with those from the cells with the t(8;14) rearrangement, also indicate that the activating effect of the immunoglobulin gene can occur whether it is located on the 5' side or the 3' side of the c-*myc* oncogene. A diagrammatic representation of our findings with the t(8;22) translocation is given in Figure 2.

We have also examined the chromosomes of the BL2 cells using an in situ hybridization procedure with the C-λ DNA probe. These analyses indicate that all the C-λ genes translocate from chromosome 22 to chromosome 8 in these Burkitt's lymphoma cells (Emanuel et al. 1983). On the contrary, we have observed, using a similar technique, that all the C-λ genes remain on the Philadelphia chromosome

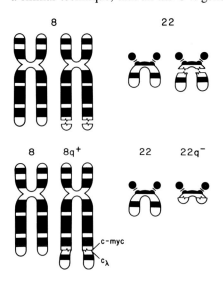

Figure 2. The t(8;22) translocation observed in BL2 Burkitt's lymphoma cells. The activated c-*myc* oncogene remains on chromosome 8, while the C-λ locus translocates to a region distal to the c-*myc* oncogene. (Reproduced from Croce et al. 1983, with permission of Proc Natl Acad Sci USA)

(22q⁻) in chronic myelogenous leukemia (CML) cells with the t(9;22) translocation that is typical of this disease (Emanuel et al. 1983). Thus, it appears that the chromosomal breakpoints in the q11 region of chromosomes 22 are different in Burkitt's lymphoma and CML, and the role of the λ immunoglobulin genes in the pathogenesis of the two diseases may also be different (Emanuel et al. 1983).

INVOLVEMENT OF THE c-*myc* ONCOGENE IN BURKITT'S LYMPHOMAS WITH THE t(2;8) TRANSLOCATION

We have also examined somatic cell hybrids between a mouse plasmacytoma and the JI Burkitt's cell line that carry the variant t(2;8) chromosome translocation for the structure and function of the human c-*myc* oncogene and κ-chain genes. Our results indicate that the c-*myc* gene is unrearranged and remains on the 8q⁺ chromosome of the JI cell line (Erikson et al. 1983b). Two rearranged immunoglobulin C-κ genes were detected, the expressed allele on the normal chromosome 2 and the excluded allele translocated from chromosome 2 to the involved chromosome 8(8q⁺) (Erikson et al. 1983b). The distribution of human V-κ and C-κ genes in hybrid clones retaining different human chromosomes indicated that C-κ is distal to V-κ on the short arm of chromosome 2 (2p) and that the chromosomal breakpoint in this Burkitt's lymphoma is within the portion of the gene complex coding for the variable region. High levels of transcripts of the c-*myc* gene were found when it resided on the 8q⁺ chromosome but not on the normal chromosome 8, demonstrating again, as in the t(8;22) rearrangement, that translocation of a light-chain gene locus to a region distal to the c-*myc* oncogene can enhance c-*myc* transcription. A diagram illustrating our findings with the JI cell line is given in Figure 3.

DISCUSSION AND CONCLUSIONS

The present findings support the hypothesis that chromosomal translocations can be one means by which genes that are important in the development of neoplasia (oncogenes) can undergo alterations in function that result in a selective growth advantage for the cell bearing such a translocation, and the progeny of that cell emerges as a neoplastic clone. Specifically, the findings in the Burkitt's tumor suggest that a chromosomal rearrangement in a B lymphocyte that places the c-*myc* oncogene adjacent to a transcriptionally active immunoglobulin gene leads to markedly increased transcription of the oncogene in circumstances in which it is not normally active. Additional support for this conclusion comes from concurrent observations with mouse plasmacytomas, in which a characteristic nonrandom chromosomal translocation involves the same immunoglobulin and *myc* genes as in the Burkitt's tumor, with the same effect of increased transcription of the c-*myc* gene (Marcu et al. 1982, Taub et al. 1982).

Although the nature and function of the *myc* gene product is not currently known, a 48,000 dalton protein has been precipitated from cells with high levels of *myc* transcripts. This is done by utilizing antibodies prepared against a synthetic peptide

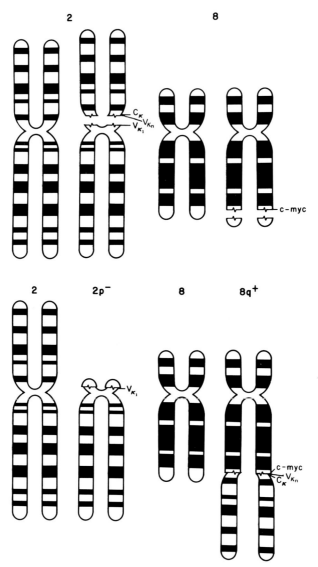

Figure 3. The t(2;8) translocation observed in JI Burkitt's lymphoma cells. The activated c-*myc* oncogene remains on chromosome 8, while the C-κ gene translocates to a region distal to the c-*myc* oncogene. (Reproduced from Erikson et al. 1983b, with permission of Proc Natl Acad Sci USA)

specific for the carboxyl terminus of the c-*myc* protein on the basis of the nucleotide sequences of *myc* DNA (Watt et al. 1983, Giallongo et al. 1983). Further study of this 48,000 dalton protein may well provide the basis for a better understanding of how increased transcription of c-*myc* in the Burkitt's tumor contributes to the abnormal growth of the neoplastic cells.

Chromosomal translocations, however, represent only one mechanism whereby various kinds of cytogenetic changes may alter gene function and contribute to tumorigenesis. Other nonrandom chromosome alterations that have been observed in various leukemias and lymphomas may reflect significant increase or decrease in oncogene dosage. This results from gains or losses of chromosomal segments or from gene amplification units observed as homogenous staining regions, abnormal banding regions, and double minutes (Yunis 1983, Nowell et al. 1983). It is also true that changes in oncogene function resulting from any of these kinds of cytogenetic alterations, as well as other critical changes in the genome not visible at the chromosome level, may themselves represent, in each instance, only one step in a complex sequence that ultimately results in the development of a clinical tumor. For instance, in the Burkitt's lymphoma, the development of the malignancy, particularly in those sections of Africa where it is endemic, may often require not only the alteration in *myc* gene expression resulting from the chromosome translocation but also EBV infection to enhance B-cell proliferation and chronic malarial infection to distort the immune system and allow the incipient neoplasm to flourish.

Nevertheless, the present results illustrate a fruitful approach to the search for human oncogenes and for the mechanisms of their activation. It is logical now to attempt to extend these studies to other non-Hodgkin's lymphomas, many of which demonstrate translocations that involve the terminal portion of 14q and either the long arm of chromosome 11 or the long arm of chromosome 18 (Fukuhara et al. 1978, Yunis et al. 1982). It appears very likely that these rearrangements involve the immunoglobulin heavy-chain locus, as in the t(8;14) translocation of the Burkitt's tumor, but at present there is no candidate oncogene that has been mapped to the relevant regions of 11q and 18q that might be activated in the same fashion as the *myc* gene in the Burkitt's lymphoma. It is possible that there are human "oncogenes" at these sites that are not represented among the retroviral oncogenes. In any event, techniques are now available to examine the structure and function of DNA sequences from these sites and to attempt to determine, in transfection experiments, their capacity to transform cells in vitro. In this connection, however, it will be important to keep in mind our studies of the 14q$^+$ chromosome from Burkitt's tumors, which indicate altered function of the *myc* gene at this site in the genome. Its contribution to neoplastic growth occurs in a lymphoid cell and not in a fibroblast. Test systems for unknown oncogenes that are important in the development of other lymphomas may also require the appropriate cell type to demonstrate their potential for oncogenesis.

REFERENCES

Croce CM, Shander M, Martinis J, Cicurel L, D'Ancona GG, Dolby TW, Koprowski H. 1979. Chromosomal location of the human immunoglobulin heavy chain genes. Proc Natl Acad Sci USA 76:3416–3419.

Croce C, Thierfelder W, Erikson J, Nishikura K, Finan J, Lenoir G, Rabbitts T, Nowell P. 1983. Transcriptional activation of an unrearranged and untranslocated c-myc oncogene by translocation of a C-lambda locus in Burkitt lymphoma. Proc Natl Acad Sci USA 80:6922–6926.

Dalla Favera R, Bregni M, Erikson J, Patterson D, Gallo RC, Croce CM. 1982a. Assignment of the human c-myc onc-gene to the region of chromosome 8 which is translocated in Burkitt lymphoma cells. Proc Natl Acad Sci USA 79:7824.

Dalla Favera R, Franchini G, Martinotti S, Wong-Staal F, Gallo RC, Croce CM. 1982b. Chromosomal assignment of the human homologues of feline sarcoma virus and avian myeloblastosis virus onc-genes. Proc Natl Acad Sci USA 79:4714–4717.

Dalla Favera R, Gallo RC, Giallongo A, Croce CM. 1982c. Chromosomal localization of the human homolog (c-sis) of the Simian sarcoma virus onc gene. Science 218:686–688.

Dalla Favera R, Martinotti S, Gallo RC, Erikson J, Croce CM. 1983. Translocation and rearrangements of the c-myc onc-gene in human undifferentiated B-cell lymphomas. Science 219:963–967.

Dalla Favera R, Wong-Staal F, Gallo RC. 1982d. *onc* gene amplificiation in promyelocytic leukaemia cell line HL-60 and primary leukaemic cells of the same patient. Nature 299:61–63.

Emanuel B, Wang E, Nowell PC, Selden J, Croce CM. 1984. Non-identical 22q11 breakpoint for the t(9;22) of CML and the t(8;22) of Burkitt's lymphoma. Cytogenet Cell Genet (In press).

Erikson J, Martinis J, Croce CM. 1981. Assignment of the human genes for immunoglobulin chains to chromosome 22. Nature 294:173–175.

Erikson J, ar-Rushdi A, Drwinga HL, Nowell PC, Croce CM. 1983a. Transcriptional activation of the c-myc oncogene in Burkitt lymphoma. Proc Natl Acad Sci USA 80:820–824.

Erikson J, Nishikura K, ar-Rushdi A, Finan J, Emanuel B, Lenoir G, Rabbitts TH, Nowell PC, Croce CM 1983b. Translocation of an immunoglobulin kappa locus to a region 3' of an unrearranged c-*myc* oncogene enhances c-*myc* transcription. Proc Natl Acad Sci USA. 80:7581–7585.

Fukuhara S, Rowley JD, Variakojis D, Sweet DL Jr. 1978. Banding studies on chromosomes in diffuse "histiocytic" lymphomas: correlation of 14q⁺ marker chromosomes with cytology. Blood 52:989–1002.

Giallongo A, Appella E, Ricciardi R, Rovera G, Croce CM. 1983. Identification of the c-*myc* oncogene product in normal and malignant B cells. Science 222:430–432.

Hamlin PH, Rabbitts TH. 1983. Translocation joins c-*myc* and immunoglobulin gamma-1 genes in a Burkitt lymphoma revealing a third exon in the c-myc oncogene. Nature 304:135–139.

Klein G. 1981. The role of gene dosage and genetic transpositions in carcinogenesis. Nature 294:313.

Lenoir GM, Preud'homme JL, Bernheim A, Berger R. 1982. Correlation between immunoglobulin light chain expression and variant translocation in Burkitt's lymphoma. Nature 298:474–476.

Malcolm S, Barton P, Murphy C, Ferguson-Smith MA, Bentley DL, Rabbitts TH. 1982. Localization of human immunoglobulin light chain variable region genes to the short arm of chromosome 2 by *in situ* hybridization. Proc Natl Acad Sci USA 79:4957–4961.

Manolov G, Manolova Y. 1972. Marker band in one chromosome 14 from Burkitt lymphoma. Nature 237:33–34.

Marcu K, Harris L, Stanton L, Erikson J, Watt R, Croce CM. 1982. Transcriptionally active c-*myc* oncogene is contained within NIARD, a DNA sequence associated with chromosomal translocations in B-cell neoplasia. Proc Natl Acad Sci USA 80:519–523.

McBride OW, Heiter PA, Hollis GF, Swan D, Otey MC, Leder P. 1982. Chromosomal location of human kappa and lambda immunoglobulin light chain constant region genes. J Exp Med 155:1480–1490.

Neel B, Jhanwar S, Chaganti R, Hayward W. 1982. Two human c-onc genes are located on the long arm of chromosome 8. Proc Natl Acad Sci USA 79:7842–7846.

Nishikura K, ar-Rushdi A, Erikson J, Watt R, Rovera G, Croce CM. 1983. Differential expression of the normal and of the translocated human c-myc oncogenes in B cells. Proc Natl Acad Sci USA 80:4822–4826.

Nowell P. 1983. Tumor progression and clonal evolution: the role of genetic instability. *In* German J ed., Chromosome Mutation and Neoplasia. Alan R. Liss, New York, pp. 413–432.

Nowell P, Finan J, Dalla Favera R, Gallo R, ar-Rushdi A, Ramanczuk P, Selden J, Emanuel B, Rovera G, Croce C. 1983. Association of amplified oncogene c-*myc* with an abnormally banded chromosome 8 in a human leukaemia cell line. Nature 306:494–497.

Taub R, Kirsch I, Morton C, Lenoir G, Swan D, Tronick S, Aaronson S, Leder P. 1982. Translocation of the c-*myc* gene into the immunoglobulin heavy chain locus in human Burkitt lymphoma and murine plasmacytoma cells. Proc Natl Acad Sci USA 79:7837–7841.

Van Den Berghe H, Paloir C, Gosseye S, Englebienne V, Cornu G, Sokal G. 1979. Variant translocation in Burkitt lymphoma. Cancer Genet Cytogenet 1:9–14.

Watt R, Stanton LW, Marcu KB, Gallo RC, Croce CM, Rovera, G. 1983. Nucleotide sequence of cloned cDNA of the human c-*myc* oncogene. Nature 303:725–728.

Yunis JJ, Oken, MM, Kaplan ME, Ensrud KM, Howe RR, Theologides A. 1982. Distinctive chromosomal abnormalities in histologic subtypes of non-Hodgkin's lymphoma. N Engl J Med 307:1231–1236.

Yunis JJ 1983. The chromosomal basis of human neoplasia. Science 221:227–236.

Zech L, Haglund V, Nilsson N, Klein G. 1976. Characteristic chromosomal abnormalities in biopsied and lymphoid-cell lines from patients with Burkitt and non-Burkitt lymphomas. Int J Cancer 17:47–57.

UT M.D. Anderson Clinical Conference on Cancer,
Vol. 27, edited by R. J. Ford, L. M. Fuller, and
F. B. Hagemeister. Raven Press, New York © 1984.

The Family of Human T-Cell Tropic Retroviruses Called HTLV and Its Role in Adult T-Cell Leukemia

Flossie Wong-Staal and Robert C. Gallo

*Laboratory of Tumor Cell Biology, National Cancer Institute, National Institutes of
Health, Bethesda, Maryland 20205*

Although retroviruses have been identified as the prime etiologic agents in many animal leukemias and lymphomas, the evidence for a human leukemia virus was slow to develop. In retrospect, the earlier studies were limited by technology that was inadequate to detect a low level virus and to effect the long-term growth of appropriate leukemic cells and by the lack of a prototype human retrovirus to use as a probe. These difficulties were not appreciated because the then available animal models all indicated abundant virus replication in the leukemic cells and substantial antigen cross-reactivity among different mammalian retrovirus core proteins so that reagents from one virus could be used to detect other viruses. However, findings in the bovine leukemia virus (BLV) system compelled us to reexamine these preconceived notions. First, although BLV is clearly the agent in bovine leukemia, the circulating leukemic cells are negative for virus, virus antigens, or even viral mRNA. Only after the cells were cultured did they express the BLV genome, and then the virus could be isolated (see Burny et al., 1980 for review). Second, once isolated, BLV was found to have no immunologic cross reactivity with other retroviruses. These are exact parallels for isolation of the first class of the human leukemia virus, HTLV.

The discovery of the T-cell growth factor (TCGF) (Morgan et al. 1976) made it possible, for the first time, to grow both normal and neoplastic mature human T cells in long-term suspension culture. T cells from normal donors can be grown only after lectin or antigen stimulation. In contrast, certain neoplastic mature T cells respond to TCGF without prior lectin or antigen activation in vitro. These cells already contain TCGF receptors, now routinely detected by a monoclonal antibody called anti-TAC (Leonard et al. 1982). It was from some of these cultured T-cell lines, established from sporadic cases in United States with a certain subtype of adult T-cell malignancy, that the first unambiguous human retrovirus, HTLV, was isolated (Poiesz et al. 1980, 1981).

There are now about 35 isolates of HTLV. Isolates have been obtained from cell lines established from patients around the world with mature T-cell malignancies.

These patients include individuals born in the United States, Israel, Japan, the Caribbean, Africa, and South America (see Popovic et al. 1984 for review). All virus isolates from Japan are indistinguishable from the prototype United States HTLV isolates. Multiple isolates have also been obtained from black patients from the Caribbean. Most of the isolates from the different patients belong to a particular strain we call HTLV-I. It has become apparent that *most* HTLV-I–positive lymphomas and leukemias fall into a clinical syndrome consisting of disease onset in adulthood, rapid disease course, associated lymphadenopathy and hepatosplenomegaly, circulating large and usually pleomorphic lymphocytes with lobulated nuclei, presence of T-cell surface phenotypic markers (usually OKT4+), and frequent hypercalcemia and skin manifestations (Gallo et al. 1983). This disease is now called adult T-cell leukemia-lymphoma (ATLL). In 1982, we isolated another T-lymphotropic human retrovirus that is distantly related to HTLV-I (Kalyanaraman et al., 1982). This isolate, which we call HTLV-II, was obtained from the cell line MO, derived from a young white male with hairy cell leukemia of a T-cell subtype (Saxon et al 1978). Since then, HTLV-II has been isolated once from a black i.v. drug user with acquired immune deficiency syndrome (AIDS) (Popovic M, Gallo R unpublished data). Very recently, we identified variants of HTLV-I from ATLL and AIDS patients (Shaw G, Hahn B, Wong-Staal F, and Gallo R unpublished data). Old World monkeys are also infected with viruses related to but distinguishable from HTLV-I. (Guo et al. 1984).

A seroepidemiological survey of patients with ATLL and normal people from endemic and nonendemic regions of Japan shows that almost all patients with the clinical diagnosis of ATLL have HTLV-specific antibodies and that a number of normal individuals from these regions are also antibody positive (Robert-Guroff et al. 1983). In collaborative studies with W. Blattner and the National Cancer Institute and N. Gibbs in Jamaica, we found an unusually high incidence of antibody to HTLV in patients from the Caribbean with lymphoid malignancies and in a small percentage of normal individuals from that area (Blattner et al. 1983). Finally, more recently related findings have been made in black patients from the southeastern United States, Africa, and South America (Saxinger et al. 1984).

In this paper, we will emphasize the recent molecular biological studies on HTLV, focusing on three aspects:

1. A molecular epidemiological survey of human leukemias using cloned HTLV probes. Even though seroepidemiological studies have already indicated an association between HTLV and ATLL, this analysis would allow detection of HTLV infection even in the absence of viral antigens or antibodies. In seropositive cases, in which the patients' diseases are not ATLL, this analysis will also tell us if HTLV plays a direct role in these other diseases.

2. The state of the provirus in fresh ATLL cells, primary T-cell lines established from these, and normal cord blood T-cell lines transformed in vitro with HTLV. These may represent different stages of leukemogenesis, in which the in vitro

transformed cells are at the initiation phase and the circulating leukemic cells are at the maintenance phase.

3. The mode of expression of viral and some relevant cellular genes in different HTLV infected cells. Through these studies, coupled with those outlined in 2, we hope to gain some insight into the molecular mechanism of leukemogenesis.

MOLECULAR EPIDEMIOLOGY OF HTLV AND HUMAN LEUKEMIAS

We have used the cloned genomes of HTLV-I and HTLV-II (Marzari et al. 1983b, Gelmann et al. 1984) to survey fresh cells and tissues of patients with various hematologic malignancies. All of the typical ATLL samples, as well as a few cases of more benign cutaneous T-cell lymphoma, were postive. All of these contain closely related, if not identical, proviruses of the HTLV-I subgroup. All other malignancies, including acute and chronic myeloid leukemias, acute lympho-cytic leukemias, and hairy cell leukemia, were negative. Thus, HTLV-I is tightly associated with mature T-cell malignancies, and HTLV-II is an extremely rare variant of HTLV, obviously not the agent generally associated with hairy cell leukemia. Table 1 lists the samples that were positive. With one exception, all fresh

Table 1. *HTLV Provirus in Fresh Tissues of ATL Patients*

Patient	Origin	Tissue	Copy number
CF	US	PBL	3
BH	US	PBL	1
HSy	US	PBL	1½
		Spleen	1½
		Thymus	1½
MA	Brazil	Skin biopsy	3
SY	Japan	PBL	1½
JT	Japan/Haiti	PBL	1½
JM	Japan	PBL	½
TY	Japan	PBL	2
FY	Japan	PBL	1½
YT	Japan	Lymph node	1
SD	Japan/US	PBL	1
SK	Japan	PBL	1
HSt	Caribbean/UK	PBL	Polyclonal
MI	Caribbean/US	PBL	3
		Thymus	3
		Lymph node	3
		Spleen	3
		Lung	Negative
		Kidney	Negative
		Brain	Negative
		Liver	Negative

ATL–adult T-cell leukemia; PBL–peripheral blood leuko-cytes.

tumor cells appear to be clonally infected. One patient (HST) with adult T-cell leukemia (ATL) who migrated to London from the Caribbean was unique in that his cells were polyclonally infected. More detailed analysis of this case is underway. The other leukemic cells contained one to three copies of proviruses that are either complete or defective. DNA from the leukemic cell of a patient (JM) who had no antibody against HTLV antigens contained a single defective provirus.

Autopsy tissues from two patients showed that the level of detectable HTLV sequences correlated with the degree of infiltration of the leukemic cells, while noninvolved tissues were negative.

Leukemic cells of two patients who were seropositive for HTLV but whose diseases were not ATLL were examined. Neither sample, a T-cell acute lymphocytic leukemia (T-ALL) and a B-cell chronic lymphocytic leukemia (B-CLL), contained detectable HTLV sequences, although cultured T cells of the latter did contain HTLV. This result indicates that HTLV does not have a direct role in these patients' diseases. However, since it has been observed that in HTLV endemic regions, patients with lymphoid malignancies had a higher percentage of HTLV positivity than normal, it is possible that in some patients HTLV-infected T cells can secrete a protein, e.g., a growth factor that primarily stimulates the abnormal proliferation of B cells or immature T cells leading to transformation by a secondary process. Alternatively, HTLV-infected individuals may be immune compromised and more prone to develop other malignancies.

CLONAL SELECTION OF HTLV-INFECTED CELLS IN VIVO AND IN VITRO

All ATL leukemic cells, as well as established T-cell lines from HTLV-positive individuals, are mono- or oligoclonally derived, as analyzed by provirus integration (Wong-Staal et al. 1983, Yoshida et al. 1982). While peripheral blood cells from healthy seropositive individuals are polyclonally infected, cell lines established from normal individuals also appear to be clonally derived (Hahn B, Gallo R, Wong-Staal F, unpublished data). These observations suggest that clonal selection occurs in vivo in the leukemic patient and in vitro for cells established from nonleukemic individuals.

To determine whether fresh and cultured cells represent similar infected cell populations, we compared DNA from fresh peripheral blood cells of a patient (SK) with his cultured T cells. As shown in Figure 1, fresh SK cells contained one predominant cell clone, as reflected by the 17 Kb EcoRI bands. The predominant clone in the fresh cells was present, at best, as a rare clone in the cultured SK cell line, which contained multiple copies of HTLV provirus, some of which were defective. Comparison of several other pairs of primary and cultured leukemic cells consistently showed one or two copies of HTLV in the fresh cells and increased copies in the cultured cells (Hahn B, Franchini G, Gallo R, Wong-Staal F, unpublished data). Digestions with the restriction endonucleases PstI, BamHI, and SstI revealed conserved internal bands between SK fresh cells and cell lines but non-

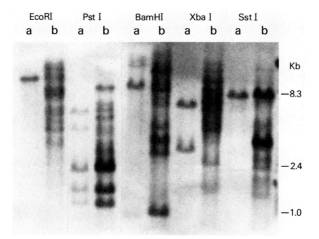

Figure 1. Comparison of HTLV proviruses in primary leukemic cells and an established cell line of an ATLL patient. High molecular cellular DNA was digested with the enzymes as indicated, electrophoresed in 0.8% agarose gels, transferred to nitrocellulose, and hybridized with a complete HTLV-I genome probe. The conditions for hybridization, washing, and autoradiography were as described (Wong-Staal et al. 1983). **(a)** Fresh leukemic cells of SK. **(b)** The SK line.

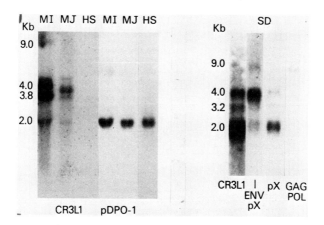

Figure 2. Expression of viral mRNA in fresh and cultured HTLV-infected cells. Poly(A) containing cellular RNA was hybridized to the probes as indicated. CR3L1 is a HTLV probe containing U3 and R sequences. pDPO-1 is an HLA class I probe. Fragments containing *gag, pol, env, pX* of HTLV established T-cell lines and HS and SD are fresh leukemic cells. (See text for description of results.)

corresponding junction bands. The clearest result was with XbaI, which cuts once in the HTLV genome. The two junction bands in fresh SK cells do not comigrate with any of the junction bands of the SK cell line.

These results suggest that the clonally expanded leukemic cells lose their proliferative advantage so that the normal T cells infected in vivo or during culture outgrow the leukemic cells. These infected normal cells may initally go through a polyclonal phase. However, a specific cell population eventually dominates in the culture. The apparent clonality of the infected cell lines established from normal people may have been a progression of this selection process in vitro. Examination of primary infected cells or cultured cells taken at different time intervals from these individuals is necessary to address this possibility.

Normal T cells infected and immortalized by HTLV in vitro are also clonal, and we consider them to be equivalent to the established cell lines from ATLL patients. These newly infected cells resemble primary transformed cells in many respects (Popovic et al. 1984) and provides a good model for studying the process of transformation initiation. The circulating leukemic cells, on the other hand, may only have to maintain the leukemic state. We shall examine the role of viral and some cellular genes in these two separate cell systems.

DETECTION OF VIRAL TRANSCRIPTS IN HTLV-INFECTED CELL LINES AND FRESH LEUKEMIC CELLS OF ATL PATIENTS

RNA obtained from the fresh lymphocytes of two ATLL patients and five established cell lines was hybridized to a long terminal repeat (LTR) probe of HTLV (Franchini G, Gallo R, Wong-Staal F, unpublished data) (Figure 2). Several species of viral mRNA were detected in all cell lines and in one of the two fresh cell samples, including a 9.0 kilobase (kb) mRNA corresponding to the HTLV genomic size, which must encode for the *gag* and *pol* proteins, and a 4 kb species, which is probably the mRNA for the *env* protein. In the one fresh cell sample (SD) we also used specific probes to define the different species. As expected, the 9.0 kb species hybridized to all the probes. The intensity of the 4 kb species increases conspicuously when hybridized with a probe containing the whole *env* gene plus 1 kb of a region identified as pX, which lies 3' to the envelope sequence and whose function is unknown (Seiki et al. 1983). This finding confirms its identity as the *env* mRNA. A 2.0 kb species was hybridized specifically to LTR and a pX probe, suggesting that the pX region is transcribed separately from *env* sequences as a subgenomic mRNA. Finally, a 3.2 kb species contains only LTR sequences and because of its size, must contain nonviral sequences covalently linked to the LTR. The nature of the presumable cell-derived sequences is not known.

RNA from one fresh sample (HSy) was not hybridized to any viral probes. As a control for the quality of HS RNA, the same filter was annealed with a plasmid probe containing the HLA class I gene. The expected 2 kb mRNA was detected in this RNA and in the two positive cell lines with comparable signal intensities.

Thus, it appears that expression of viral proteins, including pX, may be necessary for the initiation, but not for maintenance, of transformation. In the latter stage, cellular genes may be activated. The most obvious candidates are growth factor genes and cellular homologues of retroviral *onc* genes.

MODE OF EXPRESSION OF THE T-CELL GROWTH FACTOR GENE AND SOME CELLULAR *onc* GENE HOMOLOGUES

The clonality of the HTLV in vivo- and in vitro-transformed cells, the presence of defective viral genomes, and the lack of a requirement for viral gene expression are features that resemble the avian leukosis virus—bursal lymphoma system (Neel et al. 1981). In the latter, activation of a cellular proto-oncogene c-*myc* is known to be responsible for neoplastic transformation. We therefore examined the possibility of gene activation as a possible mechanism of leukemogenesis by HTLV. All HTLV infected cells express a high density of the TCGF receptor (Waldmann et al. 1983).Therefore, an attractive model would be expression of TCGF in these same cells, which would result in autostimulation. Using a cloned TCGF gene (Clark et al. 1984) as a probe, we detected an extremely low level of transcripts in a few HTLV-positive cell lines but not in most (Arya et al. 1984). TCGF is not expressed in the fresh leukemic cells (Franchini G, Gallo R, Wong-Staal F, unpublished data). Therefore, a simple autostimulation mechanism cannot be operative either in initiation or maintenance of leukemia. However, it is possible that the TCGF receptor expressed on these cells has been altered so that it now recognizes another growth factor or that, in its altered state, it is activated without binding to any factor. There is some evidence that the TCGF receptor expressed in HTLV-infected T cells may be qualitatively different from that of normal cells (W. Greene, personal communication). Therefore, the receptor for TCGF is a natural focus for future efforts to understand the mechanism of transformation by HTLV.

We have also examined the possibility of *onc* gene activation after HTLV infection (Franchini G, Gallo R, Wong-Staal F, unpublished data). Using cloned probes of *sis, myc, myb, fes, abl, src, rasH, rasK*, we failed to find consistent activation of any *onc* gene in either the in vitro infected cells or fresh leukemic cells, thus negating a requisite role of the *onc* genes tested in either initiation or maintenance of transformation. However, it is of interest to note that a significant number of HTLV infected cell lines express c-*sis*, (Westin et al. 1982, Wong-Staal et al. 1984) a gene not normally expressed in hematopoietic cells. Since c-*sis* codes for a growth factor (PDGF), which normally acts on fibroblasts, smooth muscle cells, and glial cells, it would be of interest to see if the *sis* product produced in these cells can aberrently stimulate their proliferation.

SUMMARY

HTLV is a family of related T-cell tropic human exogenous retroviruses consisting of at least two distinct subgroups. Members of subgroup I are highly conserved, if not identical, isolates obtained worldwide, while subgroup II consists of only two isolates so far. HTLV-I infection is closely associated with adult T-cell leukemia and lymphoma, but the disease spectrum of HTLV-II has not been defined.

HTLV does not carry an *onc* gene and causes tumors that are clonally derived. Therefore, it falls into the class of chronic leukemia viruses. However, it is the only known chronic leukemia virus that can efficiently immortalize fresh human cells in vitro. We believe that in vitro immortalization represents a first stage (initiation) of neoplastic transformation, while the circulating leukemic cells represent a later stage, involving maintenance of the transformed state. We found that viral expression may be necessary for initiation but not maintenance of transformation. A simple autostimulation mechanism involving TCGF production in the transformed cells has been ruled out at both early and late stages, and there is no evidence of consistent activation of a known *onc* gene. However, the TCGF receptor and c-*sis* are genes we want to investigate further. Whether HTLV activates these or other cellular genes by provirus insertion during the initiation phase and the kind of events that lead to establishment of leukemia are questions of great interest.

ACKNOWLEDGMENT

We are grateful to our colleagues who contributed to this work, especially Drs. G. Franchini and B. Hahn for permission to cite their unpublished data. We also thank A. Mazzuca and N. Gustat for editorial assistance.

REFERENCES

Arya SK, Wong-Staal F, Gallo RC. 1984. Expression of T-cell growth factor gene in human T-cell leukemia-lymphoma virus infected cells. Science 223:1086–1087.

Blattner WA, Kalyanaraman VS, Robert-Guroff M, Lister TA, Galton DAG, Sarin PS, Crawford MH, Catovsky D, Greaves M, Gallo RC. 1982. The human type-C retrovirus HTLV in Blacks from the Caribbean region, and relationship to adult T-cell leukemia/lymphoma. Int J Cancer 30:257–264.

Burny A, Bruck C, Chantrenne H, Cleuter Y, Dekezel D, Ghysdael J, Kettemann R, Leclercq M, Leunen J, Mammerickx M, Potelle D. 1980. Bovine leukemia virus: Molecular biology and epidemiology. *In* Klein G., ed., Viral Oncology. Raven Press, New York, pp. 231–280.

Clark SC, Arya SK, Wong-Staal F, Matsumoto-Kobayashi M, Kay RM, Kaufman RJ, Brown EL, Showmaker C, Copeland T, Oroszlan S, Smith K, Sarngadharan MG, Lindner SG, Gallo RC. 1984. Human T-cell growth factor: Partial amino acid sequence of the proteins expressed by normal and leukemic cells, molecular cloning of the mRNA from normal cells, analysis of gene structure and expression in different human cell types. Proc Natl Acad Sci USA 81:2543–2547.

Gallo RC, Kalyanaraman VS, Sarngadharan MG, Sliski A, Vonherheid EC, Maeda M, Nakao Y, Yamada K, Ito Y, Gutensohn N, Murphy S, Bunn PA, Catovsky D, Greaves MF, Blayney DW, Blattner W, Jarrett WFH, zur Hausen H, Seligman M, Brouet JC, Haynes BF, Jegasothy BV, Jaffe E, Cossman J, Broder S, Fisher RI, Golde DW, Robert-Guroff M. 1983. Association of the human type-C retrovirus with subset of adult T-cell cancers. Cancer Res 43:3892–3899.

Gelmann EP, Franchini G, Manzari V, Wong-Staal F, Gallo RC. 1984. Molecular cloning of a new unique T-leukemia virus (HTLV-II$_{Mo}$). Proc Natl Acad Sci USA 81:993–997.

Guo HG, Wong-Staal F, Gallo RC. 1984. Novel viral sequences related to human T-cell leukemia virus in T-cells of a seropositive baboon. Science 223:1195–1197.

Kalyanaraman VS, Sarngadharan MG, Robert-Guroff M, Miyoshi I, Blayney D, Golde D, Gallo RC. 1982. A new subtype of human T-cell leukemia virus (HTLV-I) associated with a T-cell variant of hairy cell leukemia. Science 218:571–573.

Leonard WJ, Depper JM, Uchiyama T, Smith KA, Waldman TA, Greene WC. 1982. A monoclonal antibody that appears to recognize the receptor for human T-cell growth factor. Nature 300:267–269.

Manzari V, Wong-Staal F, Franchini G, Colombini S, Gelmann EP, Oroszlan S, Staal SP, Gallo RC. 1983. Human T-cell leukemia-lymphoma virus, HTLV: Molecular cloning of an integrated defective provirus and flanking cellular sequences. Proc Natl Acad Sci USA 80:1574–1578.

Morgan DA, Ruscetti FW, Gallo RC. 1976. Selective *in vitro* growth of T-lymphocytes from normal human bone marrows. Science 193:1007–1008.

Neel BG, Hayward WS, Robinson HL, Fang J, Astrin SM. 1981. Avian leukosis virus induced tumors have common proviral integration sites and synthesize discrete new RNA's: Oncogenesis by promoter insertion. Cell 23:323–334.

Poiesz BJ, Ruscetti FW, Gazdar AF, Bunn PA, Minna JD, Gallo RC. 1980. Isolation of type-c retrovirus particles from cultured and fresh lymphocytes from a patient with cutaneous T-cell lymphoma. Proc Natl Acad Sci USA 77:7415–7419.

Poiesz BJ, Ruscetti FW, Retiz MS, Kalyanaraman VS, Gallo RC. 1981. Isolation of a new type-C retrovirus (HTLV) in primary uncultured cells of a patient with Sezary T-cell leukemia. Nature 294:268–271.

Popovic M, Wong-Staal F, Sarin P, Gallo RC. 1984. Biology of human T-cell leukemia/lymphoma virus HTLV: Transformation of T-cells *in vivo* and *in vitro*. *In* Klein G., ed., Advances in Viral Oncology. Raven Press, New York pp. 44–70.

Robert-Guroff M, Kalyanaraman VS, Blattner, WA, Popovic M, Sarngadharan MG, Maeda M, Blayney D, Catovsky D, Bunn PA, Shibata A, Nakao Y, Ito Y, Aoki T, Gallo RC. 1983. Evidence for human T-cell lymphoma-leukemia virus infection of family members of human T-cell leukemia-lymphoma patients. J Exp Med 157:248–258.

Saxinger WC, Lange-Wantzin G, Thomsen K, Lapin B, Yakovleva I, Li YW, Guo HG, Robert-Guroff M, Blattner WA, Ito Y, Gallo RC. 1984. Human T-cell leukemia virus: A diverse family of related exogenous retroviruses of human and old world primates. *In* Gallo RC, Essex M, Gross L, eds., Human T-cell leukemia viruses. Cold Spring Harbor Press, New York pp. 323–330.

Saxon A, Stevens RH, Golde DW. 1978. T-lymphocyte variant of hairy cell leukemia. Ann Intern Med 88:323–326.

Seiki M, Hattori S, Hirayama Y, Yoishida M. 1983. Human adult T-cell leukemia virus: Complete nucleotide sequence of the provirus genome integrated in leukemia cell DNA. Proc Natl Acad Sci USA 88:3618–3622.

Waldmann T, Broder S, Greene W, Sarin PS, Goldman C, Frost K, Sharrow S, Depper J, Leonard W, Uchiyama T, Gallo RC. 1983. A comparison of the function and phenotype Sezary T-cells adult T-cell leukemia cells. Clin Res 31:547A.

Westin EH, Wong-Staal F, Gelmann EP, Dalla-Favera R, Papas TS, Lautenberger JA, Eva A, Reddy EP, Tronick SR, Aaronson SA, Gallo RC. 1982. Expression of cellular homologues of retroviral *onc* genes in human hematopoietic cells. Proc Natl Acad Sci USA 79:2490–2494.

Wong-Staal F, Hahn B, Manzari V, Colombini S, Franchini G, Gelmann EP, Gallo RC. 1983. A survey of human leukemias for sequences of a human retrovirus. Nature 302:626–628.

Yoshida M, Miyoshi I, Hinuma Y. 1982. Isolation and characterization of retrovirus from cell lines of human adult T-cell leukemia and its implication in the disease. Proc Natl Acad Sci USA 79:2031–2035.

UT M.D. Anderson Clinical Conference on Cancer,
Vol. 27, edited by R.J. Ford, L.M. Fuller, and
F.B. Hagemeister. Raven Press, New York © 1984.

Immunoglobulin Gene Rearrangements as B-Cell–Associated Clonal Markers in Human Lymphoid Neoplasms

Andrew Arnold, Ajay Bakhshi, Jeffrey Cossman, Elaine S. Jaffe, Thomas A. Waldmann, and Stanley J. Korsmeyer

Metabolism Branch and Laboratory of Pathology, National Cancer Institute, National Institutes of Health, Bethesda, Maryland 20205

The elucidation of the specific cellular lineage to which lymphoid neoplasms belong has been of crucial importance in advancing our understanding of the biology and pathogenesis of these malignancies. The analyses of cell surface markers have been the predominant means by which the cellular type and stage of differentiation have been assigned to individual neoplasms (Aisenberg 1978, Rudders et al. 1981). Furthermore, the determination of clonality within malignant expansions of cells has been of great conceptual importance in the investigation of their etiologies. The demonstration of a monoclonal population has also served as a central piece of information to help distinguish benign from malignant cell proliferation (Faguet et al. 1978).

A wide variety of lineage-associated cell surface markers are usually sufficient to classify a lymphoid neoplasm as a B or T cell. At times however, such marker analysis can be inconclusive. This is frequently because of an admixture of large numbers of nonneoplastic cells with the neoplastic cells of a lymphomatous tissue. In addition, malignancies representing cellular stages that are early in differentiation may not yet express surface markers solely restricted to a given lineage. Finally, purely technical factors, such as the presence of extraordinarily avid Fc receptors, can result in ambiguous findings. Beyond assigning a B- or T-cell classification to a neoplasm, the determination of whether such cells are monoclonal may be even more difficult. In fact, the determination of clonality is predominantly limited to B-cell tumors that display the presence of only one light-chain isotype, κ or λ (Levy et al. 1977). Other clonal markers that may be useful, even in T cells, are specific cytogenetic abnormalities or the presence of one of two distinguishable glucose-6-phosphate dehydrogenase (G6PD) isoenzymes in a female patient (Rowley and Fukuhara 1980, Fialkow et al. 1973). However, the latter markers are frequently not applicable or available in many cases.

Because of the frequent difficulties in ascertaining the cellular lineage and clonality of a neoplasm, we turned to a recombinant DNA approach. Specifically, we have utilized the DNA rearrangement of Ig genes as a sensitive marker for clonality and a specific marker for B-cell lineage.

THE GENERATION OF UNIQUE CLONAL MARKERS BY REARRANGEMENT OF IMMUNOGLOBULIN DNA SEGMENTS

The process of making a functional Ig gene creates a clonal marker specific to that particular B cell. This is generated by the act of DNA rearrangement, which combines, at the DNA level, the separated gene segments responsible for the final Ig molecule (Brack et al. 1978, Seidman et al. 1979). One such Ig gene rearrangement is shown schematically in Figure 1, in which one of many available variable (V_κ) regions is juxtaposed with one of five joining (J_κ) segments (Hieter et al. 1980). This completed rearrangement of V_κ/J_κ codes for the entire variable portion of the κ-chain molecule. This rearranged allele of κ can then be transcribed into RNA, and the recombined V_κ/J_κ and constant (C_κ) information assembled at the RNA level. It is however, the phenomenon of V/J joining at the DNA level that generates a marker that is unique to an individual cell. This results from a change in the location of restriction endonuclease sites that surround the κ gene (Figure 1). A restriction endonuclease is an enzyme that reproducibly cuts DNA and does so only at a specific site where a select set of nucleic acid bases are aligned. Such endonuclease digestion results in restriction DNA fragments of reproducible length. A DNA rearrangement such as V_κ/J_κ joining alters the location of such restriction sites and thus generates an altered size of the restriction fragment containing the κ gene. Therefore rearranged Ig genes are found on different size DNA restriction fragments when compared with their germline or embryonic form (Figure 1) (Korsmeyer et al. 1981).

A polyclonal population of normal B cells is comprised of many different cells that contain numerous different Ig gene rearrangements. Correspondingly, such a

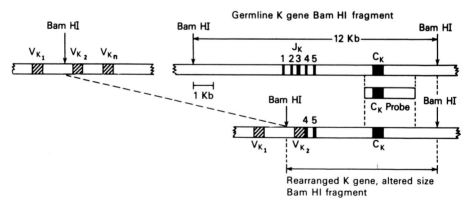

Figure 1. A germline rearranged κ gene allele. A single variable κ segment (V_κ 2) is rearranged to join a single joining κ segment ($J_{\kappa4}$). This rearrangement introduces a new 5′ BamHI site so that the BamHI restriction endonuclease fragment recognized by the constant κ (C_κ) probe is of different size than the 12 kilobase (12,000 base pair) germline BamHI fragment.

mixture of cells will have numerous different size DNA restriction fragments that contain these rearranged genes. When analyzed using the Southern blot analysis, none of the rearranged genes in this collective population is discernible because they are below the threshold of sensitivity (Korsmeyer et al. 1982). In contrast, a monoclonal expansion of B cells represents the progeny of a single cell and will thus have multiple copies of the same DNA rearrangement, which is unique to that cell. This rearrangement is clearly detectable as a distinct band on the autoradiogram of a Southern blot. As we will discuss, such detectable Ig gene rearrangements serve as sensitive as well as specific markers for clonal B cells.

IMMUNOGLOBULIN GENE CONFIGURATION IN HUMAN HEMATOPOIETIC MALIGNANCIES

The rearrangement of heavy- plus light-chain genes is mandatory in mature B cells in order to produce Ig. Consistently, all known B-cell malignancies studied have displayed clonal rearrangements of heavy- and light-chain genes. This includes over 30 cases composed of chronic lymphocytic leukemia, Waldenstrom's macro-globulinemia, multiple myeloma, hairy cell leukemia, B-cell follicular and diffuse lymphomas, Burkitt's lymphoma, as well as Epstein-Barr virus–transformed normal B-cell lines (Korsmeyer et al. 1983b). At least one, and frequently both, heavy-chain genes were rearranged in order to effectively assemble variable (V_H), diversity (D_H) and joining (J_H) segments of the variable portion of the molecule (Ravetch et al. 1981). It is important to note that κ-producing B cells had at least one κ gene rearrangement, while their λ genes remained in the germline form. In contrast, λ-producing B cells that displayed the obligate λ gene rearrangements had either rearranged or deleted their κ genes (Hieter et al. 1981b, Hieter et al. 1981a, Korsmeyer et al. 1982). These findings are the result of an ordered sequence of Ig gene rearrangments in humans in which heavy-chain gene rearrangement precedes light-chain genes and κ rearranges before λ (Korsmeyer et al. 1981).

Twenty-five known T-cell malignancies, including T-cell–type acute lympho-blastic leukemia, T-cell–type chronic lymphocytic leukemia, Sezáry cell syndrome, adult T-cell leukemia, as well as T-cell–type diffuse and lymphoblastic lymphomas, all retained germline light-chain genes (κ and λ). Furthermore, most malignancies (23/25) also displayed germline heavy-chain genes, although several exceptions do exist. Malignancies of nonlymphoid hematopoietic cells, including acute myelogen-ous leukemia, acute and chronic myeloid phases of chronic myelogenous leukemia, promyelocytic leukemia, monocytic leukemia, and a histiocytelike case of diffuse lymphoma, retained germline heavy- and light-chain genes. Therefore, the presence of heavy- plus light-chain gene rearrangements is a finding apparently restricted to cells of B-cell lineage (Arnold et al. 1983).

IMMUNOGLOBULIN GENE REARRANGEMENTS IN AN UNDIFFERENTIATED MALIGNANCY

Of the nine cases we examined, histologic and cell surface marker analyses did not enable us to classify the malignant cells as either a lymphoma or an undifferentiated carcinoma in Case 1 (Figure 2). Surface staining with the monoclonal antibodies B1, BA-1, BA-2, Lyt3, and T-200 were negative. In addition there was no detectable TdT (terminal deoxynucleotydl transferase), HLA-DR, or cytoplasmic or surface Ig. Furthermore, electron microscopic examination revealed no signs of epithelial differentiation. However, the DNA from these malignant cells of a pleural effusion revealed clonal heavy- and κ light-chain gene rearrangements (Arnold et al. 1983). Non–B-cell hematopoietic malignancies and a variety of carcinomas retained germline heavy- and light-chain genes. This DNA information is therefore strong evidence favoring a diagnosis of a B-cell lymphoma when the histology was unclear.

CLONAL POPULATIONS OF B CELLS IN SOME T-CELL–PREDOMINANT LYMPHOMAS

Our attention was directed to several lymphomas (Cases 2, 3, and 4) with predominances of T cells and small numbers of B cells present in the biopsies (Table 1). In addition, one of these patients (Case 3) with diffuse histology had a recurrence following an initial diagnosis of follicular lymphoma. We questioned whether clonal B cells might exist within these lymphomatous tissues. Initial experiments indicated that Ig gene rearrangments could be detected within the total

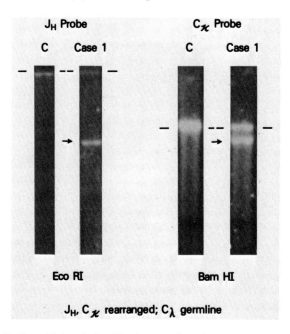

Figure 2. The Southern blot analysis of the Ig genes from Case 1 when probed with a heavy-chain joining (J_H) probe and a κ constant ($C_κ$) probe. An *arrow* indicates the rearranged alleles while *dash marks* denote the germline positions of these genes in nonlymphoid control DNA (C) and the case. The patient had gastric mass and malignant pleural effusion. Histopathology, cytology: large cell lymphoma versus undifferentiated carcinoma.

Table 1. *Histology, Cell Surface Phenotype, and Immunoglobulin Gene Configuration*

Case	Histology	B1	Lyt3	Surface Ig H-chain	κ	λ	Ig genes
2	Diffuse mixed cell lymphoma	13%	73%	Neg	Neg	Neg	J_H rearranged $C_κ$ rearranged
3	Follicular and diffuse mixed cell lymphoma	26%	89%	None predominant (G 5%, A 23%, M 28%, D 14%)	Neg	Neg	J_H rearranged $C_λ$ rearranged
4	Diffuse large cell lymphoma	15%	77%	None predominant (G 7%, M 14%, D 8%)	12%	9%	J_H rearranged
5	Follicular large cell lymphoma	B1 n.d. BA − 1 = 6% BA − 2 = 0	32%	None predominant (G 27%, A 11%, M 26%, D 20%)	11%	4%	J_H rearranged $C_κ$ doubly rearranged
6	Diffuse large cell lymphoma	36%	47%	Minority G 7% and M 39%	15%	28%	J_H rearranged
7	Follicular small cleaved cell lymphoma	65%	17%	None predominant (G 3%, M 19%, D 14%)	11%	18%	J_H doubly rearranged $C_κ$ rearranged
8	Follicular small cleaved cell lymphoma	70%	23%	None predominant (G 16%, M 24%, D 25%)	12%	14%	J_H rearranged $C_λ$ rearranged
9	Diffuse large cell lymphoma	93%	2%	Neg	Neg	Neg	$C_λ$ rearranged

H-chain–heavy chain; n.d.–not done; G–IgG; A–IgA; M–IgM; D–IgD.
Reactivity with monoclonal antibodies B1 and Lyt3 are presented as representative B- and T-cell antigens, respectively, except Case 5 in which BA-1 and BA-2 data are shown. Surface Ig is listed as negative (Neg) when less than 10% of cells bore Ig. All cases (except 9) were analyzed with J_H, $C_κ$ and $C_λ$ probes and the rearrangements seen are listed.

DNA from a mixture of cell types if monoclonal B cells constituted only 5%-10% of the cells present. In spite of the T-cell majority (73%-89%) in these three tissues, clonally rearranged Ig genes were present in all three cases. Cases 2 and 3 actually had heavy- and light-chain rearrangements indicating that clonal populations of B cells were present (Arnold et al. 1983). There are no applicable markers at this time to exclude the simultaneous presence of a clonal T-cell population in these tissues. The balance of the information however, suggests that these are B-cell malignancies with a large number of infiltrating nonneoplastic T cells.

ESTABLISHMENT OF MONOCLONALITY AND CELLULAR LINEAGE IN LYMPHOMAS WITH NONDEFINITIVE SURFACE MARKER ANALYSIS

Immunoglobulin surface analysis revealed five cases (Cases 5-9) in which no single heavy- or light-chain isotype was predominant (Table 1). T cells, as well as

B cells, were present in various proportions in each case. Despite this, Cases 5, 7, 8, and 9 had clonal light-chain gene rearrangements indicating a commitment to producing a single light chain at the DNA level (Table 1). Thus, these lymphomas also appear to be comprised of clonal B-cell proliferations (Arnold et al. 1983). Case 6 revealed a heavy-chain gene rearrangement but no light-chain gene rearrangement. While this finding established its clonal nature, a B- versus T-cell origin could not be unequivocally determined for Case 6 because some T cells may have recombined heavy-chain genes. It is possible that this malignancy corresponds to a B-cell precursor in which heavy-chain genes are rearranged but light-chain gene rearrangement has not been initiated (Korsmeyer et al. 1983a).

DETECTION OF CLONAL B CELLS IN
LYMPHOPROLIFERATIVE LESIONS

The diagnostic choice between a benign and malignant lymphoid proliferation in the setting of an immunodeficient host is frequently difficult to make on histologic grounds alone. In such cases, the demonstration of clonality, often based on the presence of a single cell surface light chain (κ or λ) has served as important information favoring malignancy (Zulman et al. 1978). A tissue biopsy of progressively enlarging lymphadenopathy revealed the histology shown in Figure 3, in a patient with Wiskott-Aldrich syndrome. The diagnosis was atypical follicular hyperplasia. Consistent with this, surface marker analysis of the cellular population revealed the presence of both κ- and λ-bearing B cells and many Lyt3-positive T cells. Despite this, DNA analysis demonstrated the presence of a minority population of clonal B cells, bearing rearranged heavy- and κ light-chain genes (Figure 3) (Arnold et al. 1983). Because another atypical follicular hyperplasia from an immunodeficient patient, as well as four sets of tonsils with reactive follicular hyperplasia showed no Ig gene rearrangements, the clonal population of cells in the patient with Wiskott-Aldrich syndrome are of concern. It is possible that these clonal B cells are still benign and under some regulatory control. Alternatively, their presence may represent the early detection of a malignancy that will ultimately become the dominant cell in these lymph nodes.

IMMUNOGLOBULIN REARRANGMENTS AS UNIQUE
CLONAL MARKERS

The specific Ig gene rearrangement pattern noted in the lymph node of the patient with Wiskott-Aldrich syndrome (Figure 3) is unique to a clone of B cells comprising a minority of the cells within the tissue. This type of marker will allow the natural history of such a cell clone to be determined by following the cells during serial examinations.

A dramatic example of the potency of DNA rearrangements as unique clonal markers was provided by a serial examination of the affected cells from a patient with chronic myelogenous leukemia (CML) (Bakhshi et al. 1983). When this patient's affected cells were examined during a chronic myelogenous phase, the

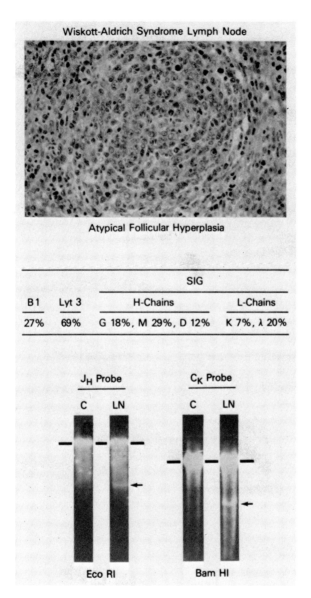

Figure 3. A lymph node biopsy from a patient with Wiskott-Aldrich syndrome had a histologic appearance of an atypical follicular hyperplasia. Cell surface marker analysis of lymphoid cells obtained from this lesion revealed a mixed population. Examination of the DNA from this lymph node (LN) revealed clonal rearrangements in a subpopulation of these cells *(arrows)* when the J_H and C_κ probes were hybridized with the EcoRI- and BamHI-digested DNA respectively. A non-lymphoid control DNA (C) displays the germline configuration *(dash marks)* of these genes.

clonal granulocytes bearing the t(9;22) Philadelphia chromosomal marker had germ-line heavy- and light-chain genes (Figure 4). During two separate lymphoid blast crises, however, the lymphoid cells displayed a new cytogenetic marker consisting of a loss of chromosome 7, 45XY-7 t(9;22). In addition, these clinically distinct lymphoid crises possessed identical heavy-chain gene rearrangments in both epi-sodes. These findings indicate that both blast crises could ultimately be traced to a common lymphoid progenitor cell that had doubly rearranged heavy-chain genes but had germline light-chain genes. The two lymphoid blast crises could be genet-ically distinguished, however. The first crisis had moved on to λ light-chain gene rearrangement, whereas the second crisis had germline light-chain genes. Thus, the immediate precursor cells, which gave rise to the separate lymphoid blast crises in the patient, varied in their extent of genetic maturation. This finding indicated that the clonally affected B-cell precursors in CML can undergo the sequential differ-entiation steps of heavy- and then light-chain rearrangement (Bakhski et al. 1983).

IMPLICATIONS

The Ig gene assembly recombines, in an apparently random fashion, a single variable and joining segment from multiple germline alternatives. The pattern of

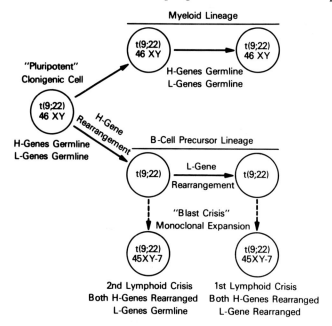

Figure 4. The pluripotent clonigenic cell, which bears the Philadelphia chromosome t(9;22) when it pursues an acute or chronic myeloid course, retains germline Ig genes. When the affected cells pursue a B-cell pathway, they are capable of sequential heavy-(H) and light-chain (L) gene rearrangement. In this particular individual, two separate episodes of lymphoid blast crisis had identical H-chain gene rearrangements as well as a unique cytogenetic marker missing chro-mosome 7. However, the first lymphoid crisis had progressed to light chain gene rearrangement, whereas the second crisis retained germline light-chain genes. (Reproduced from Bakhshi et al. 1983 with permission of *New England Journal of Medicine*.)

heavy- and light-chain gene rearrangement generated is thus specific for an individual B cell and can serve as a unique, clonal marker identifying the progeny of that cell. In addition the simultaneous presence of heavy- plus light-chain rearrangements is relatively restricted to B cells and thus serves as a lineage-associated marker. This specificity is complemented by the sensitivity of this methodology, which allows clonal B cells to be identified even if they contribute only 5% of the total DNA that is being analyzed (Arnold et al. 1983). The cases presented here offer evidence for the value of this technology.

Since Ig gene rearrangement is a marker at the DNA level, it does not require the final expression of the antibody product for its detection. Ig gene rearrangements are initiated early in B-cell development thus making this method of value even in B-cell precursors, which express no surface Ig (Korsmeyer et al. 1983). Furthermore, sufficient DNA is readily obtained from either fresh or frozen specimens making the procedure possible on routinely available clinical material. Such a sensitive and specific marker will enable clonal populations of B cells to be followed over time and their natural history to be determined. The sensitivity of this approach may be of particular use when an Ig rearrangement serves as a tumor-specific marker. It may allow the early detection of recurrences following therapy when no other tumor markers are available.

Although Ig gene rearrangements are predominantly restricted to cells of B-lymphoid lineage, other malignancies frequently possess DNA rearrangements as well. One example of this is the chromosomal translocations that are specifically associated with a number of malignancies (Rowley 1980). These recombinations between nonhomologous chromosomes involve certain genetic loci and result in changes in the location of restriction endonuclease sites within the DNA. As these translocation sites become better defined, it should be possible to identify molecular rearrangements in the DNA in many of them. This approach should generate genetic markers unique to the individual tumors from a wide variety of malignancies. The application of these molecular genetic approaches should improve our ability to understand, identify, classify, and follow neoplastic cells.

REFERENCES

Aisenberg AC. 1978. Cell surface markers in lymphoproliferative disease. N Engl J Med 304:331–336.

Arnold A, Cossman J, Bakhshi A, Jaffe E, Waldmann TA, Korsmeyer SJ. 1983. Immunoglobulin gene rearrangements as unique clonal markers in human lymphoid neoplasms. N Engl J Med 309:1593–1599.

Bakhshi A, Minowada J, Arnold A, Cossman J, Jensen JP, Whang-Peng J, Waldmann TA, Korsmeyer SJ. 1983. Lymphoid blast crises of chronic myelogenous leukemia represent stages in the development of B-cell precursors. N Engl J Med 309:826–831.

Brack C, Hirama N, Lenhard-Schuller R, Tonegawa S. 1978. A complete immunoglobulin gene is created by somatic recombination. Cell 15:1–14.

Faguet GB, Webb HH, Agee JF, Ricks WB, Sharbaugh AH. 1978. Immunologically diagnosed malignancy in Sjogren's pseudolymphoma. Am J Med 65:424–429.

Fialkow PJ, Klein E, Klein G, Clifford P, Singh S. 1973. Immunoglobulin and glucose-6-phosphate dehydrogenase as markers of cellular origin in Burkitt lymphoma. J Exp Med 138:89–102.

Hieter PA, Hollis GF, Korsmeyer SJ, Waldmann TA, Leder P. 1981a. Clustered arrangement of immunoglobulin λ constant region genes in man. Nature 294:536–540.

Hieter PA, Korsmeyer SJ, Waldmann TA, Leder P. 1981b. Human immunoglobulin κ light-chain genes are deleted or rearranged in λ-producing B-cells. Nature 290:368–372.

Hieter PA, Max EE, Seidman JG, Maizel JV Jr, Leder P. 1980. Cloned human and mouse kappa immunoglobulin constant and J region genes conserve homology in functional segments. Cell 22:197–207.

Korsmeyer SJ, Arnold A, Bakhshi A, Ravetch JV, Siebenlist U, Hieter PA, Sharrow SO, LeBien TW, Kersey JH, Poplack DG, Leder P, Waldmann TA. 1983a. Immunoglobulin gene rearrangement and cell surface antigen expression in acute lymphocytic leukemias of T-cell and B-cell precursor origins. J Clin Invest 71:301–313.

Korsmeyer SJ, Greene WC, Cossman J, Hsu Su-M, Neckers LM, Marshall SL, Jensen JP, Bakhshi A, Leonard WJ, Jaffe ES, Waldmann TA. 1983b. Rearrangement and expression of immunoglobulin genes and expression of Tac antigen in hairy cell leukemia. Proc Natl Acad Sci USA 80:4522–4526.

Korsmeyer SJ, Hieter PA, Ravetch JV, Poplack DG, Waldmann TA, Leder P. 1981. Developmental hierarchy of immunoglobulin gene rearrangements in human leukemic pre-B cells. Proc Natl Acad Sci USA 78:7096–7100.

Korsmeyer SJ, Hieter PA, Sharrow SO, Goldmann CK, Leder P, Waldmann TA. 1982. Normal human B-cells display ordered light chain gene rearrangements and deletions. J Exp Med 156:975–985.

Levy R, Warnke R, Dorfman RF, Haimovich J. 1977. The monoclonality of human B-cell lymphomas. J Exp Med 145:1014–28.

Ravetch JV, Siebenlist U, Korsmeyer SJ, Waldmann TA, Leder P. 1981. Structure of the immunoglobulin μ locus: Characterization of embryonic and rearranged J and D genes. Cell 27:583–591.

Rowley JD. 1980. Chromosome abnormalities in cancer. Cancer Genet Cytogenet 2:175–198.

Rowley JD, Fukuhara S. 1980. Chromosome studies in non-Hodgkin's lymphomas. Sem Oncol 7:255–266.

Rudders RA, Ahl ET Jr, DeLellis RA. 1981. Surface marker and histopathologic correlation with long term survival in advanced large-cell non-Hodgkin's lymphoma. Cancer 47:1329–35.

Seidman JG, Max EE, Leder P. 1979. A κ-immunoglobulin gene is formed by site specific recombination without further somatic mutation. Nature 280:370–5.

Zulman J, Jaffe R, Talal N. 1978. Evidence that the malignant lymphoma of Sjorgen's syndrome is a monoclonal B-cell neoplasm. N Engl J Med 299:1215–1220.

UT M.D. Anderson Clinical Conference on Cancer,
Vol. 27, edited by R. J. Ford, L. M. Fuller, and
F. B. Hagemeister. Raven Press, New York © 1984.

Approaches to Understanding the Role of Normal Lymphocyte Homing Mechanisms in the Spread of Human Lymphoid Neoplasms

Eugene C. Butcher, Sirpa Jalkanen, Lynne Herron,
and Robert Bargatze

*Department of Pathology, Stanford University Medical Center, Stanford, California
94305, and The Veterans Administration Medical Center, Palo Alto, California 94304*

Normal lymphocytes are uniquely mobile cells, circulating continuously from one lymphoid organ to another during certain phases of their life cycle. The non-Hodgkin's lymphomas—neoplasms of lymphocytes—frequently appear to share this propensity to migrate. Although some lymphomas demonstrate metastasis by mechanisms similar to those of many nonlymphoid malignancies (i.e., by local lymphatic spread or by formation of distant solid metastases), other lymphoid neoplasms demonstrate a unique capacity to disseminate via the blood stream to involve many distant lymphoid organs. It is interesting to hypothesize that such patterns of hematogenous lymphoid dissemination may be determined by the same homing mechanisms utilized in the circulation and traffic of normal lymphocyte populations. In this chapter, we describe two approaches that we have initiated to analyze the expression of normal lymphocyte migration mechanisms by neoplastic human lymphocytes and to understand the role of these lymphocyte homing mechanisms in the dissemination of lymphomas and leukemias.

BACKGROUND: THE CONTROL OF LYMPHOCYTE TRAFFIC BY LYMPHOCYTE–ENDOTHELIAL CELL INTERACTIONS

Normal lymphocytes utilize specific cell to cell interactions to regulate their migration and positioning. One of the most important of these involves the specific recognition by normal recirculating lymphocytes of endothelial cell determinants expressed in high levels by the specialized high endothelial venules (HEV) in lymph nodes and in the mucosa-associated lymphoid organs (appendix and Peyer's patches). Lymphocyte recognition of and binding to HEV leads to selective lymphocyte entry into these lymphoid organs from the blood (Gowans and Knight 1964, reviewed in Butcher 1984). The ability of lymphocytes to bind to HEV has been studied extensively in murine model systems, using an in vitro assay in which viable lymphocytes bind specifically to HEV when incubated on frozen sections of mouse or rat lymph nodes or Peyer's patches (Stamper and Woodruff 1976, Butcher et al. 1979). The binding of lymphocytes to HEV in this in vitro assay correlates extremely well with their ability to home to lymphoid organs in vivo and with their ability to participate in the recirculating lymphocyte pool.

The capacity of lymphocytes to bind to HEV is exquisitely regulated during lymphocyte development and differentiation (reviewed in Butcher 1984). Pre-B cells in the bone marrow and the vast majority of thymocytes express only very low levels of homing receptors, and bind poorly to HEV. Upon migrating from the primary lymphoid organs as mature but "virgin" B and T cells, however, lymphocytes join the circulating lymphocyte pool and are capable of binding well to HEV. Antigenic stimulation appears to lead to a transient phase of suppression of HEV-binding capacity. In the B-cell lineage, antigen-specific dividing blasts accumulate within germinal centers, and in this site, they undergo little exchange with the surrounding circulating pool of IgD$^+$ B lymphocytes (Parrott 1966). When isolated from stimulated lymph nodes or Peyer's patches by virtue of their unique phenotype (surface peanut agglutinin-binding, surface IgD$^-$), germinal center cells fail to bind to HEV and are unable to migrate normally from the blood into lymphoid organs in vivo (Reichert et al. 1983). Within the T-cell lineage, antigen-activated T blasts may also undergo a sessile stage of differentiation during which they are incompetent to migrate or bind to HEV (Sprent 1980). Cloned murine T cells of suppressor or helper phenotype appear to be uniformly unable to interact with HEV or to circulate in vivo and, in fact, the ability to bind HEV appears to be rapidly lost following T-cell activation with concanavalin A or in a mixed leukocyte culture (Dailey et al. 1983). Presumably this stage of suppression of migration mechanisms relates to the need for stimulated cells to differentiate and proliferate under local microenvironmental controls prior to reentering the circulatory system.

Following this period of homing receptor suppression and local differentiation, many lymphoblasts appear to reexpress HEV-binding ability and the capacity to traffic in vivo, so that when they leave the site of antigenic stimulation as differentiated effector cells or effector-precursor cells, they are able to specifically traffic from the blood to other lymphoid sites or to sites of inflammation. For example, immunoblasts draining into efferent lymph from stimulated lymphoid organs are competent to home to specific lymphoid tissues (Gowans and Knight 1965, Griscelli et al. 1969, Smith et al. 1980), and in selected cases bind to HEV as well (Butcher et al. 1982). Included in such immunoblastic populations may be Ig-containing immunoblast precursors of plasma cells, as well as specific T effector or effector-precursor cell populations. Antigen stimulated lymphocytes also give rise to populations of memory lymphocytes, and these also recirculate extensively, probably more rapidly than virgin B- and T-lymphocyte populations. The migratory properties of specific tissue effector cells have not often been studied, but it seems likely that mature plasma cells may again repress the surface characteristics associated with lymphocyte circulation.

In summary, the HEV-binding ability and migratory properties of lymphocytes are modulated as a function of development, antigen stimulation, and specific microenvironments. Thus particular stages of normal lymphocyte differentiation, many of which have specific neoplastic counterparts, are characterized by well-defined HEV-binding and migratory characteristics.

RELATIONSHIP BETWEEN THE SPREAD OF LYMPHOID NEOPLASMS AND THE MIGRATORY PROPERTIES OF THEIR NORMAL LYMPHOCYTE COUNTERPARTS

Many human lymphomas or leukemias appear to mimic or to represent malignant transformation of cells at particular stages of B- or T-cell differentiation, and a consideration of the clinical presentation and behavior of non-Hodgkin's lymphomas suggests that the rate and mode of dissemination of these lymphoid neoplasms not infrequently reflects the migratory potential of their normal counterparts. For example, large cell follicular lymphomas, which exhibit the surface and morphologic phenotype of large germinal center cells (a sessile lymphocyte population), may involve solitary lymphoid sites with local lymphatic spread. On the other hand, well differentiated B-cell malignancies with similarities to circulating small IgD$^+$ B cells, such as chronic lymphocytic leukemia or well-differentiated lymphoma, often disseminate widely via the bloodstream to involve lymphoid organs more generally. Such correspondence between the spread of lymphomas and the traffic patterns of their normal lymphocyte counterparts is far from absolute, however, and, in fact, exceptions to such correlation are very common. Clearly, the morphologic or antigenic phenotype of a lymphoma or leukemia is not an adequate predictor of its tendency to utilize normal lymphocyte modes of dissemination. *Direct assay of lymphoid malignancies for the expression of normal lymphocyte homing mechanisms might, however, permit more accurate predictions about their means of spread.*

The potential prognostic significance of direct assays of migratory competence is suggested by preliminary studies of a well-defined class of lymphoid malignancies that occur spontaneously in AKR mice. These AKR lymphomas are of thymic origin and are, in general, morphologically similar, yet they demonstrate diverse patterns of presentation and of dissemination on passage into adoptive syngeneic recipients. Preliminary studies of a small series of these related lymphomas suggest that *HEV-binding lymphomas* (N = 8) tend toward early hematogenous dissemination, involving all secondary lymphoid organs symmetrically with little or no local involvement at subcutaneous sites of injection, whereas the predominant manifestation of *nonbinding lymphomas* (N = 3) is massive local growth with local lymphatic spread and only late dissemination to distant lymphoid sites (Bargatze R, Weissman IL, Butcher EC, unpublished data). Although preliminary, these studies suggest that the expression of surface receptors for HEV, receptors required for the circulation of normal lymphocytes, may also help determine or at least be correlated with the patterns of dissemination of lymphoid malignancies. The role of lymphoid homing receptors in controlling the in vivo behavior of lymphomas and leukemias clearly requires more extensive and critical analysis in murine model systems, but even more important, it must be examined in humans.

AN IN VITRO FUNCTIONAL ASSAY OF HUMAN LYMPHOCYTE MIGRATORY POTENTIAL

The ability of lymphocytes to recognize and bind to endothelial cells is intrinsic to the migration of lymphocytes from the blood stream into lymphoid organs, and therefore is necessary for the overall process of lymphocyte traffic and for the vascular dissemination of lymphocyte populations. The in vitro model of lymphocyte binding to HEV in lymph node frozen sections has provided a direct functional assay for this essential recognition step in murine systems. We have been able to adapt this assay to allow analysis of the HEV-binding properties of human lymphocytes on mouse HEV and, more recently, on human HEV also. Preliminary analyses of normal lymphocyte populations suggest that, as in the mouse, the expression of HEV-binding ability and thus of migratory competence is closely regulated during human lymphocyte differentiation. For example, human thymocytes bind poorly in comparison to human peripheral blood lymphocytes or tonsillar cells.

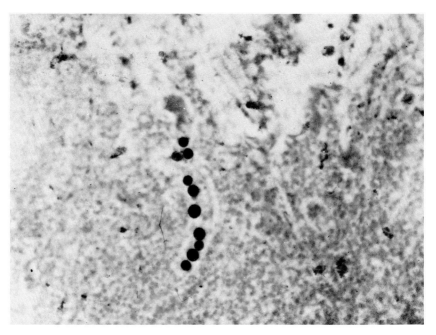

Figure 1. Cells of a B-lymphoblastoid cell line (1BW4) binding to high endothelial venules (HEV) in the frozen section assay. (Cells are incubated with agitation on fresh frozen sections, and HEV-adherent cells are cross linked to the tissue section by placing the slides in 1% glutaraldehyde in phosphate-buffered saline.) Thionine stains the whole bound cells more darkly than the fragmented cells in the frozen section. × 200.

Initial studies of several in vitro human T-cell lines and B-lymphoblastoid lines have revealed a spectrum of HEV-binding in these transformed human lymphocyte populations (Figure 1, Table 1). These preliminary data suggest that human lymphoid malignancies may indeed vary in their expression of normal lymphocyte traffic mechanisms. In the future we will use this in vitro assay to study a series of non-Hodgkin's lymphomas for correlation of their HEV-binding ability with their in vivo growth patterns.

A MOLECULAR APPROACH: MONOCLONAL ANTIBODIES AGAINST HUMAN LYMPHOCYTE HOMING RECEPTORS FOR HEV

The production of monoclonal antibodies against human lymphocyte surface molecules mediating lymphocyte recognition of HEV might allow assessment of the expression of such homing receptors in simple immunofluorescence or immunoperoxidase analyses. If the surface expression of these molecules correlated well with HEV-binding ability, such antireceptor antibodies might offer an attractive alternative approach to characterizing the migratory potential of normal and neoplastic human lymphocytes. In fact, we have recently isolated a monoclonal antibody, LSRE-1 (9B5), that appears to define the human lymphocyte surface receptor or receptors for HEV. Produced from a fusion of Sp2/0 murine myeloma cells with spleen cells from a rat immunized with human peripheral blood and tonsillar lymphocytes, LSRE-1 defines a human lymphocyte surface antigen whose expression correlates well with the migratory properties and probable HEV-binding characteristics of defined normal lymphocyte subpopulations. For example, the putative homing receptor is expressed only at very low levels by most cortical thymocytes, but the vast majority of peripheral small T cells and mature, IgD$^+$ B cells that participate in the recirculating lymphocyte pool stain brightly with the antibody. Germinal center cells, which represent a nonmigratory stage of B-cell activation in vivo in the mouse, fail to stain with LSRE-1. Furthermore, the antigen defined by LSRE-1 demonstrates striking biochemical similarities to a mouse lymphocyte

Table 1. *High Endothelial Venule Binding Abilities of Selected Human B-Lymphoblastoid Cell Lines*

Sample cell	HEV binding ability (arbitrary units)*	Sample cell	HEV binding ability (arbitrary units)*
Daudi	0.03	KCA	0.2
LBF	1.9	PBL control†	1.7
1BW4	1.2		

*Sample populations were incubated 30 min at 6°C on fresh frozen tissue sections of lymph nodes, and bound cells were fixed to HEV by placing the slides in 1% glutaraldehyde in phosphate-buffered saline. Details of assay and quantitation of HEV binding are described in Butcher et al. 1979.

†Ficoll-purified normal peripheral blood lymphocytes (PBL) are included for comparison.

surface receptor for lymph node HEV, which we have previously described. This mouse lymphocyte homing receptor is defined by a monoclonal antibody, MEL-14 (Gallatin et al. 1983). Like MEL-14 in the murine system, LSRE-1 immuno-precipitates an 80-90kd surface glycoprotein from circulating human lymphocytes. The mouse and human antigens also share a highly acidic isoelectric point (pI≈4.25). While in the murine system MEL-14 can directly inhibit lymphocyte recognition of lymph node HEV, pretreatment of human lymphocytes with LSRE-1 does not directly block HEV binding, which suggests that the antigenic determinant defined is not in the recognition domain of the putative HEV receptor. However, the LSRE-1 antigen can be serologically linked to the HEV recognition function. Rat anti–human lymphocyte serum pretreatment effectively blocks the ability of human lymphocytes to bind to HEV, and this functional blocking activity can be specifically removed by absorption of the antiserum with the purified receptor molecule, affinity isolated from lymphocyte membrane lysates on an LSRE-1 antibody column (Jalkanen S, Bargatze R, Butcher EC, unpublished data). While short of formal proof, these findings strongly support the proposal that LSRE-1 defines a specific lymphocyte surface molecule responsible for HEV recognition and binding and hence required for lymphocyte migration.

Preliminary immunofluorescence studies of B- and T-cell lines in vitro indicate (as suggested by the functional assays just described) that transformed cells demonstrate substantial differences in levels of expression of the putative homing receptor. Studies of the expression of the LSRE-1–defined homing receptor by non-Hodgkin's lymphomas in vivo have just been initiated, however, and thus at present we do not know whether receptor expression will correlate with the morphologic or antigenic phenotype of lymphomas or with patterns of presentation or spread. It is already clear, however, that the antibody will be useful for examining these questions. As shown in Figure 2, LSRE-1 permits direct immunohistologic analysis of homing receptor expression by in vivo lymphoid malignancies, and the few such studies performed to date have already confirmed the expected diversity in expression of this functionally important surface molecule. The availability of this immunohistologic approach to assessing the migratory potential of lymphoid cells should not only facilitate analysis of the role of homing receptors in the dissemination of lymphoid neoplasms but may also permit study of the importance of these receptors in controlling the traffic of normal lymphocytes in inflammatory and autoimmune conditions.

Figure 2.   Immunoperoxidase staining of two non-Hodgkin's lymphomas with an antibody against the putative human lymphocyte surface receptor for HEV.   Top. Chronic lymphocytic leukemia in a lymph node. Most cells stain intensely. Note the presence of several positive lymphocytes in the lumen of a long HEV. ×250. Bottom. Large cell follicular lymphoma. The malignant follicular cells are negative (as are normal germinal center blasts), but the populations of normal B and T cells surrounding the malignant follicles are largely receptor positive. ×50.

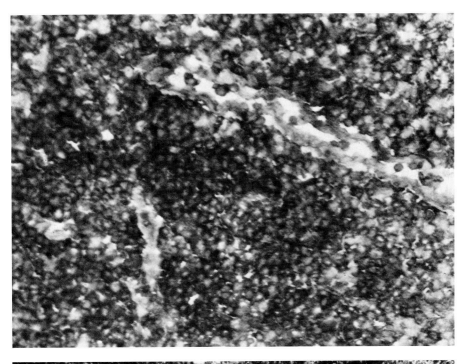

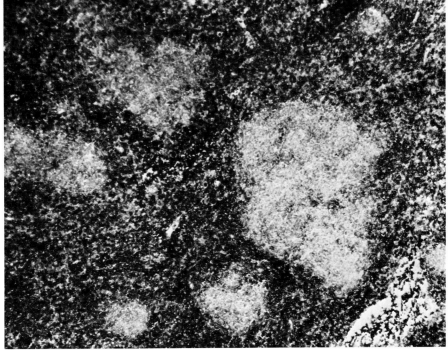

CONCLUSION AND SUMMARY

The ability of lymphocytes to recognize and bind to specialized lymphoid organ endothelial cells is an essential controlling element in the process of lymphocyte migration from blood into lymphoid tissue and thus in the process of lymphocyte circulation and traffic. This recognition event is controlled by specific lymphocyte surface molecules or receptors for endothelial cell determinants. We have proposed that the expression of these homing receptors and of endothelial cell interaction ability by non-Hodgkin's lymphomas may play an important role in determining their propensity for hematogenous dissemination to distant lymphoid sites. In this chapter, we have defined two approaches that will allow us to test this proposal. In the first, we have adapted an in vitro model of lymphocyte–endothelial cell recognition and binding, previously utilized in murine systems, to the functional assay of the endothelial cell recognition capacity of normal and neoplastic human lymphocytes. In the second we have produced a monoclonal antibody that appears to define the human lymphocyte surface homing receptor or receptors for lymphoid organ endothelial cells. Thus, we have established both functional and antigenic assays of the expression of normal lymphocyte homing mechanisms by the non-Hodgkin's lymphomas. These assays will permit critical analysis of the role of these mechanisms in the dissemination of lymphoid malignancies.

ACKNOWLEDGMENT

This investigation supported by grants CA34233 and CA34709 awarded by the National Cancer Institute, United States Department of Health and Human Services.

Dr. Butcher is a scholar of the Leukemia Society of America.

We thank M. Beers for excellent secretarial assistance, R. Coffin for photographic assistance, and C. Butnut and D. Chestnut for their encouragement and support.

REFERENCES

Butcher EC. 1984. The regulation of lymphocyte traffic. Current Topics in Microbiology and Immunology, Springer-Verlag, Heidelberg. (In press.)

Butcher EC, Kraal G, Stevens SK, Weissman IL. 1982. Selective migration of murine lymphocyte and lymphoblast populations and the role of endothelial cell recognition. Adv Exp Med Biol 149:199–206.

Butcher EC, Scollay RG, Weissman IL. 1979. Lymphocyte adherence to high endothelial venules: characterization of a modified in vitro assay, and examination of the binding of syngeneic and allogeneic lymphocyte population. J Immunol 123:1996.

Dailey MO, Gallatin WM, Weissman IL, Butcher EC. 1983. Surface phenotype and migration properties of activated lymphocytes and T cell clones. In Parker JW, O'Brien RL, eds., Intercellular Communication in Leukocyte Function, J Wiley and Sons, Ltd, New York pp. 641–644.

Gallatin WM, Weissman IL, Butcher EC. 1983. A cell surface molecule involved in organ specific homing of lymphocytes. Nature 303:30–34.

Gowans JL, Knight EJ 1964. The route of recirculation of lymphocytes in the rat. Proc R Soc Lond (Biol) 159:257.

Griscelli C, Vassalli P, McCluskey RT. 1969. The distribution of large dividing lymph node cells in syngeneic recipient rats after intravenous injection. J Exp Med 130:1427–1451.

Parrott DMV. 1966. The integrity of the germinal center: An investigation of the differential localization of labeled cells in lymphoid organs. *In* Cottier H, ed., Germinal Centers in Immune Responses, Springer Verlag, New York pp. 168–175.

Reichert RA, Weissman IL, Butcher EC. 1983. Germinal center cells lack homing receptors necessary for normal lymphocyte recirculation. J Exp Med 157:813–827.

Smith ME, Martin AF, Ford WL. 1980. Migration of lymphoblasts in the rat: Preferential localization of DNA-synthesizing lymphocytes in particular lymph nodes and other sites. Monogr Allergy 16:203–232.

Sprent J. 1980. Antigen-induced selective sequestration of T lymphocytes: Role of the major histocompatibility complex. Monogr Allergy 16:233–244.

Stamper HB Jr, Woodruff JJ. 1976. Lymphocyte homing into lymph nodes: in vitro demonstration of the selective affinity of recirculating lymphocytes for high endothelial venules. J Exp Med 144:818–820.

UT M.D. Anderson Clinical Conference on Cancer, Vol. 27, edited by R. J. Ford, L. M. Fuller, and F. B. Hagemeister. Raven Press, New York © 1984.

Biologic Features of Pediatric Non-Hodgkin's Lymphoma

Ian Magrath, Jeffrey Cossman,* David Benjamin, Hauke Sieverts, and Timothy Triche*

Pediatric Branch and Laboratory of Pathology, Division of Cancer Treatment, National Cancer Institute, National Institutes of Health, Bethesda, Maryland 20205*

Non-Hodgkin's lymphomas account for approximately 5% of the malignant neoplasms in children younger than 16 years in the United States. According to the SEER (Surveillance, Epidemiology, and End Results) figures for 1973-1977, non-Hodgkin's lymphomas that arise in the first two decades of life account for only 3.3% of all non-Hodgkin's lymphomas occurring in Caucasians (Table 1). Yet, the study of childhood lymphoid neoplasms has provided insights into several aspects of tumor biology that far outweigh their seemingly minor importance, when judged numerically.

In this very brief overview, we would like to emphasize four tenets that have been largely substantiated in recent years and which, we believe, provide not only a rational basis for the comprehension of lymphoid neoplasia in children but also a model for the understanding of other neoplasms and a basis for the development of novel means of intervention, whether the aim is prevention or therapy.

These four tenets, which apply to childhood non-Hodgkin's lymphomas are:

1. The neoplastic cells have the characteristics of lymphocyte precursor cells.
2. A failure of cellular differentiation is a critical component of pathogenesis.
3. Clinical behavior patterns are a consequence of the phenotypic characteristics of the cells.
4. Specific genetic changes involving proto-oncogenes are the immediate cause of the abnormal cellular behavior.

CHILDHOOD NON-HODGKIN'S LYMPHOMAS AND LYMPHOCYTE PRECURSOR CELLS

Even when considered purely from a histological perspective, it is apparent that lymphoid neoplasms of well-differentiated lymphoid cells or cells of germinal follicular origin are extremely rare in childhood (Berard et al. 1981, Magrath 1981). Childhood non-Hodgkin's lymphomas are almost always diffuse and conform to one of three major histological classes, although numerous terms have been applied

Table 1. *Number of Cases Diagnosed in 1973–*
1977 (Caucasian Males and Females, USA)

Age Group (years)	Hodgkin's (%)	NHL (%)
<5	6 (0.2)	39 (0.5)
5–9	30 (1.1)	63 (0.8)
10–14	119 (4.3)	86 (1.0)
15–19	300 (11)	79 (1.0)
>20	2,301 (83)	7,828 (97)
All ages	2,756	8,095

NHL–Non-Hodgkin's lymphoma.

by lymphoma taxonomists (Table 2). Considerably more insight into the nature of these major subclasses is gained by examination of their immunological phenotype and comparison with the characteristics of known normal lymphoid cells.

The presence or absence or terminal deoxynucleotide transferase (TdT) at once divides the tumors into two main groups and correlates very well with the morphological appearance. With very rare exceptions, tumors that are composed of cells indistinguishable from the lymphoblasts of acute lymphoblastic leukemia (ALL) express TdT. Those with Burkitt's-like or large cell morphology do not (Berard et al. 1981). Moreover, within the group with lymphoblast morphology, even where there is no bone marrow involvement, all of the cellular phenotypes described in ALL may occur, although the majority of these tumors are of T-cell lineage (Roper et al. 1983, Bernard et al. 1981).

TdT-Positive Tumors with Lymphoblastic Morphology

As discussed by Dr. Korsmeyer, in acute lymphoblastic leukemias expressing the common ALL antigen, HLA/DR, or both but lacking immunoglobulin or T-cell antigen expression, immunoglobulin genes are rearranged (Korsmeyer et al. 1983). These tumors are, therefore, the neoplastic counterparts of early lymphoid cells committed to B-cell differentiation. Neoplasms with pre-B phenotype (i.e., cytoplasmic immunoglobulin, usually μ-chains) represent the next differentiation step (Figure 1). Both of these phenotypes have been reported in lymphoblastic tumors of the skin, bone, or lymph nodes, without bone marrow involvement (Table 3) (Link et al. 1983, Cossman et al. 1983). The majority of lymphoblastic lymphomas, however, have been clearly identified, on the basis of monoclonal T-cell antibodies, as being of thymocyte origin. These tumors appear predominantly to be the neoplastic counterparts of intermediate (T6, T4 and T8) and late thymocytes (T4 *or* T8, T1, T3) (Figure 2, Table 4) (Bernard et al. 1981, Roper et al. 1983). It should be pointed out that the phenotype of the malignant cells does not always correlate with published data on normal cell phenotypes. Some tumors may represent "forbidden clones" that would normally be destroyed in the thymus, but atypical patterns such as the possession of "early" and "late" antigens not normally expressed

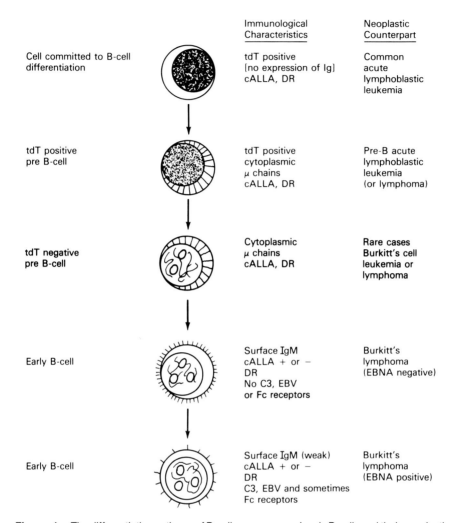

	Immunological Characteristics	Neoplastic Counterpart
Cell committed to B-cell differentiation	tdT positive [no expression of Ig] cALLA, DR	Common acute lymphoblastic leukemia
tdT positive pre B-cell	tdT positive cytoplasmic μ chains cALLA, DR	Pre-B acute lymphoblastic leukemia (or lymphoma)
tdT negative pre B-cell	Cytoplasmic μ chains cALLA, DR	Rare cases Burkitt's cell leukemia or lymphoma
Early B-cell	Surface IgM cALLA + or − DR No C3, EBV or Fc receptors	Burkitt's lymphoma (EBNA negative)
Early B-cell	Surface IgM (weak) cALLA + or − DR C3, EBV and sometimes Fc receptors	Burkitt's lymphoma (EBNA positive)

Figure 1. The differentiation pathway of B-cell precursors and early B-cells and their neoplastic cell counterparts.

together may also be observed because of the abnormalities of cellular differentiation. The relationship between T-lymphoblastic lymphoma and T-ALL is still not entirely clear and distinctions are often arbitrary. Early thymocyte neoplasms, however, appear to present predominantly as ALL, whereas neoplasms with phenotypic characteristics of more mature thymocytes may present with or without bone marrow involvement (Bernard et al. 1981, Roper et al. 1983, Reinherz et al. 1979). It is possible that the blurring of a clear relationship between phenotype and clinical presentation is a consequence of differentiation occurring within the malignant clone.

Table 2. *Histologic Designations of Childhood Non-Hodgkin's Lymphoma*

	Lymphoblasts indistinguishable from ALL	Indistinguishable or very similar to African Burkitt's cells	Large cells similar to histiocytes
Rappaport (Nathwani 1979)	Lymphoblastic lymphoma	Undifferentiated lymphoma, Burkitt's and non-Burkitt's	Histiocytic lymphoma
Lukes and Collins (1975)	ML of convoluted lymphocytes	ML of small noncleaved cell	ML of large follicle center cell. Immunoblastic sarcoma
Kiel (Lennert and Mohri 1978)	ML lymphoblastic, convoluted cell and unclassified types	ML lymphoblastic, Burkitt's type	ML centroblastic. ML immunoblastic
Non-Hodgkin's Classification Project (1982)	ML lymphoblastic	ML small noncleaved cell	ML large cells. ML large cell, immunoblastic

ALL—acute lymphoblastic leukemia; ML—malignant lymphoma.

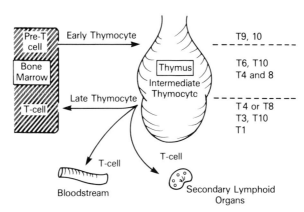

Figure 2. Representation of T-cell differentiation demonstrating the cellular origins of T-cell neoplasia.

TdT-Negative Tumors with Burkitt's-Like Morphology

The vast majority of undifferentiated lymphomas (lymphomas of small non-cleaved cells) express surface IgM, as well as a number of other B-cell markers, such as B1, I_A, or DR locus antigens (Magrath 1984). In the United States these neoplasms express low levels of complement (C3) and Fc receptors. African Burkitt's lymphoma may express higher levels of C3 and Fc receptors (Berard et al. 1981). This may be significant since Epstein-Barr virus (EBV) receptor expression correlates with C3 receptor expression (Magrath et al. 1980, 1981). The lack of EBV receptors in tumors seen in the United States presumably accounts for the

Table 3. *Phenotypes of Selected Cases of Lymphoblastic Lymphomas*

Age/Sex	Primary site	Marrow	T-cell Ags	E-rosettes	I$_A$	J5	TdT	cIg	Designation
16/F	Pleura	—	6,8,11	4%	—	+ +	+ +	ND	T
20/M	Node	—	3,9,11	16%	—	—	+ +	ND	T
14/M	Mediastinum	—	3,11	92%	—	—	+ +	ND	T
8/F	Tibia	—	—	—	+ +	+ +	+ +	—	Non-T, non-B
16/M	Node	Focal	—	—	+ +	+	+ +	+ +	Pre-B
4/F	Tibia	—	—	—	+ +	+ +	+ +	+ +	Pre-B

ND–Not done; − −negative; + −positive.

absence of EBV from this tumor, in spite of the fact that 75% of patients possess antibodies to EBV. A proportion of undifferentiated lymphomas, perhaps half, also express the common ALL antigen (Magrath 1981).

It is highly probable that these tumors are the neoplastic counterparts of early B cells. Not only is their expression of IgM, rather than other heavy-chain classes, suggestive of this, but rare tumors with Burkitt's morphology, and some Burkitt's cell lines, actually have a pre-B phenotype (Ganick and Finlay 1980, Kaneko et al. 1980). These tumors are still TdT negative and thus appear to be the malignant counterparts of the majority population of pre-B cells in normal bone marrow, which also lack TdT. In contrast, the pre-B phenotype of ALL appears to conform to the minority of normal pre-B cells, which are TdT positive.

TdT-Negative Large Cell Lymphomas

No clear differences in immunological markers have been described between large cell and undifferentiated lymphomas in childhood. Rarely, however, large cell lymphomas with T-cell markers, often occurring in the thymus, have been described (Levitt et al. 1982). The biological significance of this is speculative.

Thus, we can conclude, on the basis of these immunological data, that the majority of childhood non-Hodgkin's lymphomas are the neoplastic counterparts of lymphocyte precursors and represent, therefore, clones of cells in which cellular differentiation failure has occurred. This conclusion is substantiated by the documentation that at least some of these neoplasms, or cell lines derived from them, including common ALL and undifferentiated lymphomas, may be induced to undergo some further differentiation in vitro (e.g., by incubation with phorbol ester) (Delia et al. 1982, LeBien et al. 1982, Cossman et al. 1982) (Figure 3). The in vitro data also indicate that the differentiation failure is not irreversible, as would be the case if major genetic changes, e.g., involving gene deletions, had occurred. In contrast, the majority of adult non-Hodgkin's lymphomas express more differentiated characteristics. They may even have documented functional activity, such as help or suppression of immunoglobulin production, as in the case of T-cell neoplasms, or the production of large amounts of antibody, as in lymphoplasmacytoid or plasmacytoid neoplasms (Magrath 1981).

Table 4. *Phenotype of Patients with T-Cell Lymphoblastic*
Lymphoma (Excludes Bone Marrow Involvement)

Thymocyte group	Bernard et al. (1981)	Roper et al. (1983)	Total
Early (T9, 10)	3 (20%)	0	3 (9%)
Intermediate (T6, 4 & 8)	9 (60%)	9 (53%)	18 (56%)
Late (T1, 3, 4 or 8)	3 (20%)	8 (47%)	11 (34%)
Total	15	17	32

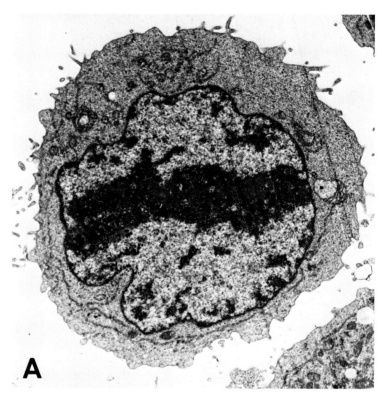

Figure 3. Ultrastructural features of 12-0-tetradecanoyl 13-acetate (TPA)-induced plasmacy-toid differentiation in an undifferentiated cell line, JD38. **A.** Control culture, identical to treated cells but unexposed to TPA. × 7,500. Nuclear detail is dominated by extended nucleolar material attached to nuclear membrane. Scattered dense heterochromatin is present throughout remainder of nucleus. The nuclear membrane is irregular. The nucleus is centrally disposed. The cytoplasm is dominated by diffusely distributed polyribosomes. Single strands of rough endoplasmic reticulum (RER) are present. Other cytoplasmic organelles, save rare mitochondria, are inevident.

IMPLICATIONS OF CELLULAR DIFFERENTIATION FAILURE

The exit of a cell from a cellular differentiation compartment can occur either by virtue of its death, a mechanism that applies to a large proportion of thymocytes

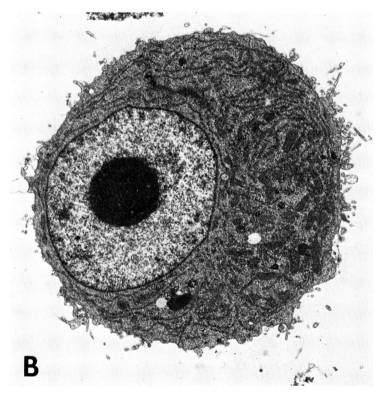

Figure 3. Cont. B. TPA-treated culture. ×6,000. The nucleus is distinguished from the un-treated nuclei by the presence of a conspicuous dense central nucleolus, similar to plasma cells. The nuclear border is regular and round but lacks marginated heterochromatin as seen in normal plasma cells. The nucleus is eccentric, typical of plasmacytoid cells. Innumerable strands of RER are distributed throughout the cytoplasm, in some areas in parallel array. Increased numbers of mitochondria are evident. Other cells also displayed a prominent Golgi apparatus. In aggregate, these features provide unmistakable morphological evidence of TPA-induced plasmacytoid dif-ferentiation. The illustrated cells are typical of the total cell population. The degree of differen-tiation varied somewhat but was, in all cases, noticeably present in the treated cells but not in the untreated cells.

and possibly to many B-cell clones, or by cellular differentiation and entry into a more mature compartment.

In the presence of a block to cellular differentiation, the latter mechanism is lost and, assuming cell proliferation continues, partially differentiated cells will initially continue to accumulate in the anatomically appropriate location (Figure 4). Thus, the development of a neoplasm appears to be a consequence of the development of a cellular differentiation block in a single clone of cells. While the mechanism of this process remains speculative, it must involve altered gene expression. The possible role of viral genetic information integrated into the cell genome cannot be excluded, particularly in view of the important role of viruses in the pathogenesis of lymphoid neoplasms in animals. Particularly exciting as an explanation for the

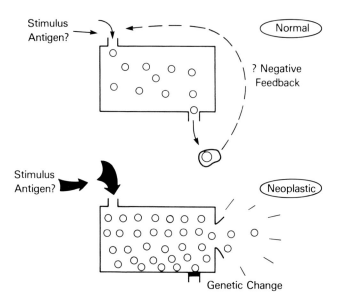

Figure 4. Basic elements in the pathogenesis of childhood lymphoid neoplasms. Predisposition as a result of environmental factors influencing specific cell populations and a genetic change giving rise to cellular differentiation block and expansion of a cellular differentiation compartment within a single clone. The possibility that a single environmental agent, e.g., a virus, may induce neoplasia of a specific target cell or cells cannot be excluded.

genetic modulation are the data discussed by Dr. Nowell (1984) regarding the characteristic chromosomal translocations seen in the TdT-negative B-cell tumors, which occur predominantly in childhood and which are surely pathogenetically implicated.

CLINICAL SIGNIFICANCE OF THESE OBSERVATIONS

Because these lymphoid neoplasms possess many or all of the phenotypic characteristics of their normal cell counterparts, their behavior, at least in terms of location and traffic, also mimics, to a considerable extent, that of their normal counterparts. This is particularly obvious in the case of lymphoblastic lymphoma, which presents, in perhaps 75% of cases, as a thymic mass. B-cell lymphomas rarely, if ever, involve the thymus but occur frequently in the gut (Magrath et al. 1983, Anderson et al. 1983). Since lymphoid precursor cells arise predominantly in the bone marrow during the postpartum period, the marrow is frequently involved in these tumors, especially when relapse occurs. Indeed, occult involvement may be the rule rather than the exception (Benjamin et al. 1983). Peripheral lymph nodes are not commonly involved, and involvement that does occur may be secondary rather than primary. This is consistent with the precursor origin of these neoplasms. Precise determinants of the distribution of either normal or neoplastic lymphoid cells have not been established, although there is good evidence that normal lymphocyte traffic is a consequence of surface antigens (Gallatin et al. 1983). In neoplasia, the simple fact of overexpansion of a cellular differentiation compartment may result in the presence of cells at abnormal sites, but which sites are normal and which are abnormal is not at all clear, since little is known of the migration patterns of normal precursor cells such as the normal cell counterparts of Burkitt's lymphoma. These cells appear to be present in very low numbers in normal individuals, which severely restricts or prohibits studies of their behavior. More is known of the anatomic locations of T-lymphocyte precursors, and in the case of T-cell lymphoblastic lymphomas, the most commonly involved sites correspond well with the location of the normal cell counterparts.

From these considerations, however, it is apparent that even when childhood lymphoid neoplasms appear to be localized, there is a high chance that neoplastic cells are widely disseminated, particularly in the marrow. Patients who die of progressive disease, whether of T- or B-cell phenotype, have a very high frequency of marrow involvement. Thus, chemotherapy is the primary treatment modality of these diseases, although the possibility remains that additional local therapy to sites of bulk disease may sometimes be of benefit.

The characterization of pediatric malignancies on the basis of immunological phenotype clearly improves the degree of diagnostic certainty and provides the possibility of further refining prognostic categories. Within the major groups of TdT-positive and TdT-negative lymphomas, however, we are not aware of data that unequivocally demonstrate that phenotype influences prognosis, although this is the case in ALL.

ALTERED EXPRESSION OF NORMAL CELLULAR GENES IN NEOPLASIA

The high frequency of occurrence of a translocation involving chromosome 8 (at or near the c-*myc* gene locus) and one of the immunoglobulin gene loci in Burkitt's lymphoma and closely related tumors (including other undifferentiated lymphomas and some large cell lymphomas) is most unlikely to be a chance or secondary phenomenon, particularly in view of the occurrence of analogous translocations in mouse plasmacytomas (Taub et al. 1982). Although altered regulation of the c-*myc* gene appears to be a necessary consequence of the translocation, there may be several mechanisms whereby this occurs, including physical relocation of either the c-*myc* gene or components of the immunoglobulin genes (Leder et al. 1983). However, this is unlikely to be the whole story, for Diamond et al. (1983) have shown the presence of DNA sequences capable of transforming mouse 3T3 cells (fibroblasts) in Burkitt's lymphoma cell lines. These sequences have been designated Blym. They are homologous with sequences in chicken bursal lymphomas but differ from other known oncogenes (Diamond et al. 1983). Weinberg and colleagues have demonstrated a transforming principle identified as N-ras in Burkitt's lymphoma

DNA (Murray et al. 1983). Further, we have recently demonstrated translocation into chromosome 8 and expression of the c-*sis* gene in a Burkitt's lymphoma cell line with a t(8;22) chromosomal translocation. C-*sis* is a proto-oncogene whose expression appears to be very limited in normal differentiated cell types. These findings are consistent with the possibility that several oncogenes are necessarily activated in the genesis of a neoplastic cell (Land et al. 1983).

In any event, there is strong evidence that alterations in the regulation or expression of cellular genes concerned in cell differentation and proliferation are a critical component of pathogenesis, and are likely, therefore, to be the immediate cause of the differentiation block. Data regarding oncogene expression in the TdT-positive lymphomas of childhood have not yet been published, but transformation of mouse 3T3 cells with DNA derived from human T-cell leukemia cell lines has been described (Souyri and Fleissner 1983).

POSSIBLE PATHOGENETIC MECHANISMS IN CHILDHOOD LYMPHOMAS

In order to comprehend the origins of lymphoid neoplasia in children, it is essential to view these neoplasms as tumors of the immune system. Whereas it is possible to envisage a single hit mechanism, such as a virus infection, in the genesis of neoplasia, it seems more probable that multiple predisposing factors are involved. Among the most important are likely to be environmental antigens. In attempting to comprehend lymphomas, it is surely of critical importance to explain why childhood lymphoid neoplasms most often involve lymphocyte precursors, while adult neoplasms more frequently involve cells that, under normal circumstances, take part in an immune response. Could this relate to the emphasis upon development of a repertoire of specific reactivities in a young individual as opposed to the secondary response to an antigen reencountered in the adult? This possibility is consistent with the fact that the primary lymphoid organs are at their peak of development in the first two decades of life. The entire immune system begins a slow but progressive involution after puberty (Yunis et al. 1978).

Whereas antigen-specific stimulation of immunologically responsive cells can only occur after the development of antigen receptor, a nonspecific feedback mechanism may also exist. In either event, environmental antigens or lymphocyte mitogens may alter the balance of lymphoid cell subsets. Increased rates of proliferation of different cell populations are not sufficient in themselves to account for neoplasia. They may, however, increase the chances of an additional cellular lesion–this time a genetic one, however perpetrated–that locks the cell into its differentiation compartment (though minor degrees of differentiation may be possible), perhaps at the same time dooming it to perpetual proliferation. The type of genetic change required to accomplish this is likely to depend upon the cell lineage and hence would be at least lineage specific. It would probably also be restricted to a specific stage along the cellular differentiation pathway. Specific cytogenetic or molecular changes may ultimately provide the most precise method of distinguishing among separate pathological entities.

Finally, a comprehension of the nature of the cellular abnormality leading to neoplastic behavior permits a consideration of novel therapeutic or even preventative approaches. Although these cells have a genetic abnormality, the cellular differentiation block may not be irreversible. We have, for example, been able to induce cellular differentiation with phorbol ester in some of our Burkitt's cell lines, which contain t(8;14) translocations (Benjamin et al. 1984). In essence, treatment approaches may be classified either as attempts to delete a neoplastic clone or attempts to alter its behavior (e.g., to induce cellular differentiation). Theoretically, both approaches may ultimately prove possible by the utilization of appropriate surface receptors via monoclonal antibody therapy or by noncytotoxic chemotherapy. Antibodies directed at tumor-specific antigens (i.e., clonal markers) such as idiotype or the T-cell receptor are particularly attractive in this regard. Whether or not such approaches will prove feasible or to be of general applicability is unclear at present, but the possibility of avoiding or minimizing cytotoxic chemotherapy would appear to justify their exploration.

REFERENCES

Anderson JR, Wilson, JF, Derek, R, Jenkin T, Meadows AT, Kersey J, Chilcote RR, Coccia P, Exelby P, Kushner J, Siegel S, Hammon D. 1983. Childhood non-Hodgkin's lymphoma. N Engl J Med 308:559–565.

Benjamin D, Magrath IT, Triche TJ, Schroff RW, Jensen JP, Korsmeyer SJ. 1984. Induction of plasmacytoid differentiation by Phorbol ester in B-cell lymphoma cell lines bearing 8;14 translocations. Proc Natl Acad Sci USA (In press).

Benjamin D, Magrath IT, Douglass EC, Corash LM. 1983. Derivation of lymphoma cell lines from microscopically normal bone marrow in patients with undifferentiated lymphomas: Evidence of occult bone marrow involvement. Blood 61:1017–1019.

Berard CW, Green MH, Jaffe ES, Magrath I, Ziegler J. 1981. A multidisciplinary approach to non-Hodgkin's lymphomas. Ann Intern Med 94:218–235.

Bernard A, Boumsell L, Reinherz EL, Nadler LM, Ritz J, Coppin H, Richard Y, Valensi F, Dausset J, Flandrin G, Lemerle J, Schlossman SF. 1981. Cell surface characterization of malignant T cells from lymphoblastic lymphoma using monoclonal antibodies: Evidence for phenotypic differences between malignant T cells from patients with acute lymphoblastic leukemia and lymphoblastic lymphoma. Blood 57:1105–1110.

Cossman J, Neckers LM, Arnold A, Korsmeyer SJ. 1982. Induction of differentiation in a case of common acute lymphoblastic leukemia. N Engl J Med 307:1251–1254.

Cossman J, Chused TM, Fisher RI, Magrath I, Bollum F, Jaffe ES. 1983. Diversity of immunological phenotypes of lymphoblastic lymphoma. Cancer Res 43:4486–4490.

Delia D, Greaves MF, Newman RA, Suterland DR, Minowada J, Kung P, Goldstein G. 1982. Modulation of T leukaemic cell phenotype with phorbol ester. Int J Cancer 29:23–31.

Diamond A, Cooper GM, Ritz, J, Lane M-A. 1983. Identification and molecular cloning of the human Blym transforming gene activated in Burkitt's lymphomas. Nature 305:112–116.

Gallatin WM, Weissman IL, Butcher EC. 1983. A cell-surface molecule involved in organ-specific homing of lymphocytes. Nature 304:30–34.

Ganick DJ, Finlay JL. 1980. Acute lymphoblastic leukemia with Burkitt cell morphology and cytoplasmic immunoglobulin. Blood 56:311–314.

Kaneko Y, Rowley JD, Check I, Variakojis D, Moohr JW. 1980. The 14q + chromosome in pre-B-ALL. Blood 56:782–785.

Korsmeyer SJ, Arnold A, Bakhshi A, Ravetch JV, Siebenlist U, Hieter PA, Sharrow SO, LeBien TW, Kersey JH, Poplack DG, Leder P, Waldmann TA. 1983. Immunoglobulin gene rearrangement and cell surface antigen expression in acute lymphocytic leukemias of T cell and B cell precursor origins. J Clin Invest 71:301–313.

Land H, Parada LF, Weinberg RA. 1983. Cellular oncogenes and multistep carcinogenesis. Science 222:771–778.

LeBien TW, Bollum FJ, Yasmineh WG, Kersey JH. 1982. Phorbol ester-induced differentiation of a non-T, non-B leukemic cell line: Model for human lymphoid progenitor cell development. J Immunol 128:1316–1320.

Leder P, Battey J, Lenoir G, Moulding C, Murphy W, Potter M, Stewart T, Taub R. 1983. Translocations among antibody genes in human cancer. Science 222:765–771.

Lennert K. 1978. Classification of non-Hodgkin's lymphomas. *In* Lennert K, Mohri N, eds., Malignant Lymphomas Other Than Hodgkins' Disease. Springer-Verlag, New York, pp. 83–110.

Levitt LJ, Aisenberg AC, Harris NL, Linggood RM, Poppema S. 1982. Primary non-Hodgkin's lymphoma of the mediastinum. Cancer 50:2486–2492.

Link MP, Hoper M, Dorfman RF, Crist WM, Cooper MD, Levy R. 1983. Cutaneous lymphoblastic lymphoma with pre-B markers. Blood 61:838–841.

Lukes RJ, Collins RD. 1975. New approaches to the classification of lymphomata. Br J Cancer 30 (Suppl II): 1–28.

Magrath IT. 1981. Lymphocyte differentiation pathways—an essential basis for the comprehension of lymphoid neoplasia. JNCI 67:501–514.

Magrath IT. 1984. Burkitt's lymphoma. *In* Molander D, ed., Diseases of the Lymphatic System. Springer Verlag, New York, pp. 103–139.

Magrath IT, Freeman CB, Pizzo PA, Gadek J, Jaffe E, Santaella M, Hammer C, Frank M, Reaman G, Novikovs L. 1980. Characterization of lymphoma-derived cell lines: Comparison of cell lines positive and negative for Epstein-Barr virus nuclear antigen. II. Surface Markers. JNCI 64:477–483.

Magrath IT, Freeman C, Santaella M, Gadek J, Frank M, Spiegel R, Novikovs L. 1981. Induction of complement receptor expression in cell lines derived from human undifferentiated lymphomas. II. Characterization of the induced complement receptors and demonstration of the simultaneous induction of EBV receptor. J Immunol 127:1039–1043.

Magrath I, Janus C, Edwards B, Spiegel R, Jaffe E, Berard C, Miliauskas C, Morris K, Barnwell R. 1984. An effective therapy for both undifferentiated (including Burkitt's) lymphomas and lymphoblastic lymphomas in children and young adults. Blood 63:1102-1111.

Murray MJ, Cunningham JM, Parada, LF, Weinberg RA. 1983. HL60 transforming sequence: A ras oncogene coexisting with altered myc genes in hematopoietic tumors. Cell 33:749–757.

Nathwani BH. 1979. A critical analysis of the classifications of non-Hodgkin's lymphomas. Cancer 44:347–384.

Non-Hodgkin's Lymphoma Pathology Classification Project. 1982. National Cancer Institute sponsored study of classification of non-Hodgkin's lymphomas: Summary and description of a Working Formulation for clinical usage. Cancer 49:2112–2135.

Nowell PC, Finan J, Erikson J, Croce CM. 1984. Burkitt's lymphoma: Chromosome translocations and oncogene activation. *In* Ford RJ, Fuller LM, Hagemeister FB, eds., UT M. D. Anderson Clinical Conference on Cancer Vol. 27. Raven Press, New York, pp. 161–169.

Reinherz EL, Nadler LM, Sallan SE, Schlossman SF. 1979. Subset derivation of T-cell acute lymphoblastic leukemia in man. J Clin Invest 64:392–397.

Roper M, Crist WM, Metzgar R, Ragab AH, Smith S, Starling K, Pullen J, Leventhal B, Bartolucci AA, Cooper MD. 1983. Monoclonal antibody characterization of surface antigens in childhood T-cell lymphoid malignancies. Blood 61:830–837.

Souyri M, Fleissner E. 1983. Identification by transfection of transforming sequences in DNA of human T-cell leukemias. Proc Natl Acad Sci USA 80:6676–6679.

Taub R, Kirsch I, Morton C, Lenoir G, Swan D, Tronick S, Aaronson S, Leder P. 1982. Translocation of the c-myc gene into the immunoglobulin heavy chain locus in human Burkitt lymphoma and murine plasmacytoma cells. Proc Natl Acad Sci USA 79:7837–7841.

Yunis EJ, Fernandes C, Good RA. 1978. Aging and involution of the immunological apparatus. *In* Good R, Day S, eds., The Immunopathology of Lymphoreticular Neoplasms. Plenum Medical Book Co., New York, pp. 53–80.

Diagnosis and Staging

UT M.D. Anderson Clinical Conference on Cancer,
Vol. 27, edited by R. J. Ford, L. M. Fuller, and
F. B. Hagemeister. Raven Press, New York © 1984.

Malignant Lymphomas: Appearance, Behavior, and Classification

Robert D. Collins and John B. Cousar

Department of Pathology, Vanderbilt Medical Center, Nashville, Tennessee 37232

The microscopic appearance of malignant lymphomas has traditionally determined classification and has therefore been predictive of behavior. Factors affecting
the microscopic appearance of malignant lymphomas, and possibly their behavior,
are increasingly subjected to analysis; these factors are briefly discussed in this
chapter. Classifications of malignant lymphomas have naturally focused on the
nature of the neoplastic cells, and very detailed information about the phenotype
and growth fraction of neoplastic cells is becoming available. However, some of
the information discussed in this paper about the reacting components of lymphomas
may be equally important. Since normal lymphocytes are influenced in division
and differentiation by a complex interaction of lymphocytes and macrophages,
information predictive of lymphoma behavior may be obtained from a detailed
analysis of the functional relationships between the nonneoplastic and the neoplastic
components of lymphomas. The type of reacting components and their distribution
in relationship to the neoplastic component are now evaluable by studies of cell
suspensions and frozen tissue section immunoperoxidase preparations. However,
very little information is available about the functional interactions of reacting cells
with neoplastic components.

APPEARANCE OF MALIGNANT LYMPHOMAS

In addition to the cytological features of neoplastic cells, pathologists have
traditionally been concerned with the growth patterns of lymphomas. Other factors
affecting the appearance of lymphomas are the mixture of reacting and neoplastic
elements and the distribution and character of the vascular and stromal elements.

Growth Pattern

Some lymphomas are recognizable on low-power microscopic examination due
to their distinctive growth; follicular center-cell (FCC) lymphomas producing follicular nodules and nodular sclerosing Hodgkin's disease (NSHD) are examples.
Neoplasms with growth patterns almost as distinctive include lymphocyte-predom-
inant Hodgkins' disease (nodular lymphocytic and histiocytic types), mantle zone

lymphomas, small cell neoplasms (chronic lymphocytic leukemia type), in which the mounding pattern is recognizable, and lymphoid neoplasms with plasmacytic differentiation. With some experience, the pathologist may recognize the low-power microscopic appearance of many lymphomas. Conversely, mistakes in classification are often made if the distinctive growth patterns are not appreciated.

Cytologic Features and Evaluation of Cell Cycle State of Predominant Cell or Extent of Differentiation

Various small lymphocytes, transformed lymphocytes, and plasma cells are easily distinguished one from the other on smears or properly prepared tissue sections. However, it is more difficult to identify small or transformed lymphocytes according to immunological phenotype. Mycosis fungoides cells are distinctive due to their cerebriform nuclear convolutions. Cleaved FCC and the convoluted cells of thymic lymphoma may also be recognized by experienced pathologists. In general, nuclear features are usually less reliable as predictors of immunological phenotype of lymphomas than is the growth pattern.

Analysis of touch preparations or tissue sections allows a semiquantitative prediction of growth fraction. Neoplasms composed chiefly of blasts, with a high mitotic index and numerous macrophages, are easily recognized as high-grade neoplasms; indolent or low-grade lymphomas, composed chiefly of small cells, are also identified with reasonable precision. The intermediate processes, with mixtures of small and transformed lymphocytes, are difficult to categorize according to growth fraction. Flow cytometric counts done on representative samples from these neoplasms will obviously be a much more precise measure of growth fraction than present microscopic analyses.

Different neoplastic lymphoid cells in an individual neoplasm may be in different stages of the cell cycle. A dividing component is present in every neoplasm, but blasts may be difficult to find in indolent processes. In such cases, small lymphocytes (in a dormant or G0 functional state) predominate, and the dividing component may be inconspicuous. In many lymphomas, there is insignificant differentiation to effector cells. For example, few FCC lymphomas contain plasma cells, although normal follicles are the sites of production of plasma cell precursors in nodes. On the other hand plasmacytic differentiation is easily recognized in immunoblastic sarcoma of B cells.

Reacting Components, Normal Nodes, and Malignant Lymphomas

Normal Nodes

B cells in nodes are found in the primary and secondary follicles; most plasma cells are found in the interfollicular areas. Most T cells are located in the para-cortical and medullary areas, although substantial numbers of T cells (Poppema et al. 1981), mostly helper T cells (TH) (Dvoretsky et al. 1982, Hsu et al. 1983), are noted in secondary follicles. Natural killer cells are confined to follicular centers

(Miller et al. 1983), while mantle zones are rich in IgD-bearing cells (Figure 1) and T cells (Stein et al. 1980). Approximately 75% of lymphocytes in the paracortex are T cells, and most of these are TH (Dvoretsky et al. 1982, Kvaloy et al. 1982). Phagocytosing macrophages are usually abundant in follicular centers, and large numbers of dendritic reticulum cells may be detected in immunostained preparations (Figure 1).

Hodgkin's Disease

Several studies of involved and uninvolved tissues from patients with Hodgkin's disease have described the percentages of T and B cells, T-cell subset analyses, and the relationship of T cells to Reed-Sternberg cells. Involved nodes or spleens have been reported as having normal percentages of T and B cells (Gajl-Peczalska et al. 1976, Han et al. 1980) or increased proportions of T cells (Payne et al. 1976, Pinkus et al. 1978, Dorreen et al. 1982, Poppema et al. 1979,1982, Baroni et al. 1982, Borowitz et al. 1982). Interestingly, in five cases of lymphocyte predominant Hodgkin's disease, the majority of lymphocytes were B cells (Poppema et al. 1979). Most studies have shown that TH cells predominate (Borowitz et al. 1982, Poppema et al. 1982), although two cases of NSHD without eosinophilia had

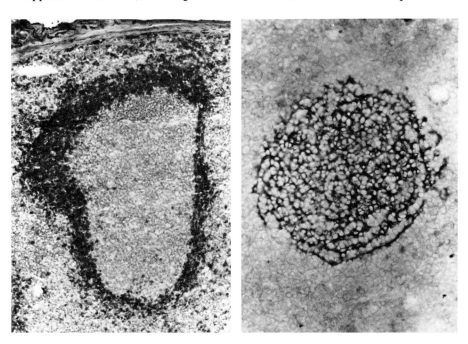

Figure 1. **Left:** Frozen tissue section from a normal lymph node immunostained for IgD. Note very heavy staining of mantle lymphocytes and very few positive cells in the follicular center or interfollicular area. **Right:** Frozen tissue section from a normal node immunostained for dendritic reticulum cells (Dako-DRC monoclonal antibody). Note intercellular meshwork staining pattern in follicular center. Reduced from × 160.

reduced TH cells (Borowitz et al. 1982). TH cells often surrounded Reed-Sternberg cells (Borowitz et al. 1982, Poppema et al. 1982). The monoclonal antibody T10 (found on activated T cells) has been detected on many lymphocytes in Hodgkin's disease (Poppema et al. 1982).

Follicular Center Cell Lymphomas

FCC lymphomas have been extensively analyzed in terms of the quantity and type of reacting elements; these studies have been facilitated by the relative ease of recognition in frozen sections of neoplastic follicular structures (Figure 2). Cell suspension studies have shown a wide range (20% to 73%) of T cells in these B-cell neoplasms (summarized in Vogler et al. 1983). Most of these cells are located in interfollicular areas (Stein et al. 1980, Dvoretsky et al. 1982, Harris et al. 1983) and are functionally TH cells (Dvoretsky et al. 1982, Miller et al. 1983), although almost equal percentages of TH and T suppressor/cytotoxic (T S/C) have been reported (Kvaloy et al. 1982). Natural killer cells, as detected by Leu 7 positivity, are apparently confined to follicular nodules (Miller et al. 1983). Mantle zones noted around some neoplastic follicular structures may contain both polytypic (Stein et al. 1980, Harris and Data 1982) and monotypic populations (Harris and Data

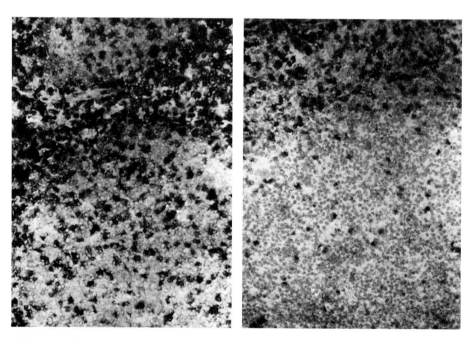

Figure 2. Frozen section of small cleaved follicular center-cell lymphoma immunostained for TH cells using anti-Leu 3a and 3b **(left)** and T S/C cells using anti-Leu 2a **(right)**. Areas adjacent to neoplastic follicles contain many anti-Leu 3a and 3b and anti–Leu-2a positive cells. Positive cells within the neoplastic follicles are primarily of TH phenotype. Reduced from ×250.

1982). FCC lymphomas may show an even distribution of T cells (Figure 3) throughout the tumor when the growth pattern is diffuse.

There are fewer detailed studies of the macrophage (Ree et al. 1981) and reticulum cell components of FCC lymphomas. Phagocytosing macrophages are occasionally seen in neoplastic follicular nodules; when present, they may contain tingible bodies, and upon examination using light and electron microscopy, they resemble similar macrophages in reactive nodes. Numerous macrophages of this type are a well-known component of Burkitt's lymphoma, as well as other lymphomas with large growth fractions. Epithelioid macrophages have also been described in FCC lymphomas but rarely in the form of granulomas. Dendritic reticulum cells have long been recognized in the ultrastructure of FCC lymphomas (Glick et al. 1975, Lennert et al. 1978); their presence has recently been confirmed using the monoclonal antibody R4/23 techniques in areas of nodular and diffuse FCC lymphomas (Naiem et al. 1983). R4/23-reacting cells were found in a kidney growth in one FCC lymphoma case but were not found in other B-cell lymphomas.

T Lymphomas

There are only a few analyses of the reacting components of T-cell lymphomas. Peripheral T-cell lymphomas characteristically contain nonphagocytic macrophages

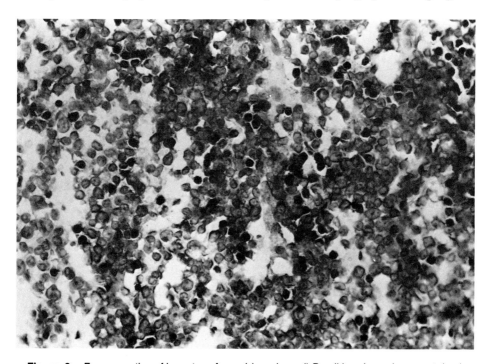

Figure 3. Frozen section of large transformed (noncleaved) B-cell lymphoma immunostained with anti-Leu 4 (pan T-cell monoclonal antibody). Note numerous positive small lymphocytes intermingled with negatively stained large transformed cells. × 400.

(Waldron et al. 1977), sometimes in the form of distinct aggregates in those neoplasms identified as Lennert's lymphoma. These macrophages do not contain Langerhans' granules. In the experience at Vanderbilt, a few cases of peripheral T-cell lymphoma have shown a preponderance of neoplastic TH cells; only a few B cells and T S/C cells have been detected using the frozen tissue section immunoperoxidase technique.

Cutaneous T-cell lymphomas typically contain macrophages in which Langerhans' granules are identified (Figure 4). Scattered Langerhans' granule-containing macrophages have been identified in the Vanderbilt series in the disseminated phases of this disease amongst the neoplastic cells in node and marrow. Ia$^+$ macrophages have been demonstrated in high numbers around epidermal aggregates of neoplastic T cells (Janossy et al. 1981). Most of these neoplasms have a helper phenotype; presumably, reactive suppressor cells have been demonstrated in frozen tissue section immunoperoxidase preparations (Figure 4).

Thymic lymphomas (convoluted lymphocytic lymphomas) contain phagocytosing macrophages and often have a "starry sky" appearance. These neoplasms occasionally contain large numbers of eosinophils. Other reacting cells have not been demonstrated.

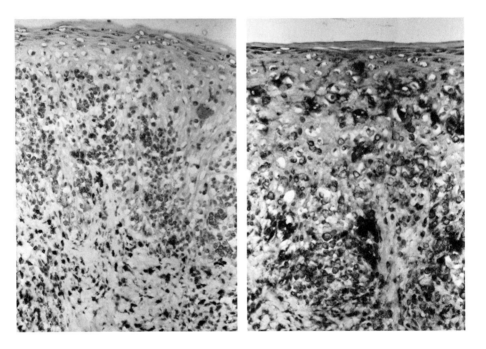

Figure 4. Frozen tissue section of skin involved by cutaneous T lymphoma of helper phenotype. **Left:** Immunostaining for T S/C cells (anti-Leu 2a). Scattered positive small lymphocytes are present in dermis at the periphery of the neoplastic infiltrate. **Right:** Immunostaining for Langerhans' cells using OKT-6 monoclonal antibody. Note positive cells with dendritic processes in epidermis and dermis. Reduced from ×250.

Stromal and Vascular Elements

Hodgkin's Disease

The connective tissue in Hodgkin's disease has been demonstrated to contain abundant filamentous and granular electron-dense material, collagen fibers, and myofibroblasts (Seemayer et al. 1980), leading these authors to conclude that the sclerosis seen in nodular sclerosing Hodgkin's disease was related to myofibroblasts.

NSHD is characterized by bands of polarizable connective tissue (Lukes 1971, Colby et al. 1981).

Follicular Center Cell Lymphomas

FCC lymphomas, particularly in the retroperitoneum and inguinal areas, may have such extensive sclerosis that the lymphoid elements are overshadowed. The distribution of sclerosis in these lymphomas may be predominantly associated with follicular nodules, may be predominantly interfollicular, or may be both. The sclerotic material does not polarize, may be periodic acid-Schiff (PAS) positive or hyaline in appearance, and has not been characterized as to collagenous type. The mechanism or significance of its deposition is not known, although similar-appearing material has been noted in reactive follicles.

T-Cell Lymphomas

Connective tissue deposition is not a prominent feature of most T-cell lymphomas. Peripheral T-cell lymphomas have a delicate compartmentalization of cells by thin strands of PAS-positive connective tissue (Waldron et al. 1977). Some of the T-cell lymphomas have also been noted to contain numerous epithelioid venules (Lennert et al. 1978).

BEHAVIOR OF MALIGNANT LYMPHOMAS

The behavior of lymphomas is determined in part by the proportion of dividing and dormant cells. Neoplasms with a large dividing pool (e.g., Burkitt's lymphoma) are likely to be aggressive and rapidly growing. Neoplasms with a large dormant pool (e.g., chronic lymphocytic leukemia) will have indolent processes, although they may be widespread at presentation.

Since differentiation and growth of lymphocytes is normally controlled, at least in part, by complex interactions between lymphocytes and monocytes, it is likely that lymphoid neoplasms are regulated similarly. *Reacting components might therefore have important regulatory capacities for growth and differentiation in lymphomas and leukemias and might be predictive of clinical behavior.*

The behavior of lymphoid neoplasms may change dramatically from a relatively indolent course to rapid clinical deterioration. Such changes in behavior are often accompanied by a change in the appearance of the neoplasm, which is usually due to loss of differentiating capacity by the neoplastic cell or a change of the predominant cell from dormant cells to rapidly dividing blasts.

CONCLUSION

The appearance of malignant lymphomas is determined by several factors: the growth pattern of the neoplasm, the cytological characteristics of neoplastic cells, the mix of neoplastic and reacting cells, and the relative percentages of dividing, dormant, and differentiated neoplastic cells. Reacting cells in malignant lymphomas include other components of the hematopoietic and lymphoid systems, as well as vascular and stromal elements. The type of these reacting elements and their distribution in relationship to the neoplastic component are now evaluable by immunoperoxidase procedures performed on frozen tissue sections. Since division and differentiation of normal lymphocytes are influenced by a complex interaction of lymphocytes and macrophages, important information predictive of lymphoma behavior will be obtained from a detailed analysis of the functional relationships of the nonneoplastic and neoplastic cellular components of lymphomas.

The mix of dividing, dormant, and differentiating neoplastic cells is perhaps the most important factor determining the appearances of malignant lymphomas and is certainly predictive of their behaviors. Neoplasms in all cases have a component of dividing cells, but the percentage of cells in division varies widely among lymphoid neoplasms and may vary in individual patients at different times. Complete differentiation to effector cells is also seen in some lymphoid neoplasms, while others may show minimal evidence of lymphocytic differentiation. Therefore, lymphoid neoplasms may have a large dividing pool (Burkitt's lymphoma), large dormant pool (chronic lymphocytic leukemia), or partial differentiation (immunoblastic sarcoma of B cells). Pathologists have traditionally determined the stage of cell cycle or degree of differentiation by cytologic differentiation; flow cytometry will provide more precise gauges of growth fraction and differentiation.

Current analyses of lymphomas in investigative centers are producing voluminous, detailed data relating to their immunologic phenotypes and growth fractions. Important information relating to underlying immunologic abnormalities, karyotypic changes, or tissue culture features is also being developed. Organization of this information into a clinically useful framework will require a classification system of lymphomas incorporating the following features: (1) organ of origin, (2) lymphoid subpopulation of origin, (3) stage of cell cycle or degree of differentiation, (4) nature of reacting component, and (5) preceding immunological abnormality. This system of classification follows the general guidelines of the two cell of origin-oriented classifications of malignant lymphomas, the Lukes-Collins and Kiel classifications (Lennert et al. 1975, Lukes and Collins 1975).

ACKNOWLEDGMENT

This investigation was supported in part by National Institutes of Health grant AM-07186.

Dr. Cousar is the recipient of an American Cancer Society Junior Faculty Clinical Fellowship.

We thank Andrea Eiring and Renee Momar for technical assistance.

REFERENCES

Baroni CD, Ruco L, Uccini S, Foschi A, Occhionero M, Marcorelli E. 1982. Tissue T-lymphocytes in untreated Hodgkin's disease. Morphologic and functional correlations in spleens and lymph nodes. Cancer 50:259–268.

Borowitz, M, Corker, BP, Metzgar, RS. 1982. Immunohistochemical analysis of the distribution of lymphocyte subpopulations in Hodgkin's disease. Cancer Treat Rep 66:667–674.

Colby, TV, Hoppe, RT, Warnke, RA. 1981. Hodgkin's disease: A clinicopathologic study of 659 cases. Cancer 49:1846–1858.

Dorreen, MS, Habeshaw, JS, Wrigley, PFM, Lister, TA. 1982. Distribution of T-lymphocyte subsets in Hodgkin's disease characterized by monoclonal antibodies. Br J Cancer 45:491–499.

Dvoretsky, P, Wood, GS, Levy, R, Warnke, RA. 1982. T-lymphocyte subsets in follicular lymphomas compared with those in non-neoplastic lymph nodes and tonsils. Hum Pathol 13:618–625.

Gajl-Peczalska, KJ, Bloomfield, CD, Sosin, H, Kersey, JH. 1976. B and T lymphocytes in Hodgkin's disease. Analysis at diagnosis and following therapy. Clin Exp Immunol 23:47–55.

Glick, AD, Leech, JH, Waldron, JA, Flexner, JM, Horn, RG, Collins, RD. 1975. Malignant lymphomas of follicular center cell origin in man. II. Ultrastructural and cytochemical studies. JNCI 54:23–36.

Han, T, Minowada, J, Subramanian, V, Barcos, M, Kim, U. 1980. Splenic T and B lymphocytes and their mitogenic response in untreated Hodgkin's disease. Cancer 45:767–774.

Harris, N, Data, RE. 1982. The distribution of neoplastic and normal B-lymphoid cells in nodular lymphomas: use of an immunoperoxidase technique on frozen sections. Hum Pathol 13:610–617.

Harris, NL, Nadler, LM, Bhan, AK. 1983. Immunohistologic characterization of non-Hodgkin's lymphoma with monoclonal antibodies. Lab Invest 48:33A.

Hsu, S-M, Cossman, J, Jaffe, ES. 1983. Lymphocyte subsets in normal human lymphoid tissues. Am J Clin Pathol 80:21–30.

Janossy, G, Thomas, JA, Pizzolo, G. 1981. Morphological, cytochemical, immunological and biochemical characterization of non-Hodgkin's lymphomas. J Cancer Res Clin Oncol 101:1–11.

Kvaloy, S, Marton, PF, Host, H, Solheim, BG, Godal, T. 1982. Distribution of T-cell subsets identified by monoclonal antibodies in cell suspensions from lymph node biopsies of human B-cell lymphomas. Scand J Haematol 28:293–305.

Lennert K, Mohri N, Stein H, Kaiserling E. 1975. The histopathology of malignant lymphoma. Br J Cancer 31:193–203.

Lennert K. 1978. Malignant Lymphomas other than Hodgkin's Disease. Histology. Cytology. Ultrastructure. Immunology. Springer-Verlag, New York.

Lukes RJ. 1971. Criteria for involvement of lymph node, bone marrow, spleen, and liver in Hodgkin's Disease. Cancer Res 31:1755–1767.

Lukes RJ, Collins RD. 1975. New approaches to the classification of the lymphomata. Br J Cancer 31:1–28.

Miller M, Tubbs R, Fishleder A, Savage R, Sebek B, Weick J. 1983. Immunoregulatory Leu-7 and T8 lymphocytes in B cell follicular lymphomas. Lab Invest 48:58A.

Naiem M, Gerdes J, Abdulaziz A, Stein H, Mason DY. 1983. Production of a monoclonal antibody reactive with human dendritic reticulum cells and its use in the immunohistological analysis of lymphoid tissue. J Clin Pathol 36:167–175.

Payne SV, Jones DB, Haegert DG, Smith JL, Wright DH. 1976. T & B lymphocytes and Reed-Sternberg cells in Hodgkin's disease lymph nodes and spleens. Clin Exp Immunol 24:280–286.

Pinkus GS, Barbuto D, Said JW, Churchill H. 1978. Lymphocyte subpopulations of lymph nodes and spleens in Hodgkin's disease. Cancer 42:1270–1279.

Poppema S, Elema JD, Halie MR. 1979. The localization of Hodgkin's disease in lymph nodes. A study with immunohistochemical, enzyme histochemical and rosetting techniques on frozen sections. Int J Cancer 24:532–540.

Poppema S, Bhan AK, Reinherz EL, McCluskey RT, Schlossman SF. 1981. Distribution of T cell subsets in human lymph nodes. J Exp Med 153:30–41.

Poppema S, Bhan AK, Reinherz EL, Posner MR, Schlossman SF. 1982. In situ immunologic characterization of cellular constituents in lymph nodes and spleen involved by Hodgkin's disease. Blood 59:226–232.

Ree HJ, Song JY, Leone LA, Crowley JP, Fanger H. 1981. Occurrence and patterns of muramidase containing cells in Hodgkin's disease, non-Hodgkin's lymphomas and reactive hyperplasia. Hum Pathol 12:49–59.

Seemayer TA, Lagace R, Schurch W. 1980. On the pathogenesis of sclerosis and nodularity in nodular sclerosing Hodgkin's disease. Virchows Arch [Pathol Anat] 385:282–291.

Stein H, Bonk A, Tolksdorf G, Lennert K, Rodt H, Gerdes J. 1980. Immunohistologic analysis of the organization of normal lymphoid tissue and non-Hodgkin's lymphomas. J Histochem Cytochem 28:746–760.

Waldron JA, Leech JH, Glick AD, Flexner JM, Collins RD. 1977. Malignant lymphoma of peripheral T-lymphocyte origin. Immunologic, pathologic and clinical features in six patients. Cancer 40:1604–1617.

Vogler LB, Glick AD, Collins RD. 1983. B cell neoplasms. Correlation of recent developments with the biology of normal B lymphocytes. Progress in Clinical Pathology, Vol. IX:197–223.

UT M.D. Anderson Clinical Conference on Cancer,
Vol. 27, edited by R.J. Ford, L.M. Fuller, and
F.B. Hagemeister. Raven Press, New York © 1984.

Immunologic Classification of B-Cell Leukemias and Lymphomas

Lee M. Nadler, Kenneth C. Anderson, David Fisher, Bruce Slaughenhoupt, Andrew W. Boyd, and Stuart F. Schlossman

Division of Tumor Immunology, Dana-Farber Cancer Institute, and The Department of Medicine, Harvard Medical School, Boston, Massachusetts 02115

Leukemias and lymphomas, which previously were not distinguishable by either morphologic or histiochemical criteria, can now be subdivided into distinct subgroups by the use of a number of cell surface markers. Traditionally, B-cell tumors have been defined by their expression of cytoplasmic immunoglobulin (cIg) (Gathings et al. 1977, Pearl et al. 1978) or monoclonal cell surface immunoglobulin (Aisenburg et al. 1972, Froland et al. 1971, Nadler et al. 1981c, Preud'homme et al. 1972). These tumors frequently express receptors for the Fc portion of human immunoglobulin (Fc) (Bianco et al. 1970, Dickler et al. 1972, Huber et al. 1969) and the third component of the complement system (C3) (Cossman and Jaffe 1981, Ross et al. 1973, Stein et al. 1978), as well as HLA-related Ia-like antigens (Ia) (Nadler et al. 1981b, Schlossman et al. 1976, Winchester et al. 1975). Although useful, the biologic and clinical utility of these conventional B-cell determinants has been limited, since they are also expressed on cells of other lineages.

More recently, several laboratories have described monoclonal antibodies directed at antigens largely restricted to normal and malignant B cells. Eight such B-cell–associated antigens have been reported from this laboratory including B1, B2, B4, and plasma cell (PC-1) which are B-cell restricted within the hematopoietic system (Anderson et al. 1984a,b, Nadler et al. 1981c,d, 1983, Stashenko et al. 1981) and common acute lymphoblastic leukemia antigen (CALLA), T1, T10, and plasma cell associated (PCA-1), which are B-cell associated, since they are also expressed on other lymphoid and myeloid cells (Anderson et al. 1983, 1984b, Reinherz et al. 1979, 1980, Ritz 1980, 1981). These B-cell surface antigens have been extensively studied on normal fetal and adult hematopoietic tissues in an attempt to define both their cellular expression and their cross-reactivities (Hokland et al. 1983, 1984, Rosenthal et al. 1983). By demonstrating that these antigens appear at distinct stages of B-cell differentiation, we have attempted to order them in B-cell ontogeny. Moreover, the expression of these antigens on B-cell tumors suggested that they might be useful in defining tumors of B lineage, as well as in demonstrating the heterogeneity of these tumors.

The B-cell–restricted antigens B1, B2, B4, and PC-1 are phenotypically and molecularly distinct from known B-cell determinants (Anderson et al. 1984a, b, Bhan et al. 1981, Oettgen et al. 1983, Nadler et al. 1981c, d, 1983, Stashenko 1980, 1981). Considerable evidence on fetal and adult normal B cells, mitogen-stimulated B cells, and malignant B cells, supports the notion that these antigens are expressed at limited stages of B-cell differentiation. The B1 antigen appears prior to the acquisition of cytoplasmic μ (cyto-μ) and remains strongly expressed on the cell surface until presecretory cIgG and plasmacytoid morphology appear (Hokland et al. 1983, 1984, Nadler et al. 1981c, 1984c, Rosenthal et al. 1983, Stashenko 1980, 1981). B2, in contrast, appears slightly later, and is lost from the cell surface when cells transform into B lymphoblasts, lose sIgD, and acquire presecretory cIgM (Nadler et al. 1981d, Rosenthal et al. 1983, Stashenko et al. 1981). The B4 antigen is expressed on all B lymphocytes, including pre-B cells, prior to the appearance of B1, CALLA, or cyto-μ (Nadler et al. 1983, 1984c). The B1, B2, and B4 antigens are all lost from the cell surface at the terminal stages of B-cell differentiation, i.e., the plasma cell. In contrast, PC-1 antigen is absent on normal and malignant B cells and is expressed exclusively on normal and malignant plasma cells (Anderson et al. 1984a).

Several B-cell–associated markers (Ia, CALLA, T1, T10, and PCA-1) are similarly expressed at distinct stages of B-cell maturation. The Ia antigen, also expressed on granulocyte precursors (colony-forming units in culture; CFU-C), monocytes, some null cells, and activated T cells, is strongly expressed on B cells from the earliest known pre-B cell and is lost at the plasma cell stage (Anderson et al. 1984a, Nadler et al. 1981b). The CALLA has a very limited expression and appears after the $Ia^+B4^+CALLA^-B1^-cyto$-μ^-pre-B cell and is lost from the cell surface prior to the appearance of surface Ig (Hokland et al. 1983, Nadler et al. 1984c, Ritz et al. 1980, 1981, Rosenthal et al. 1983). Surface Ig, the classical cell surface determinant of B cells, is acquired after cyto-μ and is largely absent on secretory B cells. The T1 antigen, originally thought to be T lymphocyte specific, is expressed on a small population of immature B lymphocytes (Caligaris-Cappio et al. 1982, Nadler et al. 1984b). Finally, the PCA-1 antigen is expressed at the terminal stages of B-cell ontogeny (lymphoplasmacytoid and plasma cell), although it also demonstrates weak cross-reactivity on granulocytes and monocytes (Anderson et al. 1983, 1984b). Although these markers are not lineage restricted, they are of considerable utility because of their restricted expression at discrete stages of B-cell differentiation.

In this chapter, we will attempt to summarize the immunologic heterogeneity of leukemia and lymphomas of B-cell origin. The enumeration of cell surface determinants, which are lineage restricted and which identify discrete stages of differentiation, now allows us to relate the malignant cells to their normal cell counterparts. By relating the malignant cell to normal B-cell differentiative steps, it may be possible to understand the heterogeneity of B-cell leukemias and lymphomas better, in addition to defining more precisely the B-cell subpopulations, ontogeny, and function. We will first review normal B-cell ontogeny, then, we will attempt to relate the stages of normal B-cell differentiation to the histopathologically defined subgroups of B-cell malignancies. It is hoped that the heterogeneity identified by these lineage-restricted differentiation antigens will allow us more precisely to understand both the biologic and clinical aspects of B-cell leukemias and lymphomas.

RESULTS AND DISCUSSION

B-Cell–Associated Surface Determinants

The human B lymphocyte expresses a large number of cell surface and cyto-plasmic determinants. The sine qua non of a B cell is either integral cell surface or cytoplasmic immunoglobulin (Aisenberg et al. 1972, Froland et al. 1978, Ga-things et al. 1977, Nadler et al. 1981a, Pearl et al. 1978, Preud'homme et al. 1972). Pre-B cells express cytoplasmic Ig heavy chains without detectable surface immu-noglobulin. True B cells express the complete Ig molecule on the surface. Following exportation of Ig to the cell surface, heavy-chain isotype diversity occurs. Finally, immunoglobulin molecules are lost from the cell surface at the time when cells become secretory and differentiate toward the plasma cell. Excluding integral cell-surface Ig, most cell surface determinants expressed on B lymphocytes are not B-lineage restricted. For example, HL-D/DR–related Ia-like antigen (Ia) are strongly expressed on B lymphocytes but are also found on monocytes, activated T cells, and myeloid precursors (CFU-C). Receptors for the Fc portion of IgG and com-plement receptor C3 are expressed at discrete stages of B-cell differentiation but are also expressed on monocytes, granulocytes, and subpopulations of T lympho-cytes. At the terminal stages of B-cell differentiation, these determinants are lost, and a new antigen, termed T10 and initially defined on stage I thymocytes, is then expressed (Figure 1). T10 expression, although not B-lineage restricted, is clearly limited to the terminal stages of differentiation.

Other than integral cell surface immunoglobulin and its isotypes, there are no other B-cell–specific surface determinants. In the past several years, several labo-

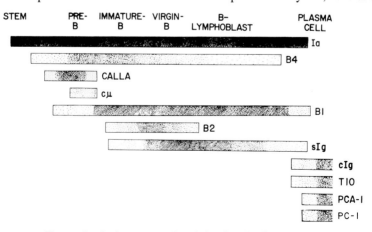

Figure 1. Antigen expression during B-cell differentiation.

ratories have reported monoclonal antibodies reactive with human B-cell antigens that are distinct from conventional human immunoglobulin and Ia-like antigens (Abramson et al. 1981, Anderson et al. 1983, 1984b, Brooks et al. 1980, 1981, Hirt et al. 1983, Iida et al. 1982, Mittler et al. 1983, Nadler et al. 1981c, d, 1983, Reinherz et al. 1979, 1980, Ritz et al. 1980, 1981, Stashenko et al. 1980, Thorley-Lawson et al. 1982, Yokochi et al. 1982). These monoclonal antibodies were derived by immunization of BALB-c mice with normal B lymphocytes, B cell lines, and B cells derived from patients with leukemias and lymphomas. We have recently characterized a panel of B-cell–associated monoclonal antibodies.

The first of the monoclonal antibodies, B1, is a nonglycosylated phosphoprotein with a molecular weight of 35,000 expressed on 95% of B cells in peripheral blood and lymphoid organs (Stashenko et al. 1980, Oettgen et al. 1983). B1 is primarily restricted to B-cell regions (follicles) of lymphoid organs (Bhan et al. 1981). Functional experiments have demonstrated that all B lymphocytes capable of being induced to secrete immunoglobulin by means of pokeweed mitogen are contained within the B1-reactive population (Stashenko et al. 1980). When cell-surface Ig-bearing B cells are stimulated in vitro to secrete immunoglobulin, the B1 antigen is lost (Stashenko et al. 1981). The loss of B1 is accompanied by the development of presecretory cytoplasmic IgG and surface T10 staining (Stashenko et al. 1981). This suggests that the B1 antigen spans B-cell differentiation and is lost at the plasma cell stage (Figure 1). A second B-cell–associated antigen, termed B2, is a glycoprotein with a molecular weight of 140,000.

In contrast to the B1 antigen, the B2 antigen is weakly expressed on peripheral blood B cells but is more strongly expressed on B cells isolated from lymphoid organs (Nadler et al. 1981d). Like B1, B2 is restricted in its expression to B cells and it is not expressed on other fractionated lymphoid cells. In an in vitro model of B-cell differentiation, pokeweed mitogen can induce B cells to lose cell-surface B2 at a time when surface IgD is also lost (Stashenko et al. 1981). Accompanying this loss of B2 is lymphoblast transformation and the development of presecretory IgM (Stashenko et al. 1981). These experiments suggest that B2 is a more restricted differentiation antigen than B1 (Figure 1).

The third B-cell–associated antigen, termed B4, is a glycoprotein demonstrating at least a bimolecular complex of 40 and 80 kd. Similar to the B2 antigen, the B4 antigen is weakly expressed on peripheral blood B cells and is more strongly expressed on B cells isolated from lymph nodes, tonsils, and spleens (Nadler et al. 1983). Like B1, however, the B4 antigen is expressed on B cells at all stages of B-cell differentiation, excluding the plasma cell (Nadler et al. 1983). The evidence that the B4 antigen is expressed prior to all previously defined determinants is derived from the fact that all non–T-cell acute lymphoblastic leukemias (ALL) studied so far expressed the B4 antigen (Nadler et al. 1984c). Preliminary studies suggest that within fetal tissues, CALLA$^+$B1$^+$cyto-μ^+ cells are a subset of the B4 population (Nadler et al. 1984c). These studies suggest that the B4 antigen is expressed on pre-B cells that precede the appearance of CALLA, B1, and cyto-μ (Nadler et al. 1984c). The expression of the B4 antigen in the pokeweed mitogen-driven system is unique from that of B1 and B2. The B4 antigen, which is initially weak in its expression, increases in intensity by day four and approximately two-thirds of B4$^+$ cells are negative at day seven. This pattern of differentiation is distinctly different from that of the B1 antigen, which is lost by seven days and the B2 antigen which is lost by four days. These observations of the expression of B4 on early lymphocytes and of its loss only at the terminal stages of B-cell differentiation argue that this antigen is in fact a pan–B-cell antigen (Figure 1). The functional nature of the B4 antigen is unknown.

Finally, we have recently defined a series of plasma cell-restricted and associated antigens (Figure 1) (Anderson et al. 1983, 1984b). The PCA-1 antigen is expressed only on plasma cells within the B-cell system but is also weakly expressed on granulocytes and monocytes. We have identified an antigen termed PC-1 that appears to be plasma cell restricted and is not seen on cells of other lineages. These antigens will provide us with a method of defining cells at the terminal stages of B-cell differentiation.

The Sequence of Normal B Cell Differentiation

In contrast to the large body of accumulated evidence for T-cell differentiation and ontogeny, the development of B cells is not well understood in either murine or human systems. The conventional pre-B cell is defined by the presence of cyto-μ heavy chains without the presence of light chains. This cell has been identified in small numbers within the fetal liver and normal adult bone marrow (Pearl et al. 1978). The pre-B cell appears to express the Ia antigen but is not known to express receptors for Fc, C3, and monkey red blood cells. Recent studies in our laboratory on both non-T cell ALL and fetal tissues suggest that several stages of pre-B cell differentiation exists prior to the cyto-μ-positive pre-B cell (Hokland et al. 1983, 1984, Nadler et al. 1984c). As seen in Figure 2, the normal adult bone marrow is thought to contain a series of stages of pre-B cell differentiation. These cells correspond to distinct populations that were isolable from human fetal liver and bone marrow. Hokland and his colleagues (1983) were able to isolate CALLA-positive cells from the fetal liver and bone marrow. By using techniques of immune rosette depletion and cell sorting, a population of cells greater than 95% CALLA positive could be isolated. Phenotypic analysis of these cells revealed that the CALLA-positive cells coexpressed the Ia antigen but lacked T cells or myeloid antigens. Of great interest was the observation that approximately 15% expressed cyto-μ (Hokland et al. 1983). These studies provided strong evidence for distinct stages of pre-B cells in the fetus. More recently, the expression of B4 on normal fetal pre-B cells suggests the existence of at least four stages of pre-B cell differentiation (Figure 2) (Nadler et al. 1984c).

The pre-B cell in the adult bone marrow matures to a resting B lymphocyte that is exported to the primary lymphoid follicle and peripheral blood. These cells express Ia, B4, B1, B2, sIgM, and sIgD (Figure 3). The resting B lymphocytes can then be triggered to differentiate. With differentiation, these cells lose the B2

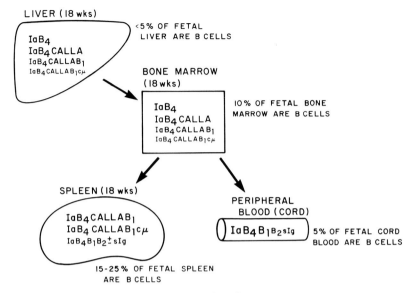

Figure 2. Fetal B-cell ontogeny.

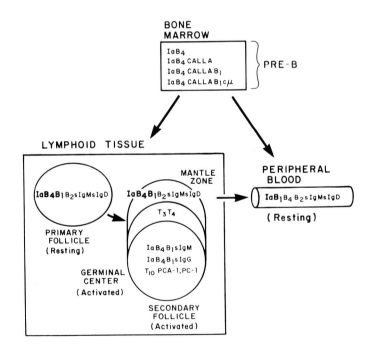

Figure 3. Adult B-cell ontogeny.

antigen and IgD. The more mature B cells acquire surface IgG and then enter the secretory phase of B-cell differentiation with the appearance of plasma cell antigens PCA-1 and PC-1 (Figure 3). The B4 antigen is weakly expressed on peripheral blood B cells and is more strongly expressed on B cells isolated from lymph nodes, tonsils, and spleens.

B-Cell Tumors

Pre–B-Cell Tumors

Leukemic cells from approximately 80% of patients with acute lymphoblastic leukemia lack cell surface Ig and T-cell antigens (Greaves et al. 1980, 1983, Ritz et al. 1980). Although the cells are devoid of conventional B- and T-cell antigens, they express a variety of cell-surface markers including the CALLA and Ia-like antigens (Greaves et al. 1980, 1983, Nadler et al. 1981a, 1984c). The cellular origin of these non–T-cell ALL has been the subject of numerous studies, which, for the most part, suggest that they are of B-cell origin. Several laboratories have demonstrated that tumor cells from approximately 20%–30% of patients with non–T-cell ALL have a pre-B cell phenotype, since they express the cyto-μ chain but lack sIg (Figure 4) (Brouet et al 1979, Greaves et al. 1979, Vogler et al. 1978).

Utilizing the B-cell–restricted and associated antigens Ia, B4, CALLA, and B1, we can now demonstrate that although they are morphologically identical, tumor cells from patients with non–T-cell ALL can be subclassified into five phenotypically defined subgroups (Figure 5) (Nadler et al. 1983, 1984c). These five subgroups

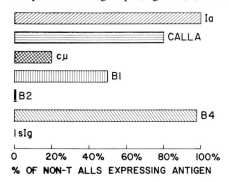

Figure 4. B-cell origin of non-T-cell acute lymphoblastic leukemia.

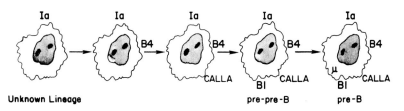

Figure 5. Spectrum of B-cell lymphoblastic leukemia.

are $Ia^+B4^-CALLA^-B1^-cyto-\mu^-$ (5%), $Ia^+B4^+CALLA^-B1^-cyto-\mu^-$ (15%), $Ia^+B4^+CALLA^+B1^-cyto-\mu^-$ (30%), $Ia^+B4^+CALLA^+B1^+cyto-\mu^-$ (35%) and $Ia^+B4^+CALLA^+B1^+cyto-\mu^+$ (15%). Examination of antigen intensity of each of these subgroups reflects the level of appearance of each antigen in B-cell ontogeny. The Ia antigen is strongly expressed on all early B-cell tumors suggesting that it appears early in pre–B-cell ontogeny. The B4 antigen, although varying from moderate to strong in intensity, is clearly positive on all non–T-cell ALL; moreover, it is expressed on non–T-cell ALL to a greater degree than any other B-cell tumor. The CALLA is moderately to strongly expressed on most non–T-cell ALL. The B1 antigen, which appears later in B-cell ontogeny, is absent on approximately 50% of these tumors and weakly to moderately expressed on the remainder. The B2 and sIg B-cell antigens, as well as the plasma cell antigens PCA-1 and PC-1, appear later in B-cell differentiation and are largely absent from non–T-cell ALL. Within each of the immunologically defined subgroups of non–T-cell ALL, there is considerable heterogeneity of expression of each of the positive antigens. For example, within the $Ia^+B4^+CALLA^+B1^+cyto-\mu^-$ subgroup, the expression of B1 varies from barely detectable to as strong as CALLA or Ia. This heterogeneity suggests that the non–T-cell ALL do not reflect distinct stages of differentiation but more likely reflect a continual neoplastic transformation of every possible step of B-cell ontogeny.

The B-cell origin of non–T-cell ALL, therefore, has been based on several lines of evidence (Figure 5). Initially, investigators demonstrated that tumor cells from approximately 15% of patients with non–T-cell ALL contained μ chains without light chains and that they corresponded phenotypically to pre-B cells. Further studies demonstrated that approximately 50% of non–T-cell ALL expressed the B1 antigen, which suggested that they were of B-cell origin (Nadler et al. 1981c). The $Ia^+CALLA^+B1^-$ non–T-cell ALL were next shown to be of B-cell origin, since they could be induced by tumor promoters or conditioned media to express B1 and cyto-μ (Nadler et al. 1982b). Almost all non–T-cell ALL express the B-cell–restricted antigen B4, which suggests that these tumors were all of B-cell origin (Nadler et al. 1983, 1984c). Korsmeyer and his colleagues (1981,1983) have recently demonstrated that all non–T-cell ALL tested (approximately 50) were of B-cell origin, since these tumor cells demonstrated gene rearrangements of the immuno-globulin heavy and light chains (Nadler et al. 1984c). Each of these subgroups of non–T-cell ALL, defined by Ia, B4, CALLA, and B1, demonstrate gene rearrange-ments for immunoglobulin heavy- and light-chain genes, confirming their B-cell origin (Nadler et al. 1984c). This genetic evidence, coupled with the expression B-cell–restricted antigens on non–T-cell ALL, suggests that these tumors phenotyp-ically correspond to discrete stages of B-cell differentiation.

The orderly acquisition of these antigens on non–T-cell ALL provides a model of pre–B-cell differentiation. The observation that all non–T-cell ALL strongly express the Ia antigen suggests that this antigen develops very early on B-cell precursors. The B4 antigen is present on 95% of these tumors. The CALLA, expressed on 80% of non–T-cell ALL, follows B4 in B-cell ontogeny. The observation that CALLA is expressed on a percentage of normal pre-B cells is based on the studies of Hokland et al. (1983,1984), which demonstrated that 50% of CALLA-positive cells isolated from fetal lymphoid organs and normal bone marrow coexpressed B1, and 20% of these cells coexpressed cyto-μ. The B1 antigen, which follows the appearance of CALLA, is expressed on only 50% of non–T-cell ALL. The B1 antigen is expressed on only the most mature non–T-cell ALL. These observations suggest that these B-cell antigens appear prior to the conventional cyto-μ pre-B cell and develop sequentially.

Early B-Cell Leukemias and Lymphomas

The next stages of B-cell development are heralded by the acquisition and loss of antigens, including B2 and the isotypes of sIg and in some cases, T1 and CALLA (Figures 1 and 6). B-cell chronic lymphocytic leukemia (CLL) appears phenotypically to correspond to a subset of normal B cells, termed the immature B cell, and is the earliest B lymphocyte to express integral sIg (Nadler et al. 1984a). The coexpression of Ia, B4, B1, B2, and sIg defines the phenotype of the immature B lymphocyte and that of B-cell CLL. Tumor cells from most patients with B-cell CLL express either very faint surface IgM or coexpress IgM and IgD and totally lack the CALLA cell surface antigen. Of great interest is the observation that the majority of patients with B-cell CLL also express the T1 antigen (Boumsell et al. 1980, Engleman et al. 1981, Hansen et al. 1980, Kamoun et al. 1981, Koziner et al. 1982, Martin et al. 1980, 1981, Royston et al. 1980, Wang et al. 1980, Wormley et al. 1981). Previous investigators have attributed this observation to the anomalous expression of this antigen on a malignant B-cell CLL. However, we have recently shown that these B-cell CLL cells correspond to a subpopulation of normal B lymphocytes that coexpress Ia, B4, B1, B2, sIg, C3b, and T1 (Iida et al. 1983, Nadler et al. 1984b). Although this represents the most common phenotype seen

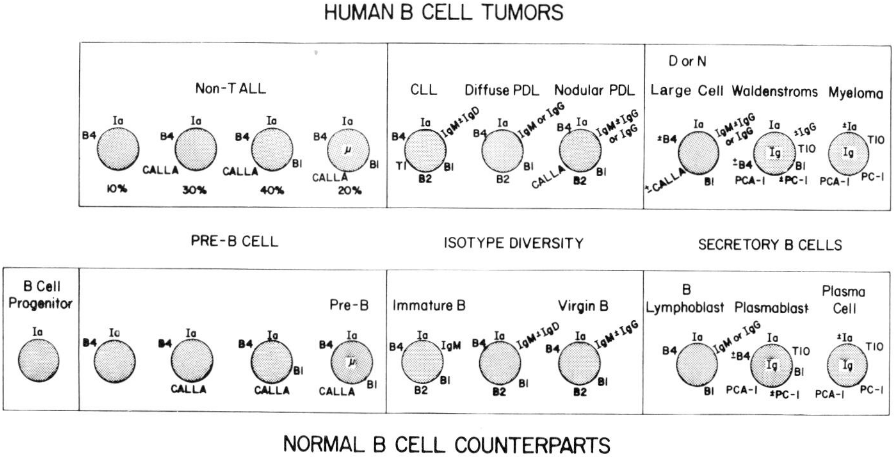

Figure 6. Correlation of human B-cell tumors with their normal cellular counterparts.

for B-cell CLL, it is clear that within this histologically defined entity, there is again heterogeneity of cell surface antigen expression. Almost every patient tested with B-cell CLL coexpresses Ia, B4, and B1; however, subgroups of CLL can be defined by the lack of sIg of B2. These observations suggests that within the morphologically defined entity termed B CLL, subgroups can be identified based upon immunologic cell surface heterogeneity. The antigen intensity on B CLL also distinguished these tumors from non–T-cell ALL prolymphocytic leukemia, B-cell lymphosarcoma cell leukemia, and B-cell lymphomas. As was true for the non–T-cell ALL, the Ia antigen can be moderately to strongly expressed on B CLL; however, the B4 antigen is more weakly expressed on B CLL than non–T-cell ALL, which suggests that B CLL cells are more differentiated. In contrast to the non–T-cell ALL on which the B1 antigen can be weak or absent, most B CLL moderately expressed B1 antigen. The CALLA is lost and the B2 antigen appears to be acquired at the B CLL stage. Both integral surface Ig and B2, however, are only weakly expressed or are absent. Plasma cell-restricted and associated (PCA-1) antigens are wholly absent on these B CLL tumors. These studies suggest that the B CLL cell is the neoplastic counterpart of a subpopulation of normal B lymphocytes and is not related to the majority of circulating B cells.

Virgin B-Cell and Transformed B-Cell Tumors

B-cell diffuse poorly differentiated lymphocytic lymphomas (PDL) of both the nodular (NPDL) and diffuse (DPDL) subtypes also correspond to the midstages of B-cell differentiation (Figure 6) (Nadler et al. 1982b, 1984a). Like B CLL, the overwhelming majority of these tumors coexpress Ia, B4, B1, B2, and sIg. In contrast to B CLL, the nodular PDL also express the CALLA and relatively few express the T1 antigen (approximately 10%). Within the PDL, the diffuse can be distinguished from the nodular subtype by the lack of cell-surface CALLA expression (Ritz et al. 1981, Nadler et al. 1984a). The intensity of the cell-surface expression of these antigens can be of further differential value. While B CLL and DPDL strongly express Ia, they lack CALLA, PCA-1, and PC-1. In contrast, the B CLL expressions of B4, B1, B2, and T1 are relatively great. The tumor cells isolated from patients with DPDL have a significantly more intense expression of B2, B4, and B1. This pattern of antigen expression suggests that NPDL and DPDL comes later in the differentiative scheme than does B CLL (Figure 6). The nodular mixed lymphomas are phenotypically identical with the NPDL, including the expression of the cell surface CALLA. These observations suggest that the nodular and diffuse PDL may be derived from distinct populations of B cells. Previous experiments in our laboratories and others have shown that the CALLA may be very weakly expressed in the germinal center cell within the secondary follicle of the normal lymph node. The observation that CALLA is on nodular lymphomas, therefore, provides further evidence that these tumors are of germinal center origin. It is important to know that there is clear-cut heterogeneity of antigen expression within the poorly differentiated lymphomas defined by the absence of sIg or B2 or both. For example, the majority of NPDL coexpress sIg and B2, but there are subgroups that lack each of these antigens. These observations on tumors corresponding to the midstages of B-cell differentiation provide further evidence that histiologically identical tumors are, in fact, heterogenous. This heterogeneity of antigen expression appears to reflect distinct stages of B-cell differentiation and suggests that these B-cell tumors are derived from unique populations of B lymphocytes.

The terminal stages of B-cell differentiation begin with the transformed (B lymphoblast) B cell and proceed to the final steps of B-cell differentiation to the plasma cell (Figure 6). The diffuse histiocytic lymphomas correlate phenotypically with the normal transformed B cell, since they coexpress Ia, B4, B1, and sIg but lack CALLA and B2. Also absent are the plasma cell antigens PCA-1 and PC-1. Although the intensity of Ia and B1 expression remains strong, the expression of B4 and sIg is weaker on diffuse histiocytic lymphoma than on NPDL, DPDL, and nodular mixed B-cell tumors. These observations suggest that the large cell lymphomas correspond to a stage of B-cell differentiation when B cells are actively dividing and entering the secretory phase of B-cell differentiation.

Secretory B-Cell Tumors

The final stage of B-cell differentiation includes the secretory pathway tumors (Waldenström's macroglobulinemia and plasma cell myelomas) (Figure 6). Waldenström's macroglobulinemia demonstrates coexpression of Ia, B4, and B1 with only one half of the tumors expressing sIg and none expressing B2 and CALLA. It is the first B-lineage tumor on which the plasma cell antigens T10 and PCA-1, as well as the plasma cell-restricted antigen PC-1, may appear (Anderson et al. 1983, 1984b). Nonetheless, the intensity of Ia, B4, B1, and sIg is less on Waldenström's macroglobulinemia than on diffuse histiocytic lymphomas and continually decreases as one moves toward the plasma cell tumors. The coexpression of Ia, B4, B1, and sIg confirms that the Waldenström's tumor is the transition from the malignant B cell to the malignant plasma cell. Finally, myelomas, as reflected by tumor cells from the bone marrow, plus plasma cell leukemias and solitary plasmacytomas wholly lack all B-cell restricted– and B-cell–associated antigens. They uniformly express T10, PCA-1, and PC-1, which suggests that they reflect neoplastic counterparts on the terminal stages of B-cell ontogeny i.e., the plasma cell. Further evidence for this notion stems from the observation that the intensity of T10, PCA-1, and PC-1 expression on myeloid plasma cell leukemias and plasmacytoma tumor cells corresponds to that of the plasma cell isolated from normal bone marrow. Both PCA-1 and PC-1 are strongly to moderately expressed on plasma cell tumors. Waldenström's macroglobulinemia and plasma cell myeloma, therefore, represent a model for the terminal phases of B-cell differentiation. The pattern of expression of B-cell antigens seen on Waldenström's macroglobulinemia with the coexpression of B1, B4, PCA-1, PC-1, supports the notion that they represent a transition from the B lymphocyte to the lymphoplasmacytoid cell. The loss of B1, B2, and B4 coupled with the acquisition of PCA-1 and PC-1 on plasma cells precisely correlates with the in vitro pokeweed mitogen-driven induction of normal B-cell differentiation in that the loss of B1 and B4 occurs concomitantly with the acquisition of cytoplasmic Ig, surface T10, PCA-1, and PC-1 staining. This stage of B-cell differentiation, to date, demonstrates considerably less heterogeneity within each of the histiologically defined subgroups and is seen at the early and midstages of B-cell differentiation.

OVERVIEW

In conclusion, cell-surface markers have identified considerably greater heterogeneity within the B-cell lymphoid neoplasms than was evident by standard morphologic and histiochemical techniques. Utilizing markers specific for lineage and stage of differentiation, it is now possible to correlate the malignant lymphocyte with its normal cell counterpart. Considering the complexity of the immune system in regard to ontogeny, differentiation, function, and migration, it is not surprising that the lymphoid malignancies reflect this degree of diversity. Moreover, the biologic and clinical heterogeneity of these diseases is clearly greater than has been identified by the presently employed histiopathologic and immunologic classification schemes. The challenge of the next several years is to integrate our understanding of the immune system with the clinical and histopathologic heterogeneity of leukemias and lymphomas in an attempt to devise a more rational classification scheme. Hopefully, this scheme will not only be biologically accurate but, more important, will identify clinically relevant subgroups.

REFERENCES

Abramson CS, Kersey JH, LeBien TW. 1981. A monoclonal antibody (BA-1) reactive with cells of human B lymphocyte lineage. J Immunol 126:83–88.

Aisenberg AC, Bloch KJ. 1972. Immunoglobulins on the surface of neoplastic lymphocytes. N Engl J Med 287:272–276.

Anderson KC, Park EK, Bates MP, Leonard RCF, Schlossman SF, Nadler LM. 1983. Antigens on human plasma cells identified by monoclonal antibodies. J Immunol 130:1132–1138.

Anderson KC, Bates MP, Slaughenhoupt B, Schlossman SF, Nadler LM. 1984a. A monoclonal antibody with reactivity restricted to normal and neoplastic plasma cells. J Immunol (In press).

Anderson KC, Slaughenhoupt B, Bates MP, Pincus G, Schlossman SF, Nadler LM. 1984b. Expression of human B cell associated antigens on leukemia and lymphomas: A model for human B cell differentiation. Blood (In press).

Bhan AK, Nadler, LM, Stashenko P, Schlossman SF. 1981. Stages of B cell differentiation in human lymphoid tissues. J Exp Med 154:737–749.

Bianco C, Patrick R, Nussenzweig V. 1970. A population of lymphocytes bearing a membrane receptor for antigen-antibody complement complexes. J Exp Med 132:702–720.

Boumsell L, Coppin H, Pham D, Raynal B, Lemerle J, Dausset J, Bernard A. 1980. An antigen shared by a human T cell subset and B cell chronic lymphocytic leukemic cells. J Exp Med 152:229–234.

Brooks DA, Beckman I, Bradley J, McNamara PJ, Thomas ME, Zola H. 1980. Human lymphocyte markers defined by antibodies derived from somatic cell hybrids. I. A hybridoma secreting antibody against a marker specific for human B lymphocytes. Clin Exp Immunol 39:477–485.

Brooks DA, Beckman I, Bradley J, McNamara PJ, Thomas ME, Zola H. 1981. Human lymphocyte markers defined by antibody derived from somatic cell hybrids. IV. A monoclonal antibody reacting specifically with a subpopulation of human B lymphocytes. J Immunol 126:1373–1387.

Brouet JC, Preud'homme JL, Penit C, Valensi F, Rouget P, Seligmann M. 1979. Acute lymphoblastic leukemia with pre-B cell characteristics. Blood 54:269–273.

Caligaris-Cappio F, Gobbi M, Bofill M, Janossy G. 1982. Infrequent normal B lymphocytes express features of B chronic lymphocytic leukemia. J Exp Med 155:623–627.

Cossman J, Jaffe ES. 1981. Distribution of complement receptor subtypes in non-Hodgkins lymphomas of B cell origin. Blood 58:20–26.

Dickler HB, Kunkel HG. 1972. Interaction of the aggregated gamma globulin with B lymphocytes. J Exp Med 136:191–196.

Engleman E, Warnke R, Fox R, Levy R. 1981. Studies of a human T lymphocyte antigen recognized by a monoclonal antibody. Proc Natl Acad Sci USA 78:1791–1795.

Froland SS, Natvig VB, Bendal P. 1971. Surface-bound immunoglobulin as a marker of B lymphocytes in man. Nature 234:251–252.

Gathings WE, Lawton AR, Cooper MD. 1977. Immunofluorescent studies on the development of pre-B cells, B lymphocytes and immunoglobulin isotype diversity in humans. Eur J Immunol 7:804–810.

Greaves MF, Verbi W, Vogler LB, Cooper M, Ellis R, Ganeshguru K, Hoffbrand V, Janossy G, Bollum FJ. 1979. Antigenic and lymphocytic leukemia. Leuk Res 3:353–362.

Greaves M, Delia D, Janossy G, Rapson N, Chessells J, Wood M, Prentice G. 1980. Acute lymphoblastic leukemia associate antigen IV. Expression on non-leukemic lymphoid cells. Leuk Res 4:15–26.

Greaves MF, Hariri G, Newman RA, Sutherland DR, Ritter MA, Ritz J. 1983. Selective expression of the common acute lymphoblast leukemia (gp100) antigens on immature lymphoid cells and their malignant counterparts. Blood 61:628–639.

Hansen JA, Martin PJ, Nowinski RC. 1980. Monoclonal antibodies identifying a novel T cell antigen and Ia antigens of human lymphocytes. Immunogenetics 10:247–260.

Hirt A, Baumgartner C, Forster HK, Imbach P, Wagner HP. 1983. Reactivity of acute lymphoblastic leukemia and normal bone marrow cells with the monoclonal antibody, Anti-Y 29/55. Cancer Res 43:4483–4485.

Hokland P, Rosenthal P, Griffin JD, Nadler LM, Daley JF, Hokland M, Schlossman SF, Ritz J. 1983. Purification and characterization of fetal hematopoietic cells that express the common acute lymphoblastic leukemia antigen (CALLA). J Exp Med 157:114–129.

Hokland P, Nadler LM, Griffin JD, Schlossman SF, Ritz J. 1984. Purification of the common acute lymphoblastic leukemia antigen (CALLA) positive cells from normal bone marrow. Blood (in press).

Huber J, Douglas SD, Fundenberg HH. 1969. The IgG receptor: an immunological marker for the characterization of mononuclear cells. Immunology 17:7–21.

Iida K, Nadler LM, Nussenzweig V. 1983. The identification of the membrane receptor for the complement fragment C3d by means of a monoclonal antibody. J Exp Med 158:1021–1033.

Iida K, Mornagh R, Nussenzweig V. 1982. Complement receptor (CR1) deficiency in erythrocytes from patients with systemic lupus erythematosis. J Exp Med 155:1427–1438.

Kamoun M, Kadin MF, Martin PJ, Nettleton J, Hansen JA. 1981. A novel human T cell antigen preferentially expressed on mature T cells and also on (B type) chronic lymphatic leukemic cells. J Immunol 127:987–996.

Korsmeyer SJ, Hieter PA, Ravetch JV, Poplack DG, Waldmann TA, Leder P. 1981. Developmental hierachy of immunoglobulin gene rearrangements in human leukemic pre-B cells. Proc Natl Acad Sci USA 78:301–313.

Korsmeyer SJ, Arnold A, Bakhshi A, Ravetch JV, Siebenlist V, Hieter PA, Sharrow SO, LeBien TW, Kersey JH, Poplack DG, Leder P, Waldmann TA. 1983. Immunoglobulin gene rearrangement and cell surface antigen expression in acute lymphocytic leukemias of T cell and B cell precursor origins. J Clin Invest 71:301–313.

Koziner B, Gebhard D, Denny T, Evans RL. 1982. Characterization of B cell type chronic lymphocytic leukemia cells by surface markers and a monoclonal antibody. Am J Med 73:802–807.

Martin PJ, Hansen JA, Nowinski RC, Brown MA. 1980. A new human T cell differentiation antigen: unexpected expression on chronic lymphocytic leukemia cells. Immunogenetics 11:429–439.

Martin PJ, Hansen JA, Siadak AW, Nowinski RC. 1981. Monoclonal antibodies recognizing normal human T lymphocytes and malignant B lymphocytes: a comparative study. J Immunol 127:1920–1923.

Mittler RS, Talle MA, Carpenter K, Rao PE, Goldstein G. 1983. Generation and characterization of monoclonal antibodies reactive with human B lymphocytes. J Immunol 131:1754–1761.

Nadler LM, Ritz J, Griffin JD, Todd RF, III, Reinherz EL, Schlossman SF. 1981a. Diagnosis and treatment of human leukemias and lymphomas utilizing monoclonal antibodies. *In* Brown EB, ed., Progress in Hematology. Grune and Stratton, Inc., New York, pp. 187–225.

Nadler LM, Stashenko P, Hardy R, Pesando JM, Yunis EJ, Schlossman SF. 1981b. Monoclonal antibodies defining serologically distinct HLA-DR related Ia-like antigens in man. Hum Immunol 1:77–90.

Nadler LM, Stashenko P, Ritz J, Hardy R, Pesando JM, Schlossman SF. 1981c. A unique cell surface antigen identifying lymphoid malignancies of B cell origin. J Clin Invest 67:134–140.

Nadler LM, Stashenko P, Hardy R, van Agthoven A, Terhorst C, Schlossman SF. 1981d. Characterization of a human B cell specific antigen (B2) distinct from B1. J Immunol 126:1941–1947.

Nadler LM, Anderson KC, Park EK, Bates MP, Leonard RCF, Reinherz EL, Schlossman SF. 1982a. Immunologic heterogeneity of human T and B cell lymphoid malignancies. In Owens AH, ed., Heterogeneity of Human Neoplasms, Academic Press, New York, pp. 53–72.

Nadler LM, Ritz J, Bates MP, Park EK, Anderson KC, Sallan SE, Schlossman SF. 1982b. Induction of human B cell antigens in non-T cell acute lymphoblastic leukemia. J Clin Invest 70:433–443.

Nadler LM, Anderson KC, Marti G, Bates MP, Park EK, Daley JF, Schlossman SF. 1983. B4, a human B lymphocyte associated antigen expressed on normal mitogen activated and malignant B lymphocytes. J Immunol 131:244–250.

Nadler LM, Bhan AK, Harris NL, Ritz J, Schlossman SF. 1984a. Nodular lymphomas correspond to discrete stages of B cell differentiation. (Unpublished data.)

Nadler LM, Hardy R, Anderson KC, Ito K, Bates MP, Slaughenhoupt B, Schlossman SF. 1984b. B cell chronic lymphocytic leukemia. I. Cell surface antigen heterogeneity and isolation of phenotypically identical normal B lymphocytes. (Unpublished data.)

Nadler LM, Korsmeyer S, Anderson KC, Boyd A, Slaughenhoupt B, Park E, Jensen J, Coral F, Mayer RJ, Sallen SE, Ritz J, Schlossman SF. 1984c. The B cell origin of non-T cell acute lymphoblastic leukemia: a model for discrete stages of neoplastic and normal pre-B cell differentiation. (Unpublished data.)

Oettgen HC, Bayard PJ, van Ewijk W, Nadler LM, Terhorst CP. 1983. Further biochemical studies of the human B cell differentiation antigens B1 and B2. Hybridoma 2:19–28.

Pearl ER, Vogler LB, Okos AJ, Christ WM, Lawton AR, Cooper MD. 1978. B lymphocytic precursors in human bone marrows: an analysis of normal individuals and patients with antibody deficiency states. J Immunol 120:1169–1175.

Preud'homme JL, Seligmann M. 1972. Surface bound immunoglobulins as a cell marker in human lymphoproliferative diseases. Blood 40:777–791.

Reinherz EL, Kung PC, Goldstein G, Schlossman SF. 1979. A monoclonal antibody with selective reactivity with functionally mature thymocytes and all peripheral human T cells. J Immunol 123:1312–1317.

Reinherz EL, Kung PC, Goldstein G, Levy RH, Schlossman SF. 1980. Discrete stages of human intrathymic differentiation: analysis of normal thymocytes and leukemic lymphoblasts of T lineage. Proc Natl Acad Sci USA 77:1588–1592.

Ritz J, Pesando JM, Notis-McConarty J, Lazarus H, Schlossman SF. 1980. A monoclonal antibody to human acute lymphoblastic leukemia antigen. Nature 283:583–585.

Ritz J, Nadler LM, Bhan AK, Notis-McConarty J, Pesando JM, Schlossman SF. 1981. Expression of common acute lymphoblastic leukemia antigen (CALLA) by lymphomas of B and T cell lineage. Blood 58:648–652.

Rosenthal P, Rimm IJ, Umiel T, Griffin JD, Schlossman SF, Nadler LM. 1983. Characterization of fetal lymphoid tissue by monoclonal antibodies. J Immunol 131:232–237.

Ross GD, Rabellino EM, Polley MJ, Grey HM. 1973. Combined studies of complement receptor and surface immunoglobulin bearing cells in normal and leukemic human lymphocytes. J Clin Invest 52:377–385.

Royston I, Magda J, Baird S, Merserve B, Griffiths J. 1980. Human T cell antigens defined by monoclonal antibodies: the 65,000 dalton antigen of T cells (T65) is also found on chronic lymphocytic leukaemic cells bearing surface immunoglobulin. J Immunol 125:725–731.

Schlossman SF, Chess L, Humphreys RE, Strominger JL. 1976. Distribution of Ia-like molecules on the surface of normal and leukemic human cells. Proc Natl Acad Sci USA 73:1288–1292.

Stashenko P, Nadler LM, Hardy R, Schlossman SF. 1980. Characterization of a human B lymphocyte specific antigen. J Immunol 125:1678–1685.

Stashenko P, Nadler LM, Hardy R, Schlossman SF. 1981. Expression of cell surface markers after human B lymphocyte activation. Proc Natl Acad Sci USA 78:3848–3852.

Stein H, Siemssen V, Lennert K. 1978. Complement receptor subtypes C3b and C3d in lymphocytic tissue and follicular lymphoma. Br J Cancer 37:520–532.

Thorley-Lawson DA, Schooley RT, Bhan AK, Nadler LM. 1982. Epstein-Barrr virus superinduces a new human B cell differentiation antigen (Blast-1) expressed on transformed lymphoblasts. Cell 30:415–425.

Vogler LB, Crist WM, Bockman DE, Pearl ER, Lawton AR, Cooper MD. 1978. Pre-B cell leukemia; a new phenotype of childhood lymphoblastic leukemia. N Engl J Med 298:872–878.

Wang CY, Good RA, Ammirati P, Dymbart G, Evans RL. 1980. Identification of a p69,71 complex expressed on human T cells sharing determinants with B type chronic lymphocytic leukemia cells. J Exp Med 151:1539–1554.

Winchester RJ, Fu SM, Wernet P, Kunkel HG, Dupont B, Jerslid C. 1975. Recognition by pregnancy serum of non-HLA alloantigen selectivity expressed on B lymphocytes. J Exp Med 141:924–929.

Wormley SB, Collins ML, Royston I. 1981. Comparative density of the human T cell antigen on T65 on normal peripheral blood T cells and chronic lymphocytic leukemia. Blood 57:657–662.

Yokochi T, Holly RD, Clark ED. 1982. B lymphoblast antigen (BB-1) expressed on Epstein-Barr activated B cell blasts, B lymphoblastoid cell lines and Burkitt's lymphoma. J Immunol 128:283.

UT M.D. Anderson Clinical Conference on Cancer,
Vol. 27, edited by R. J. Ford, L. M. Fuller, and
F. B. Hagemeister. Raven Press, New York © 1984.

Immunologic Studies in Non-Hodgkin's Lymphoma

Richard J. Ford, Jr., Nicola M. Kouttab, and Frances M. Davis

Department of Pathology, The University of Texas M. D. Anderson Hospital and Tumor Institute at Houston, Houston, Texas 77030

The non-Hodgkin's lymphomas (NHL) are a heterogeneous group of human T- and B-cell lymphoid tumors (Ford and Maizel 1982). The tumors are found primarily in lymph nodes, the spleen, and other lymphoid organs, but they also occasionally enter the peripheral blood and become leukemic. NHL have been hypothesized to represent "frozen" stages in lymphocyte differentiation, in which monoclonal populations of neoplastically transformed lymphoid cells proliferate without concomitant differentiation (Salmon and Seligmann 1974). Although these tumors have been described extensively (Ford and Maizel 1982, Lukes and Collins 1975), relatively little is known about the biology of the neoplastic cells and the differences or similarities to their normal lymphoid cell counterparts. Such studies could provide important information on tumor cell biologic characteristics and eventually may correlate clinical behavior with biologic or immunologic parameters.

TUMOR CELL PHENOTYPING

One of the major problems in experimental studies with human lymphoid tumors is defining the malignant cell population and then separating the tumor cells from the normal or reactive lymphoid cells, which are virtually always present in these lesions (Dvoretsky et al. 1982, Harris and Data 1982). A helpful, but not definitive, immunologic marker in the B-cell lymphomas, which represent the majority of human NHL, is the cell surface immunoglobulin (SIg) light chain, which can generally identify a monoclonal population of lymphoma cells (Levy et al. 1977). However, anti-idiotype antibody is needed for definitive clonal definition of the neoplasm (Hough et al. 1976). Unfortunately, such clonally restricted cell surface markers have not been described in the T-cell–type NHL. Still, the most definitive marker of lymphoid neoplasia remains cytogenetic abnormalities, usually involving the number 14 chromosome (Yunis 1983).

Recently, we have used antisera to the human malignancy-associated nucleolar antigen (HMNA), originally described in nonlymphoid tumors (Davis et al. 1979), to identify lymphoma cells. This rabbit heteroantiserum is made against purified HeLa cell nucleoli and subsequently absorbed extensively with normal cells. When this antisera was used in standard indirect immunofluorescence assays on frozen sections of morphologically defined NHL lesions, we found that the anti-HMNA antisera stained the nucleoli of the histopathologically malignant neoplastic cell populations (Ford et al. 1984). A variety of reactive lymphoid hyperplasias and normal lymph nodes, spleens, and tonsils did not show positive staining with this antisera. Also, normal peripheral blood mononuclear cells (PBMC) and purified T-, B- and monocyte-cell populations derived from PBMC (Table 1) were negative. In addition mitogen-stimulated normal T- (PHA) or B- (protein A-sepharose) cell populations did not show anti-HMNA fluorescent staining. These mitogen-stimulated normal lymphocyte populations, continually propagated in vitro with their homologous growth factors, T-cell growth factor (TCGF) and B-cell growth factor (BCGF), also did not show positive reactivity with anti-HMNA antisera. The only HMNA-positive nonneoplastic lymphoid cell populations that we have identified so far are some Epstein-Barr virus (EBV)-transformed lymphoblastoid cell lines and one patient with the atypical lymphoid hyperplasia associated with an acquired immune deficiency-like syndrome (AIDS) (Guarda et al. 1983). This latter case

Table 1. *HMNA Reactivity of Neoplastic and Normal Human Lymphoid Cells*

Cell type*	No. of cases	No. of HMNA cases+
NHL-small B cell type (PDL + WDL)	35	35
NHL-mixed B cell type	7	7
NHL-small B cell type	8	8
NHL-diffuse large B cell type	20	20
NHL-diffuse large T cell type	4	4
NHL-hairy cell type	7	7
Normal lymph nodes, various areas	22	0
Normal tonsils	4	0
Reactive lymph nodes	8	1
Purified PBMC T cells	4	0
Purified PBMC B cells	5	0
Cultured growth factor dependent normal T cells	4	0
Cultured growth factor dependent normal B cells	4	0
Mitogen stimulated PBMC	6	0

*Modified Rappaport classification, determined on paraffin-embedded, hematoxylin and eosin-stained 6 μ-tissue sections.

+Reactivity determined by rabbit anti-HMNA antisera in an indirect immunofluorescence assay. In NHL specimens, correlation was made between morphology and pattern of tumor involvement. HMNA-positive cells usually accounted for 60%–90% of cells in frozen sections of cytopreps of NHL specimens.

HMNA–human malignancy-associated nucleolar antigen; NHL–non-Hodgkin's lymphoma; PBMC–peripheral blood mononuclear cells.

may, in fact, represent incipient lymphoid neoplasia because AIDS can eventuate in lymphoid neoplasia (Ziegler et al. 1982).

These data suggest that the HMNA is an important marker for neoplastic lymphoid cells. When combined with other phenotypic parameters, such as SIg light-chain typing, monoclonal antibody-defined cell surface antigens, and cytogenetics one can provide quite definitive evidence that putative lymphoid tumor cell populations actually contain neoplastic cells. This methodology now allows us to critically evaluate tumor cell suspensions that have had reactive or normal cell components removed by various cell separation procedures such as sheep red blood cell (SRBC) rosetting to remove T lymphocytes or plastic adherence to remove cells of the monocyte-macrophage accessory cell lineage.

Figure 1 shows a B-cell–type NHL, which has been T- and adherent-cell depleted. The putative tumor cell population was greater than 98% κ light-chain positive and greater than 95% positive for HMNA. Other markers performed on the lymphoma cell population included cell surface IgM, and the B-cell antigens B1 and B4 (Nadler et al. 1983). The T-cell (SRBC rosette positive) population, on the other hand, were greater than 95% negative for both κ light chain and HMNA. These findings, along with the additional data obtained on other HMNA-positive lymphoma cell populations with cytogenetic abnormalities, indicate that purified lymphoma cell preparations can be prepared for experimental studies in vitro.

GROWTH FACTOR STUDIES ON NHL CELLS

One of the major areas of interest in studying the biology of NHL cells is the control of tumor cell proliferation. A major question relates to the lack of spontaneous proliferation in vitro of freshly explanted lymphoma cells of either the T- or B-cell type. Although flow cytometric studies often indicate a significant proportion of cells in S phase (Shackney et al. 1980), little proliferation is noted when thymidine incorporation studies are done on the tumor cell populations. Since most NHL tumors contain neoplastic cells that share many similarities with their normal T- and B-cell counterparts, we were interested to ascertain if the factors controlling normal lymphoid cell proliferation would also stimulate neoplastic cells from NHL lesions.

Table 2 shows that purified populations of small B-cell–type NHL cells incorporated little ^{3}H-thymidine (^{3}H-Tdr) after 72 hours in vitro. When the tumor cell populations were stimulated with anti-IgM (μ-chain specific)-conjugated agarose beads (Bio-Rad Laboratories, Richmond, CA), increased incorporation of ^{3}H-Tdr was observed. When greatly purified BCGF was added, either alone or in concert with anti-μ beads, increased ^{3}H-Tdr incorporation was found. Similar increases in thymidine incorporation were also observed when the B-cell mitogen *Staphlococcus* protein A conjugated to sepharose beads (Pharmacia Laboratories, Piscataway, NJ) was used to stimulate the lymphoma cells in vitro. The amount of thymidine incorporation observed in 12 cases of small B-cell–type NHL however, suggests

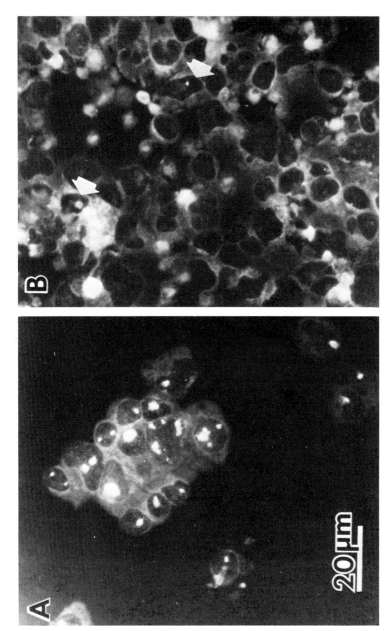

Figure 1. Cytocentrifuge preparations of fractionated cell suspensions from a small-cell (B-cell type) NHL. T cells were depleted by SRBC-rosetting and macrophages were depleted by plastic adherence. When stained with rabbit anti-HMNA by indirect immunofluorescence, virtually all the putative lymphoma cells (**A**) are positive for HMNA, while the rosette-positive T-cell population (**B**) is essentially negative, except for an occasional positive cell (arrows) that probably represents tumor cells that were trapped with the reactive T cells when the Ficoll-Hypaque density gradient separation was performed.

Table 2. *Growth Factor-Mediated Proliferation in Human B-Cell (Small Cell Type) Lymphomas*

Histopathology DX*	Cell surface and HMNA phenotype†	Bkg. CPM‡	BCGF§	α-Mu‖	α-Mu +BCGF	PA-S¶
WDL	μδκ, B1, B2, HMNA+	3500	15435	5192	17120	6364
WDL	μκ, B1, B2, B4, HMNA+	1670	10866	846	18640	11754
WDL	μδκ, B1, B2, HMNA+	1420	8009	5166	31944	10646
N-PDL	μκλ, B1, B2, HMNA+	902	5017	1625	5364	29340
N-PDL	μκ, B1, B2, HMNA+	868	5768	1256	6842	22636
N-PDL	μγκ, B1, B2, HMNA+	320	2708	3296	6573	5880

*Diagnosis (DX) according to the modified Rappaport classification.

†Tumor cell suspensions formed E_n rosettes and adherent cells were depleted prior to phenotyping using monoclonal Abs and HMNA by immunofluorescence. An antigen was considered present if >80% of the tumor cells were positive.

‡Cells were cultured for 96 hours at 37°C and labelled with 0.5 μCi of ^{3}H-Tdr (6Ci/mMole) for the final 24 hours. ^{3}H-Tdr incorporation is the mean of triplicate culture wells.

§Greatly purified BCGF preparations were obtained from DEAE and gel filtration purified PHA stimulated LyCm. 10% v/v factor preparations were added to 0.2×10^6 cells/well.

‖Anti-μ agarose beads (Bio-Rad) were added at a concentration of 15 μg/ml final concentration.

¶Protein A-sepharose beads (Pharmacia) were added at a concentration of 5% v/v.

CPM–counts per minute; BCGF–B-cell growth factor; WDL–well-differentiated lymphocytic lymphoma; N-PDL–nodular poorly differentiated lymphocytic lymphoma.

(See Table 1 for other abbreviations.)

that only about 10% of the tumor cells are being stimulated by the anti-Ig or the growth factor. The pattern of reactivity seen in these experiments usually implied that the stimulation observed with the anti-μ beads and the growth factor was additive rather than synergistic as seen when normal B cells are stimulated similarly (Maizel et al. 1983).

There are two particular points of interest here: (1) the majority of the ^{3}H-Tdr incorporation was seen with BCGF alone, which suggests that the responding neoplastic cells are already in the activated state and apparently possess a receptor for the growth factor; (2) there may be a relatively small number of apparently inactive tumor cells that can be directly activated by anti-μ alone and then recruited into the proliferating pool of lymphoma cells in the presence of BCGF. It should be noted however, that we cannot exclude that this small percentage of anti-μ–sensitive cells does not represent residual normal B cells expressing the same light chain as the neoplastic clone. This possibility implies that normal or reactive B cells might contribute to the overall proliferative response observed in the tumor cell preparation and that this minor normal subpopulation required conventional activation (Ford et al. 1981, Maizel et al. 1982).

DISCUSSION

The biology of NHL has been a difficult area to study principally because of the lack of experimental systems on which to study the neoplastic cells in vitro.

Previously, the only cells available for investigation were the B-cell lymphoblastoid cell lines derived from Burkitt's lymphomas that contain the EBV genome (Nilsson, 1979). Several other NHL cell lines have been reported (Epstein and Kaplan 1974) but they have been the exception rather than the rule; most attempts to grow NHL cells in vitro have not met with success.

The studies reported here indicate two important findings. The first is that it is possible to identify, with confidence, the neoplastic clone in the NHL by using clonal markers such as light-chain type (and ultimately idiotype, if such reagents are available), cell lineage markers defined by monoclonal antibodies to cell surface antigens, and tumor cell markers such as HMNA. Given this ability to phenotype NHL cells with precision and reproducibility, one can then use fairly standard lymphoid cell separation techniques to achieve purified lymphoma cell preparations. These NHL cell preparations can then be studied in vitro, utilizing the specialized methodologies employed by cellular immunologists to address fundamental questions about the immunobiology of the human lymphoma cells.

The second important finding relates to the apparent ability of at least some NHL cells within the tumor cell populations to respond to the homologous growth factor for the normal cell counterpart of the NHL cell. These data imply that most NHL cells do not represent autonomous immortal transformed cells that have simply lost normal growth control mechanisms. The sensitivity of at least a subpopulation of the apparently neoplastic cells in NHL to normal immunoregulatory molecules, such as lymphoid cell growth factors, suggests that some degree of immunoregulatory control is possible in these tumor cell populations. The lack of spontaneous proliferative activity observed in lymphoma cells in vitro is puzzling, as is the relatively small percentage of tumor cells that incorporate thymidine in response to growth factor. These data may indicate that only a small percentage of the tumor cells present in a lymphomatous lesion actually represent the proliferating pool of neoplastic cells. We have found that the majority of the lymphoma cells that have been generated by the small proliferating tumor cell pool may have become functionally inert. These cells are not capable of proliferating either spontaneously or in response to mitogens, growth factors, or even nonspecific mitogenic stimuli, such as phorbol ester or calcium ionophore (data not shown), even though a proportion of them apparently have an S-phase DNA content.

These studies are preliminary and the results may not be representative for all types of NHL. What is important however is the indication that experimental studies on fresh human lymphoma cells are feasible and may provide important insights, which should ultimately provide useful clinical information about the biology of NHL.

ACKNOWLEDGMENT

This investigation was supported in part by grants CA31479 and CA36243 awarded by the National Cancer Institute, United States Department of Health and Human Services and by the King Faisal Foundation.

We would like to thank Tammy Hazelrigs and Linda Kimbrough for help with manuscript preparation.

REFERENCES

Davis FM, Gyorkey F, Busch RK, Busch H. 1979. Nucleolar antigen found in several human tumors but not in the non tumor tissue studies. Proc Natl Acad Sci USA 76:892–899.

Dvoretsky P, Wood GS, Levy R, Warnke RA. 1982. T lymphocyte subsets in follicular lymphomas compared with those in non-neoplastic lymph nodes and tonsils. Hum Pathol 13:618–625.

Epstein AL, Kaplan HS. 1981. Biology of human malignant lymphomas. I. Establishment in continuous cell culture, and heterotransplantation of diffuse histiocytic lymphomas. Cancer 34:1851–1872.

Ford RJ, Cramer M, Davis FM. 1984. Identification of human lymphoma cells by antisera to malignancy-associated nucleolar antigens. Blood (In press).

Ford RJ, Maizel AL. 1982. Immunobiology of lymphoreticular neoplasms. *In* Twomey J, ed., The pathophysiology of human immunological disorders. Urban and Schwartzenburg, Baltimore pp. 199–217.

Ford RJ, Mehta SR, Franzini D, Montagna R, Lachman L, Maizel AL. 1981. Soluble factor activation of human B lymphocytes. Nature 294:261–263.

Guarda LA, Bulter JJ, Mansell P, Hersh EM, Reuben J, Newell GR. 1983. Lymphadenopathy in homosexual men. Morbid anatomy with clinical and immunologic correlations. Am J Clin Pathol 79:559–566.

Harris N, Data RE. 1982. The distribution of neoplastic and normal B lymphoid cells in nodular lymphomas. Hum Pathol 13:610–617.

Hough BW, Eady RP, Harblin TJ, Stevenson FK, Stevenson GT. 1976. Anti-idiotype sera raised against surface immunoglobulin of human neoplastic lymphocytes. J Exp Med 144:960–962.

Levy R, Warnke R, Dorfman RF, Haimovich J. 1977. The monoclonality of human B cell lymphoma. J Exp Med 145:1014–1022.

Lukes RJ, Collins RD. 1975. New approaches to the classification of the lymphomata. Br J Cancer 31(Suppl 2):1–16.

Maizel AL, Morgan JW, Mehta SR, Kouttab N, Bator JM, Sahasrabuddhe CG. 1983. Long term growth of human B cells and their use in a microassay for B-cell growth factor. Proc Natl Acad Sci USA 80:5047–5051.

Nadler LM, Anderson KC, Marti G, Bates M, Park E, Daley JF, Schlossman SF. 1983. B_4, a human B lymphocyte-associated antigen expressed on normal, mitogen-activated, and malignant B lymphocytes. J Immunol 131:244–250.

Nilsson K. 1979. The nature of lymphoid cell lines and their relationship to the virus. *In* Epstein MA, Achong BG, eds., The Epstein-Barr Virus, Springer-Verlag, New York, pp. 225–266.

Salmon S, Seligmann M. 1974. B cell neoplasia in man. Lancet 2:1229–1231.

Shackney SE, Skramstad KS, Cunningham RE, Lincoln TL, Lukes RJ. 1980. Dual parameter flow cytometry studies in human lymphomas. J Clin Invest 66:1281–1294.

Yunis JJ. 1983. The chromosomal basis of human neoplasia. Science 221:227–236.

Ziegler JL, Miner RC, Rosenbaum E, Lennette E, Shillitoe E, Casavant C, Drew WL, Mintz L, Fershow J, Greenspan J, Beckstead J, Yamamoto K. 1981. Outbreak of Burkitt's-like lymphoma in homosexual men. Lancet 2:631–633.

UT M.D. Anderson Clinical Conference on Cancer,
Vol. 27, edited by R. J. Ford, L. M. Fuller, and
F. B. Hagemeister. Raven Press, New York © 1984.

T-Cell Malignancies: Can Pathologic and Clinical Features Be Predicted from the Tumor Cell Phenotype?

Marshall E. Kadin

*Departments of Laboratory Medicine and Pathology, University of Washington,
Seattle, Washington 98105*

T-cell malignancies are highly varied in appearances, phenotypic markers, and clinical characteristics. Nevertheless, within this superficial heterogeneity are found major categories of T-cell malignancies that are relatively homogeneous in clinicopathology and tumor cell phenotype. The present study examines the consistency of the correlation among pathology, immunology, and clinical features in the author's and others' reported experience. T-cell malignancies are thus grouped into those disorders primarily affecting the mediastinum, skin, lymph nodes, or spleen (Figure 1). Exceptions to this scheme and their possible significance are noted.

MATERIALS AND METHODS

Malignant cells were isolated from heparin-treated blood and bone marrow or from cell suspensions from lymph node and spleen by Ficoll-Hypaque density gradient centrifugation, as previously described (Kadin et al. 1981). The viability of cell suspensions so obtained was usually greater than 90%, as determined by exclusion of trypan blue dye. Cells were morphologically examined in Wright's Giemsa stained preparations and cytochemically with special stains for cytoplasmic

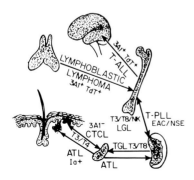

Figure 1. Proposed origin and spread of T-cell malignancy. T-PLL–T-cell prolymphocytic leukemia; T-ALL–T-cell acute lymphoblastic leukemia; LGL–lymphocytosis or leukemia of large granular lymphocytes; ATL–adult T-cell leukemia; TGL–T-gamma lymphoma; CTCL–cutaneous T-cell lymphoma; EAC–erythrocyte, antibody, complement; NSE–nonspecific esterase; NK–natural killer cell.

enzymes acid alpha-naphthyl butyrate esterase and alpha-naphthyl acetate esterase (ANAE), myeloperoxidase (MPO), and acid phosphatase (AcP), with and without tartrate inhibition, and for glycogen with the periodic acid-Schiff (PAS) stain (Kadin et al. 1981). Nuclear enzyme terminal deoxynucleotidyl transferase (TdT) was examined by immunofluorescence of acetone-fixed cytocentrifuge preparations using an antibody against TdT from Bethesda Research Laboratories (Rockville, MD).

Tumor cell suspensions were examined for spontaneous rosetting with sheep erythrocytes (ER), for IgGFc receptors using trypsin-treated ox erythrocytes coated with rabbit anti-ox erythrocyte IgG (EA), for complement receptors using trypsin-treated sheep erythrocytes coated with IgM plus complement (EAC) (Kadin et al. 1978). Tissues were embedded in 7.5% gelatin and rapidly frozen in isopentane cooled to $-70°C$. Frozen tissue sections were cut approximately 5 μ thick, adhered to glass slides, and fixed for 5 min in cold acetone. After storage overnight at $-20°C$, they were studied for surface antigens using the avidin-biotin complex (ABC) immunoperoxidase technique developed by Hsu et al. (1981).

Monoclonal antibodies used to define sIg, Ia, and B- and T-cell differentiation antigens are listed in Table 1. These antibodies were used to study cell suspensions by indirect immunofluorescence using a phase contrast fluorescence microscope or

Table 1. *Monoclonal Antibodies and Their Reactivities*

Antibody clone(s)	Antigen(s) recognized	Reactive cells	Reference
9.6 (T11)	E-rosette receptor p55	All E-rosetting T cells	Kamoun 1981
10.2 (Leu 1)	p65–67	Thymocytes, all T cells except some cytotoxic/suppressor T cells	Martin 1980
3A1	p40	Thymocytes, all T cells except some helper T cells	Haynes 1979
T4 (Leu 3a)	p62	Thymocyte subpopulations, helper T cells	Ledbetter 1981
T8 (Leu 2a)	ND	Thymocyte subpopulations, cytotoxic/suppressor T cells	Evans 1981
T6	p44–12	Cortical thymocytes, Langerhans' cells	McMichael 1979
T3	p19	Mature thymocytes, peripheral T cells	Reinherz 1979
7.2	Framework region of Ia p29–34	B cells, dendritic cells, macrophages, activated T cells	Hansen 1980
HNK (Leu 7)		Human natural killer cells	Abo 1981
Tac	Interleukin-2 receptor	Activated and functionally mature T cells	Uchiyama 1981
T9	Transferrin receptor	Proliferating cells	Trowbridge 1981

ND–not done; HNK–human natural killer cells.

to study frozen tissue sections by the ABC immunoperoxidase technique. In each instance, an irrelevant mouse myeloma protein of the appropriate class was substituted for the primary antibody as a negative or background control. All slides were evaluated for staining without knowledge of the antibody used.

RESULTS

Tumor cells from 19 patients with T-cell lymphoblastic malignancy were characterized by rosettes and monoclonal antibodies as shown in Table 2. All cases were positive for TdT. As expected, E rosette-forming lymphoblasts were positive with monoclonal antibody 9.6 (T11) directed against the ER receptor, whereas lymphoblasts not forming E rosettes were not stained by antibody 9.6. Antibody 10.2 (Leu 1) identified 10 of 11 cases in the ER$^+$ group but only 6 of 9 cases in the ER$^-$ group. Only antibody 3A1 identified all cases of T-cell lymphoblastic malignancy regardless of E rosette-forming ability or reactivity of tumor cells with one or more of the other T-cell monoclonal antibodies. In one case (patient 12, Table 2), the T-cell nature of lymphoblasts was confirmed only by the formation of EAC rosettes, a pre–T-cell property, and focal staining with acid phosphatase, a T-cell characteristic. Lymphoblasts from other patients showed variable reactivity with monoclonal antibodies directed against T cell-specific antigens T4, T8, T6, and T3. In contrast to mature or postthymic T-cell malignancies, there was frequently coexpression of T4 and T8 antigens (5 of 19 cases), but neither T4 nor T8 antigen was expressed together with T3 antigen (19 of 19 cases). T6, a thymocyte-specific antigen, was expressed in 6 of 19 cases, more often in ER$^+$ (5 of 11 cases) than in ER$^-$ (1 of 8 cases). Ia-antigens defined by antibody 7.2 were never found in these cases of T-cell lymphoblastic malignancy.

Table 3 reveals that there were no significant differences in the clinical features of patients whose early prethymic T-cell lymphoblasts failed to form E rosettes and patients with E rosette-forming lymphoblasts. Figure 2 shows the lymphoblastic morphology in one case of pre–T-cell acute lymphoblastic leukemia (ALL). A round nuclear morphology, without appreciable nuclear convolutions, was more often found in the E rosette-negative pre–T-cell group.

Patient number 20, in Table 4, illustrates the value of surface markers in the distinction of thymic-derived T-cell ALL from postthymic T-cell leukemia. The patient, an 11-year-old girl, presented with a mediastinal mass, peripheral lymphadenopathy, hepatosplenomegaly, and a white blood cell (WBC) count of 350,000/mm^3. The bone marrow contained 40% ER$^+$ lymphoblasts, and the patient was enrolled in a treatment protocol for T-cell ALL. However, review of the peripheral blood morphology and results of a peripheral lymph node biopsy revealed that the patient actually had postthymic nonlymphoblastic T-cell lymphoma-leukemia, similar to adult T-cell malignancy, described initially in Japan (Uchiyama et al. 1977). Indeed, the young patient's leukemic cells had polylobated nuclei (Figure 3), and the lymph node revealed a diffuse mixed or pleomorphic lymphoma and sparing B-cell follicles, instead of the uniform small cell type characteristic of lymphoblastic

Table 2. *Monoclonal Antibody Phenotype of T-Cell Lymphoblastic Malignancy*

	Patient																		
	E-rosette positive											E-rosette negative							
Antibody	1	2	3	4	5	6	7	8	9	10	11	12	13	14	15	16	17	18	19
9.6 (ERA)	+	+	+	+	+	+	+	+	+	+	+	0	0	0	0	0	0	0	0
10.2 (Pan T)	+	+	+	+	+	+	+	+	0	+	+	0	+	+	+	0	+	0	+
3A1	+	+	+	+	+	+	+	+	+	+	+	+	+	+	+	+	+	+	+
T4 (HI)	0	0	0	+	+	+	+	+	+	+	0	0	0	0	0	+	+	+	0
T8 (CS)	0	0	0	0	0	+	0	0	+	0	0	0	0	0	0	0	0	+	0
T6 (CT)	0	0	0	0	0	0	+	+	+	+	0	0	0	0	0	0	0	0	0
T3 (MT)	0	0	0	0	0	0	0	0	0	+	+	0	0	0	0	0	0	0	+
7.2 (Ia)	0	0	0	0	0	0	0	0	0	0	0	0	0	0	0	0	0	0	0

ERA—E-rosette associated; HI—helper inducer T cell; CS—cytotoxic suppressor T cell; CT—cortical or common thymocyte; MT—medullary or mature thymocyte.

Table 3. *Clinical Profiles of Patients with T-Cell Lymphoblastic Leukemia/Lymphoma*

	E-rosette positive	E-rosette negative
Number of cases	11	8
Mean age (yr)	14	14
Sex ratio (M/F)	11/0	6/2
Mean WBC count (mm³)	183,000	154,000
Mediastinal mass	7/11	5/8
CNS or testicular disease	2/6*	4/8

*Adequate data only available on 6 patients.

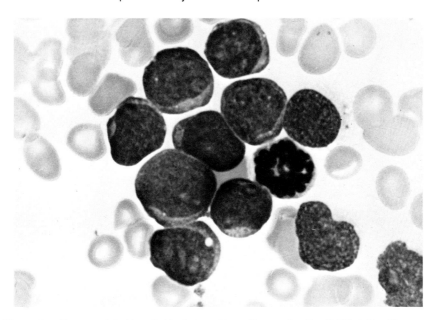

Figure 2. Nonconvoluted lymphoblasts from E-rosette negative T-cell ALL defined by monoclonal antibodies. Stained with Wright's Giemsa, × 1200.

lymphoma. Absence of TdT and expression of mature T-cell phenotype T3⁺ T4⁺ confirmed the postthymic nature of the process.

Six white adult patients with similar postthymic T-cell malignancies were studied (patients 21-26, Table 4). They all had circulating pleomorphic cells and peripheral lymphadenopathy. Involved lymph nodes contained diffuse mixed or pleomorphic lymphoma. Three patients developed skin lesions, in two, biopsy results proved malignancy. The leukemic infiltrate involved the epidermis in each case. Serologic studies confirmed the presence of antibodies against the human T-cell leukemia virus (HTLV) (Hinuma et al. 1981, Posner et al. 1981) in each of two cases studied. The T-cell phenotype was that of the mature helper T cell (T3⁺ T4⁺) in three

Table 4. *Monoclonal Antibody Phenotype of Node-Based Pleomorphic T-Cell Lymphoma*

Antibody	Patient						
	20	21	22	23	24	25	26
9.6 (T11)	+	+	+	+	+	+	+
10.2 (Leu 1)	+	+	+	+	+	0	+
3A1	+	0	0	0	+	+	0
T4	+	+	+	+	0	0	0
T8	0	0	0	0	0	0	0
T6	0	0	0	0	0	0	0
T3	+	+	+	+	+	0	0
Ia	0	0	+	0	+	+	+

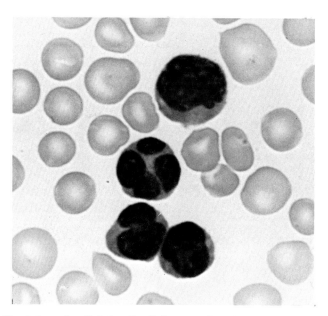

Figure 3. Circulating cells with helper T-cell phenotype in node-based pleomorphic T-cell malignancy. Stained with Wright's Giemsa, × 1200.

cases (patients 21-23, Table 4), but the leukemic cells lacked T4 antigen in the other three cases (patients 24-26, Table 4). 3A1, Ia, and Tac antigens were often expressed by leukemic cells in these cases of adult T-cell leukemia (ATL), similar to Japanese, Caribbean, and European cases of ATL (Hattori et al. 1980, 1981, Takatsuki et al. 1982, Catovsky et al. 1982, Tricot et al. 1983).

Circulating cells in patients with the Sézary syndrome were of the mature helper T-cell phenotype (T3$^+$ T4$^+$) but usually lacked 3A1, Ia, and Tac antigens (patients 27-30, Table 5). In one unusual case (patient 31, Table 5), the patient lacked antibodies against HTLV but did not develop skin lesions until five months after

Table 5. *Monoclonal Antibody Phenotype of Cutaneous T-Cell Lymphoma*

Antibody	Patient											
	27	28	29	30	31	32	33	34	35*	36*	37	38
9.6 (T11)	+	+	+	+	+	0	+	+	+	+	+	+
10.2 (Leu 1)	+	+	+	+	+	+	+	+	+	+	+	+
3A1	0	0	0	0	+	0	0	0	0	+	0	0
T4	+	+	+	+	+	+	+	+	+	+	0	0
T8	0	0	0	0	0	0	0	0	+	+	+	0
T6	0	0	0	0	0	0	0	0	0	0	0	0
T3	+	+	+	+	+	+	+	+	+	+	+	+
Ia	0	0	0	0	0	0	+	0	0	+	0	+

*Contains mixture of T4$^+$ and T8$^+$ cells.

the discovery of Sézary cells in the blood; 3A1 antigen was detected on the majority of circulating cells. In patient number 32, typical Sézary cells did not express the ER receptor or react with antibody 9.6.

Skin lesions of patients with the Sézary syndrome or mycosis fungoides, often referred to collectively as cutaneous T-cell lymphoma (CTCL), were more heterogeneous. They commonly included a mixture of T4$^+$ and T8$^+$ cells. In some instances intraepidermal groups of cells corresponding to Pautrier microabscesses expressed a phenotype similar to that of tumor cells circulating in the blood (patients 28, 29, 32, 34, & 37, Table 5). However, in other cases (patients 35 and 36, Table 5), where only scattered T4$^+$ or T8$^+$ cells were found in the epidermis, it was not possible to establish the definite phenotype of the tumor cells. In one case (patient 37, Table 5), an unexpected phenotype, T4$^-$ T8$^+$ 3A1$^-$, was clearly demonstrated for tumor cells infiltrating the epidermis. In another case (patient 38, Table 5), a patient with rapidly growing skin tumors and immunoblastic transformation of tumor cells also had tumor cells that showed little or no expression of T4 antigens. In this case, there was a clear predominance of cells expressing Leu 1, T11, T3, T9, and Ia antigens. There were almost no T8$^+$ or 3A1$^+$ cells. Expression of Tac antigens was infrequent in CTCL.

As shown in Table 6, most spleen-based T-cell malignancies were of the T3$^+$ T8$^+$ (cytotoxic/suppressor) or T3$^+$, T8$^+$, HNK$^+$ (human natural killer cell) phenotypes. The first two patients recognized (patient 39 and 40, Table 6) had lymphoid tumor cells with a curious property of erythrophagocytosis (Figure 4). Erythrophagocytosis seemed to be mediated by an IgGFc receptor, since the phagocytic cells formed EA rosettes (Figure 5). We termed this tumor erythrophagocytic T-gamma lymphoma (Kadin et al. 1981). The tumor cells formed E rosettes but did not react with antibody Leu 1 and lacked ANAE, similar to a population of T-gamma cells in normal blood. An intrasinus component of tumor cell infiltration was prominent in the liver, lymph nodes, and spleen. This sinus pattern and tumor cell erythrophagocytosis caused a superficial resemblance of T-gamma lymphoma to malignant histiocytosis (histocytic medullary reticulosis).

Table 6. *Monoclonal Antibody Phenotype of Spleen-Based T-Cell Lymphoma/Leukemia*

Antibody	Patient									
	39	40	41	42	43	44	45	46	47	48
9.6 (T11)	+	+	0	+	+	+	0	+	+	+
10.2 (Leu 1)	0	0	0	+	+	+	0	+	+	+
3A1	ND	ND	+	ND	+	ND	+	ND	ND	ND
T4	0	0	0	0	0	0	0	0	+	+
T8	+	+	+	+	+	+	+	+	0	0
T6	0	0	0	0	0	ND	0	0	0	0
T3	+	+	+	+	+	+	+	+	+	+
Ia	0	0	0	0	0	0	0	0	0	0
HNK	ND	ND	ND	+	+	+	+	+	ND	ND

(See Table 1 for abbreviations.)

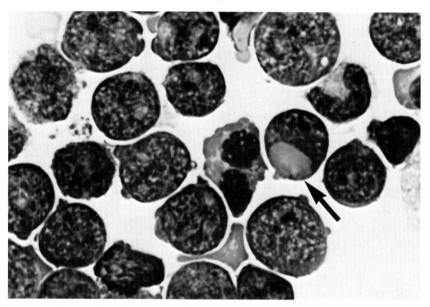

Figure 4. Spleen cells in T-gamma lymphoma. *Arrow* points to erythrocyte ingested by T-gamma cell. Stained with Wright's Giemsa, × 1200.

Six patients with leukocytosis of large granular lymphocytes (LGL) (Figure 6) were identified (patients 41-46, Table 6). Four of these patients had marked neutropenia (polymorphonuclear neutrophils <500/mm³) and three had recurrent infections. However, the results of their bone marrow biopsies showed the bone marrow to be normal or hypercellular with little evidence of diminished granulo-cytopoiesis to account for the neutropenia. The sixth patient with LGL (patient 46, Table 6) was a woman with pure red cell aplasia. Her bone marrow showed only

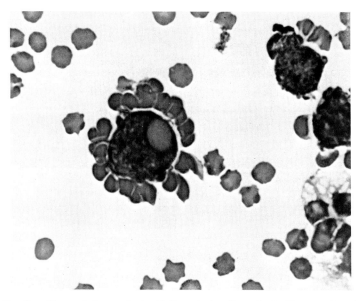

Figure 5. Rosetting and phagocytosis of IgG-coated erythrocytes by T-gamma lymphoma cell. Stained with Wright's Giemsa, × 1200.

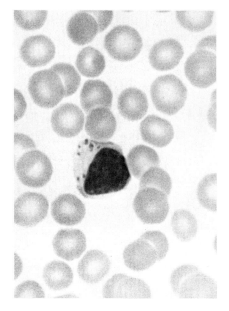

Figure 6. Large granular lymphocyte in spleen-based leukemia of suppressor and killer cell phenotype. Stained with Wright's Giemsa, × 1200.

the earliest recognizable erythroid precursors. This was the only patient with large numbers of lymphoid cells in the bone marrow. Five of the six patients with excess LGL had clinical splenomegaly but none had peripheral lymphadenopathy. In four cases (patients 42-44, and 46, Table 6), the LGL formed E rosettes, and in two cases (patients 45 and 46, Table 6), the LGL formed EA-gamma rosettes as well, but no erythrophagocytosis was demonstrated. The LGL were always T3+ T4−. In all cases more than 30% of cells expressed T8 antigen, and in five of six cases studied for HNK cell antigen (Leu 7), more than 30% of cells were positive. Immunoperoxidase studies of the enlarged spleens removed from two patients revealed that the major tumor cell infiltrate (T3+, T8+, NK+) was in the red pulp cords.

Two elderly patients (patients 47 and 48, Table 6) with massive splenomegaly had T-cell prolymphocytic leukemia (PLL), which demonstrated a single discrete nucleolus in most leukemic cells (Figure 7). These were the only cases of splenic T-cell malignancy with a T4+ helper T-cell phenotype. Unlike the node-based helper T-cell lymphomas, the malignant cells in T-cell PLL expressed receptors for complement (EAC). They also showed strong focal staining for ANAE that was not found in T8+ splenic malignancies. T-cell PLL was clinically similar to B-cell PLL, and patients presented with very high peripheral WBC counts, bone marrow failure, and hypersplenism (Lampert et al. 1980); lymphadenopathy was relatively inconspicuous, and no mediastinal mass or skin lesions were found.

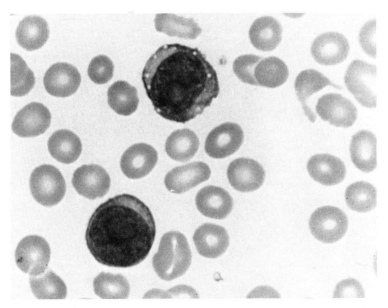

Figure 7. T-cell prolymphocytic leukemia with prominent nucleoli and helper T-cell phenotype from patient with massive splenomegaly. Stained with Wright's Giemsa, × 1200.

DISCUSSION

These results demonstrate a marked heterogeneity among T-cell malignancies but also show a remarkable correlation among morphology, clinical behavior, and immunologic phenotype, in most cases. It appears that immunocytochemical analysis of tumor cells usually enables one to predict the major organs of tumor involvement and the histopathology of the lesions in T-cell malignancies. Tumor cells of immature thymic phenotype (TdT$^+$, 3A1$^+$, Ia$^-$, ER$^+$ or ER$^-$, and coexpressing T4, T8, and T6 antigens) were usually associated with a mediastinal mass, bone marrow, and central nervous system (CNS) involvement. Tumor cells of mature helper phenotype (TdT$^-$ T3$^+$ T4$^+$) were commonly derived from enlarged lymph nodes and were often associated with skin lesions. When leukemic cells were Tac$^+$, Ia$^+$, or 3A1$^+$, cellular morphology was frequently pleomorphic and associated with rapid tumor growth. Absence of these antigens was generally associated with chronic cutaneous disease. The cytotoxic/suppressor or NK cell phenotype (T3$^+$ T8$^+$ NK$^+$) was characteristic of spleen-based T-cell malignancies. T-cell prolymphocytic leukemia with massive splenomegaly and a T4$^+$ EAC$^+$ phenotype was the only exception to this rule.

T-cell lymphoblastic malignancies were characterized by mediastinal mass and diffuse small cell high-grade lymphoma with early leukemic dissemination and common CNS or extranodal involvement. No significant clinical differences were found between patients with early prethymic T lymphoblasts that failed to form E rosettes and patients with E rosette-forming tumor cells. Antibody 3A1 was the only antibody that revealed the true T-cell lineage of lymphoblasts from both groups of patients. A similar result was recently reported with antibody 4H9 (Link et al. 1983). Antibodies 4H9 and 3A1 both detect the same antigen with a molecular weight of 40,000. Unlike postthymic T-cell malignancies, lymphoblasts of T-cell lymphoblastic leukemia-lymphoma were always positive for TdT and negative for Ia antigens. In this study of 19 patients with T-cell lymphoblastic malignancy, we did not try to distinguish sharply between surface markers of tumor cells in lymphoblastic lymphoma and those in lymphoblastic leukemia, as others have done (Bernard et al. 1981).

As reported by Haynes et al. (1981), we also found that the phenotype of leukemic Sézary cells in CTCL was typically that of a mature helper T cell, Leu 1$^+$ 3A1$^-$, T3$^+$, T4$^+$, T8$^-$. The phenotype of skin tumors (mycosis fungoides) in CTCL appeared to be less homogeneous. The exact phenotype of the malignant cells was sometimes difficult to determine because of the variable admixture of T8$^+$ nonmalignant T cells and Ia$^+$ dendritic (Langerhans') cells. Nevertheless, in one atypical case, it was clear that tumor cells infiltrating the epidermis were T8$^+$ T4$^-$. In another case, marked by rapid growth of skin tumors, blastlike tumor cells were Leu 1$^+$, T3$^+$, Ia$^+$ but both T4$^-$ and T8$^-$. Others have reported the association of blastlike tumor cells with Ia antigens and loss of either Leu 1 or T4 antigens in advanced lesions of CTCL (Wood et al. 1982, Willemze et al. 1983). We have simulated the blastic transformation and loss of T4 antigens of CTCL cells in vitro by treatment with phorbol ester (Kadin et al. 1983). Some authors suggest that cutaneous T-cell lymphomas with a noncerebriform cytology, tumor Ia expression, lack of mature helper T-cell phenotype, and nonepidermotropic histology should be classified as non-Hodgkin's cutaneous lymphomas other than mycosis fungoides (Wood et al. 1983).

Many of the Japanese cases of ATL are Ia$^+$ and involve the skin. We recognized several nonendemic cases of ATL that were Ia$^+$ and several that lacked a mature helper T-cell phenotype. Skin involvement was either epidermotropic or nonepidermotropic and when studied, serum antibodies against the human T-cell leukemia virus were found. In our study, it seemed possible to distinguish nonendemic ATL from CTCL by the more frequent expression of 3A1, Ia, and Tac antigens on circulating leukemic cells in ATL patients.

We studied a group of patients with spleen-based T-cell malignancies that most often were comprised of T-gamma or T8/NK (cytotoxic-suppressor/natural killer) cells. The proposed splenic origin of these tumors is consistent with the observation that the spleen is the only adult lymphoid organ that has a high percentage of T-gamma cells (Gupta et al. 1978, Moretta et al. 1978). Patients with disease that we designated as T-gamma lymphoma had tumors of medium-size lymphoid cells with capacity for erythrophagocytosis; they had few circulating leukemic cells. The pattern of splenic red pulp and sinus infiltration and tumor cell erythrophagocytosis led to an initial mistaken diagnosis of malignant histiocytosis. Tumor cell formation of E rosettes, expression of several different T-cell antigens (T11, T3, and T8), and lack of nonspecific esterase indicated that this was a T-cell lymphoma rather than malignant histiocytosis (Kadin et al. 1981).

Another group of patients with splenomegaly had more chronic illness characterized by severe neutropenia or, in one case, pure red cell aplasia and lymphocytosis of large granular lymphocytes (Starkebaum et al. 1983, Loughran et al. 1983, Abkowitz et al. 1983). In these cases the tumor cells bore overlapping markers of T-gamma, cytotoxic/suppressor, or NK cells. Leukemic infiltration of the splenic red pulp was proven by immunoperoxidase studies of the spleen, in two cases. The probability that this disease originates in the spleen is supported by the recently reported presence of a significant percentage of splenic, but not bone marrow or blood, lymphocytes in S and G_2/M phases of the cell cycle (Palutke et al. 1983).

Two patients with massive hypersplenism and T-cell prolymphocytic leukemia had tumor cells with a helper-inducer T3$^+$, T4$^+$ phenotype (Corwin et al. 1983). The presence of complement receptors on the leukemic cells was a unique feature not found in node-based helper T-cell malignancies. In the spleen, there was mainly red pulp infiltration without expansion of the white pulp that distinguished these cases histologically from B-cell prolymphocytic leukemia (Lampert et al. 1980).

Together, these studies indicate an overall consistency of phenotypes distinguishing major categories of T-cell malignancies. Variations in phenotypes within individual categories may be of both biological and prognostic significance. Because of the low frequency of T-cell malignancies, a larger cooperative prospective trial is recommended to test the hypothesis that immunocytochemical analysis is predictive of clinical behavior and histopathology in these disorders.

ACKNOWLEDGMENT

I wish to thank Drs. Jan Abkowitz, Tom Loughran, and John Olerud for allowing me to study their patients; Drs. Ih-Jen Su and Kaori Nasu for valuable advice and assistance; and Kate Coleman, Terri Rowe, and Diane Sako for technical assistance. This study was supported by grant CH-254 from the American Cancer Society.

REFERENCES

Abkowitz JL, Kadin ME, Powell JS, Adamson JW. 1983. T cell suppression of erythropoiesis in a patient with pure red cell aplasia (PRCA). (Abstract) Blood 62(Suppl 1)41a.

Abo T, Balch CM. 1981. A differentiation antigen of human NK and K cells identified by a monoclonal antibody (HNK-1). J Immunol 127:1024–1029.

Bernard A, Boumsell L, Reinherz E, Nadler L, Ritz J, Coppin H, Richard Y, Valensi F, Dausset J, Flandrin G, Lemerle J, Schlossman S. 1981. Cell surface characterization of malignant T cells from lymphoblastic lymphoma using monoclonal antibodies: Evidence for phenotypic differences between malignant T cells from patients with acute lymphoblastic leukemia and lymphoblastic lymphoma. Blood 57:1105–1110.

Catovsky D, Rose M, Goolden AWG, White JM, Bourikas G, Browhell AI, Blattner WA, Greaves MF, Galton DAG, McCluskey DR, Lampert I, Ireland R, Bridges GM, Gallo RC. 1982. Adult T-cell lymphoma-leukaemia in Blacks from the West Indies. Lancet i:639–643.

Corwin DJ, Kadin ME, Andres TL. 1983. T cell prolymphocytic leukemia: 2 cases having a postthymic helper phenotype with complement receptors and 14q+ chromosome abnormality. Acta Haemat 70:43–49.

Evans RL, Wall DW, Platsoncas CD, Siegal FP, Fikrig SH, Testa CM, Good RA. 1981. Thymus dependent membrane antigens in man: Inhibition of cell mediated lympholysis by monoclonal antibodies to the TH₂ antigen. Proc Natl Acad Sci USA 78:544–548.

Gupta S, Good RA. 1978. Subpopulations of human T lymphocytes III. Distribution and quantitation in peripheral blood, cord blood, tonsils, bone marrow, thymus, lymph nodes, and spleen. Cell Immunol 36:263–70.

Hansen JA, Martin PJ, Nowinski RC. 1980. Monoclonal antibodies identifying a novel T cell antigen and Ia-antigens of human lymphocytes. Immunogenetics 10:247.

Hattori T, Uchiyama T, Takatsuki K, Uchino H. 1980. Presence of human B-lymphocyte antigens on adult T-cell leukemia cells Clin Immunol Immunopathol 17:287–295.

Hattori T, Uchiyama T, Toibana T, Takatsuki K, Uchino H. 1981. Surface phenotype of Japanese adult T-cell leukemia cells characterized by monoclonal antibodies. Blood 58:645–647.

Haynes BF, Eisenbarth GS, Fauci AS. 1979. Human lymphocyte antigens: Production of a monoclonal antibody that defines functional thymus-derived lymphocyte subsets. Proc Natl Acad Sci USA 76:5829–5833.

Haynes BF, Metzgar RS, Minna JD, Bunn PA. 1981. Phenotypic characterization of cutaneous T-cell lymphoma. Use of monoclonal antibodies to compare with other malignant T cells. N Engl J Med 304:1319–1323.

Hinuma Y, Nagata K, Hanaoka M, Nakai M, Matsumoto T, Kinoshita K, Shirakawa S, Miyoshi I. 1981. Adult T-cell leukemia: Antigen in an ATL cell line and detection of antibodies to the antigen in human sera. Proc Natl Acad Sci USA 78: 6476–6480.

Hsu SM, Racine L, Fanger H. 1981. A comparative study of PAP method and avidin-biotin-peroxidase method for studying polypeptide hormones with radioimmunoassay antibodies. Am J Clin Pathol 75:734–738.

Kadin ME, Kamoun M, Lamberg J. 1981. Erythrophagocytic T gamma lymphoma. A clinicopathologic entity resembling malignant histiocytosis. N Engl J Med 304:648–653.

Kadin ME, Nasu K, Su I, Sako D. 1983. Blastic transformation and surface membrane phenotypic change in cutaneous T cell lymphoma and adult T cell leukemia. Correlation of *in vivo* and *in vitro* observations with TPA and PHA. (Abstract) Blood 62(Suppl 1)192a.

Kadin ME, Stites DP, Levy R, Warnke R. 1978. Exogenous immunoglobulin and macrophage origin of Reed-Sternberg cells in Hodgkin's disease. N Engl J Med 299:1208–1214.

Kamoun M, Martin PJ, Hansen JA, Brown MA, Siadak AW, Nowinski RC. 1981. Identification of a human T lymphocyte surface protein associated with the E-rosette receptor. J Exp Med 153:207–212.

Lampert I, Catovsky D, Marsh GW, Child JA, Galton DAG. 1980. The histopathology of prolymphocytic leukaemia with particular reference to the spleen: a comparison with chronic lymphocytic leukaemia. Histopathology 4:3–19.

Ledbetter JA, Evans RL, Lipinski M, Cunningham-Rundles C, Good RA, Herzenberg LA. 1981. Evolutionary conservation of surface molecules that distinguish T-lymphocyte helper/inducer and T-cytotoxic/suppressor subpopulations in mouse and man. J Exp Med 153:310–323.

Link M, Warnke R, Finlay J, Amylon M, Miller R, Dilley J, Levy R. 1983. A single monoclonal antibody indentifies T cell lineage of childhood lymphoid malignancies. Blood 62:722–728.

Loughran TP Jr, Kadin ME, Starkebaum G, Abkowitz JL, Clark EA, Disteche C, Slichter SJ. 1983. NK-cell proliferation associated with chromosomal abnormalities, multiple auto-antibodies, and immune-mediated peripheral blood cytopenias. (Abstract) Blood 62(Suppl 1):97a.

McMichael AJ, Pilch JR, Galfre G, Mason DY, Fabre JW, Milstein C. 1979. A human thymocyte antigen defined by a hybrid myeloma antibody. Eur J Immunol 9:205–210.

Martin PJ, Hansen JA, Nowinski RC, Brown MA. 1980. A new human T cell differentiation antigen: unexpected expression on chronic lymphocytic leukemia cells. Immunogenetics II:429–439.

Moretta L, Ferrarini M, Cooper MD. 1978. Characterization of human T-cell subpopulations as defined by specific receptors for immunoglobulins. Contemp Top Immunobiol 8:19–53.

Palutke M, Eisenberg L, Kaplan J, Hussain M, Kithier K, Tabaczka P, Mirchandani I, Tenenbaum D. 1983. Natural killer and suppressor T-cell chronic lymphocytic leukemia. Blood 62:627–634.

Posner LE, Robert-Guroff M, Kalyanaraman VS, Poiesz BJ, Ruscetti FW, Fossieck B, Bunn PA, Jr, Minna JD, Gallo RC. 1981. Natural antibodies to the human T cell lymphoma virus in patients with cutaneous T cell lymphomas. J Exp Med 154:333–346.

Reinherz EL, Kung PC, Goldstein G, Schlossman SF. 1979. A monoclonal antibody with selective reactivity with functionally mature human thymocytes and all mature peripheral T cells. J Immunol 123:1312–1317.

Starkebaum G, Martin PJ, Singer JW, Lum LG, Price TH, Kadin ME, Raskind WH, Fialkow PJ. 1983. Chronic lymphocytosis with neutropenia: evidence for a novel, abnormal T-cell population associated with antibody-mediated neutrophil destruction. Clin Immunol Immunopathol 27:110–123.

Takatsuki K, Uchiyama T, Ueshima Y, Hattori T, Toibana T, Tsudo M, Wano Y, Yodoi J. 1982. Adult T cell leukemia: proposal as a new disease and cytogenetic, phenotypic, and functional studies of leukemic cells. In GANN Monograph on Cancer Research No 28. Adult T cell leukemia and related diseases. Plenum Press, New York, pp. 13–22.

Tricot GJK, Broeckaert-Van Orshoven A, Den Ottolander GJ, De Wolf-Peeters C, Meyer CJLM, Verwilghen RL, Jansen J. 1983. Adult T-cell leukemia: a report on two white patients. Leuk Res 7:31–42.

Trowbridge I, Omary B. 1981. Human cell surface glycoprotein related to cell proliferation is the receptor for transferrin. Proc Natl Acad Sci USA 78:3039–3043.

Uchiyama T, Broder S, Waldmann TA. 1981. A monoclonal antibody (Tac) reactive with activated and functionally mature T cells. I Production of anti-Tac monoclonal antibody and distribution of Tac (+) cells. J Immunol 126:1393–1397.

Uchiyama T, Yodoi J, Sagawa K, Takatsuki K, Uchino H. 1977. Adult T cell leukemia: clinical features and hematologic features of 16 cases. Blood 50:481–492.

Willemze R, De Graaff-Reitsma CB, Cnossen J, Van Vloten WA, Meijer CJLM. 1983. Characterization of T-cell subpopulations in skin and peripheral blood of patients with cutaneous T-cell lymphomas and benign inflammatory dermatoses. J Invest Dermatol 80:60–66.

Wood GS, Burke JS, Horning S, Doggett RS, Levy R, Warnke R. 1983. The immunologic and clinicopathologic heterogeneity of cutaneous lymphomas other than mycosis fungoides. Blood 62:464–472.

Wood GS, Deneau DG, Miller RA, Levy R, Hoppe RT, Warnke RA. 1982. Subtypes of cutaneous T-cell lymphoma defined by expression of Leu-1 and Ia. Blood 59:876–882.

UT M.D. Anderson Clinical Conference on Cancer,
Vol. 27, edited by R.J. Ford, L.M. Fuller, and
F.B. Hagemeister. Raven Press, New York © 1984.

The Clinical Utility of Cell Surface Markers in Malignant Lymphoma

Clara D. Bloomfield, Kazimiera J. Gajl-Peczalska,*
Glauco Frizzera,* and Tucker W. LeBien*

*Section of Medical Oncology, Department of Medicine and, *Department of
Laboratory Medicine and Pathology, University of Minnesota Health Sciences Center,
Minneapolis, Minnesota 55455*

For patients with malignant lymphoma, lymphoid cell markers have a number of potential clinical uses. First, they may be useful for diagnosis. In particular, among the lymphoproliferative disorders, they may allow us to separate those that are malignant from those that are benign. Moreover, among morphologically undifferentiated malignancies, they may allow us to identify those that are lymphoid. Second, lymphoid cell markers may have prognostic utility; that is, they may allow us to divide the lymphomas into groups with distinctive histologic and clinical characteristics, responses to treatment, and expected survival rates. Finally, lymphoid cell markers may be therapeutically useful. Not only may they separate patients who are curable by means of current therapeutic approaches from those who require new approaches, but lymphoid cell surface markers may allow us to kill tumor cells using specific monoclonal antibodies directed against these surface antigens.

For more than 10 years we have been analyzing lymphocyte markers in biopsy specimens from patients with malignant lymphoma. One of the goals of these studies has been to define the clinical usefulness of these markers. In this chapter, we review our results from the viewpoint of the prognostic utility of lymphoid markers in patients with newly diagnosed lymphoma.

PATIENTS AND METHODS

Between September 1973 and May 1983, we studied 211 patients consecutively admitted to the University of Minnesota Hospitals with diagnoses of non-Hodgkin's lymphoma and with accessible lymphomatous tumor masses. Patients were diagnosed as having lymphoma on the basis of lymph node or other tumor mass histologic findings, using standard criteria. For this study, the histologic diagnosis used was that obtained from the pretreatment lymph node or other tumor masses studied for lymphocyte markers. In each instance, a portion of the tumor studied for immunologic markers was also fixed in B5 and histologic classification was done using the International Working Formulation for Clinical Usage (Non-Hodgkin's Lymphoma Pathology Classification Project 1982).

At diagnosis, all patients were extensively evaluated and assigned to a clinical stage according to the Ann Arbor classification (Carbone et al. 1971). One hundred sixty-seven (79%) patients underwent complete pathological staging. The remaining patients were staged clinically; in these patients pathologic staging was incomplete, usually because liver biopsy was not performed in patients who were otherwise classified stage I or II.

Initial therapy generally consisted of irradiation of involved and adjacent fields for patients with stages I or II disease and combination chemotherapy for patients with stages III or IV disease. Among patients who received treatment at the University of Minnesota, response was classified as complete remission when there was total disappearance of all symptoms and clinically detectable disease and the pathological documentation of disappearance of lymphoma from the bone marrow or liver, if one or both were initially involved. Patients who did not achieve complete remission were classified as failures. Remission duration was calculated from the date remission was achieved to the date of relapse or last follow-up; survival was calculated from the date of diagnosis to the date of death or last follow-up. All patients have been followed at least five months since diagnosis.

Immunologic Phenotyping

Immunologic phenotyping in all patients was based on studies of both single-cell suspensions and tissue frozen sections. All patient specimens were studied for SIg (surface immunoglobulin) and CIg (cytoplasmic immunoglobulin) and receptors for C'3 (complement), Fcγ and E (unsensitized sheep erythrocytes). The 96 most recent patients were also studied for TdT (terminal deoxynucleotidyl transferase) and with a panel of monoclonal antibodies (Gajl-Peczalska et al. 1982).

Our techniques for immunological analysis have been described in detail (Bloomfield and Gajl-Peczalska 1980, Gajl-Peczalska et al. 1982). In brief, suspensions of viable neoplastic cells were studied for the presence of SIg using immunofluorescence with monospecific antisera against heavy and light chains, for receptors for E by rosette formation with E, for C'3 by the erythrocyte-antibody (IgM)-complement rosette assay, and for Fcγ using immunofluorescence with fluorescein-ated aggregated human IgG. When two or more heavy or light chains were found on the surface of lymphoid cells, the cells were treated with polyvalent antiserum, incubated at 37°C for 24 hours, or subjected to both procedures and then studied for the presence of newly synthesized SIg. In the rosette assays, cytocentrifuge preparations were stained with Wright's Giemsa, and the proportion of malignant cells forming rosettes was determined.

Cryostat sections of the tumor masses were prepared from a portion of the same neoplastic tissue from which suspensions were made. Serial cryostat sections were studied for histological features by staining with hematoxylin-eosin and for the presence of immunoglobulin (SIg and CIg), C'3, and Fcγ using the methods described above for cell suspensions.

Surface antigens were studied by indirect immunofluorescence in both cell suspensions and cryostat sections using monoclonal antibodies and TdT. Frozen sections were routinely double stained to determine whether cells positive for monoclonal antibodies were also positive for monotypic SIg or CIg. The following surface antigens were studied: HLA-DR (Ia-like), BA-1 (Abramson et al. 1981), BA-2 (Kersey et al. 1981), BA-3 (LeBien et al. 1982), T101 (Royston et al. 1980), OKT11, OKT8, OKT6, OKT4, OKT3, and OKM1/OKM2 (Kung et al. 1979, Reinherz and Schlossman 1980).

Lymphomas were divided into four major immunologic groups based on the expression of SIg, CIg, E, and C'3. Cases were designated B lymphoma if the malignant cells demonstrated monotypic SIg or CIg and the absence of E, T lymphoma if the malignant cells formed rosettes with E, C'3 lymphoma if the malignant cells had C'3 receptors in the absence of monotypic SIg or CIg and E, and "null" lymphoma if malignant cells were negative for SIg, CIg, E, and C'3.

Statistical Methods

Clinical findings at presentation and histologic diagnosis were compared among the different immunologic phenotypes. Hypotheses of no difference were tested (at $\alpha = 0.05$) by use of the Pearson χ^2 statistic for two-way frequency tables (discrete variables) and by use of the rank test of Kruskal and Wallis (for continuous variables). Durations of initial remission and survival for the various immunologic groups were plotted from life tables calculated using the method of Kaplan and Meier. For remission duration analysis, patients dying while in complete remission were censored. Since 61% of the responding patients were still in remission and 58% of the total study population was still alive at the time of analysis, differences in remission duration and survival were tested for groups of at least five patients by use of the generalized Wilcoxon (Breslow modification) or Savage (Mantel-Cox modification) test. These two tests differ in the way they weight observations; the Breslow test gives greater weight to early observations and is less sensitive to late events that occur when few patients remain alive or in remission.

RESULTS

Prognostic Utility of Routine Lymphocyte Markers in Lymphoma (SIg, CIg, C'3, E)

Two hundred one of the 211 cases could be classified into one of the four major immunologic groups. One hundred fifty-six (74%) had B lymphoma, 18 (9%) had T lymphoma, 14 (7%) had C'3 lymphoma, and 13 (6%) had "null" lymphomas. In 10 cases (5%) the immunologic group was indeterminable. The histologic and clinical features of these four immunologic groups are shown in Table 1.

The majority of the patients were treated with intensive radiotherapy or chemo-

Table 1. *Histology and Clinical Features by Immunologic Phenotype in Lymphoma*

	No. pts	B (n = 156)	T (n = 18)	Null (n = 13)	C'3 (n = 14)	P
			Percentage of positive cases			
Histology						
A. Small lymphocytic	31	17	17	8	7	
B. Follicular small cleaved cell	52	31	0	8	21	
C. Follicular mixed small cleaved and large cell	13	8	0	0	0	
D. Follicular large cell	14	7	0	8	14	
E. Diffuse small cleaved cell	7	3	6	8	0	
F. Diffuse mixed small and large cell	13	3	33	15	0	<.001
G. Diffuse large cell	47	22	0	54	43	
H. Diffuse large cell immunoblastic	9	4	6	0	14	
I. Lymphoblastic	5	0	28	0	0	
J. Small noncleaved cell	6	4	0	0	0	
Other	4	1	11	0	0	
Stage						
I, IIA	32	16	11	23	21	
I, IIB	5	2	0	8	7	
IIIA	27	13	11	15	27	NS
IIIB	9	5	6	0	7	
IVA	82	43	50	15	29	
IVB	45	23	22	39	7	
First treatment			Percentage achieving complete remission			
All evaluable patients	167	60	47	56	75	NS
CHOP or CHOP-BLEO	73	67	40	67	60	NS
Mean age (yr)		58	46	64	66	.01
			Percentage male			
Sex		55	78	77	21	.006

(See text for components of chemotherapeutic regimens.)

therapy. Forty percent were treated with CHOP (cyclophosphamide, doxorubicin, vincristine, and prednisone) with or without bleomycin (CHOP-Bleo) or other equally intensive four- or five-drug combinations. The remission rate was similar for all immunologic groups whether only the patients treated with CHOP or CHOP-Bleo or the other patients were considered (Table 1). Survival was similar among the four major immunologic groups (Figure 1).

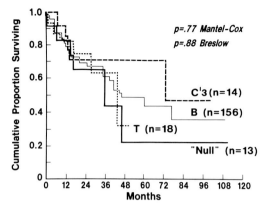

Figure 1. Survival of 201 patients with malignant lymphoma according to immunologic groups determined by study of pretreatment tumor masses.

Prognostic Utility of Routine Lymphocyte Markers Among Diffuse Large Cell Lymphomas

The prognostic utility of histologic classification of lymphoma has been repeatedly demonstrated. We have been particularly interested in whether immunologic classification adds useful prognostic information to that from histology (Bloomfield et al. 1976, Bloomfield et al. 1979). This question is especially important among diffuse large cell lymphomas, since 30%-50% of these patients may be cured with current therapeutic approaches. At the present time, there is no known way to separate, at diagnosis, those patients likely to be cured from patients unlikely to be long-term disease-free survivors. We have considered whether lymphocyte markers might help in this regard.

We studied a subset of 58 newly diagnosed patients with diffuse large cell lymphoma; 49 were classified as G-malignant lymphoma, diffuse large cell and 9 as H-malignant lymphoma, large cell, immunoblastic. The patients ranged in age from 8 to 87 years (median 65); 59% were female. By stage, 26% had I or IIA, 5% I or IIB, 10% IIIA, 9% IIIB, 26% IVA, and 24% IVB disease. Twenty-one percent had extranodal disease.

The immunologic phenotype was B in 40 patients (69%), C'3 in 8 (14%), "null" in 7 (12%), T in 1 (2%), and indeterminable in 2 patients (3%). The clinical features of the 3 larger immunologic groups are shown in Table 2. The only significant differences were found in the sex distributions; the B-lymphoma group contained about equal numbers of males and females, but the "null"-lymphoma group contained mostly males, and the C'3-lymphoma group had all females. Of interest, the majority of the "null"- and C'3-lymphoma patients had early disease (I-IIIA) compared to 30% for B-lymphoma patients. In all three immunologic groups, the majority of patients achieved complete remission.

Remission duration and survival curves were very similar for the "null"- and C'3-lymphoma groups. Thus, they have been combined for this analysis. For both remission duration (Figure 2) and survival (Figure 3) the patients with B lymphoma

Table 2. *Histologic and Clinical Features by Immunologic Phenotype in Diffuse Large Cell Lymphomas*

	B (n = 40)	Null (n = 7)	C'3 (n = 8)	P
Histology (no. cases)				
G. Diffuse Large Cell	34	7	6	NS
H. Diffuse Immunoblastic	6	0	2	
Stage (no. cases)				
I,II,IIIA	3,6,3	3,0,1	3,0,1	
I,IIIB	2,4	0,0	1,0	NS
IVA,IVB	12,10	1,2	2,1	
First treatment				
Number complete remissions/ number treated	17/32 (53%)	3/5 (60%)	6/8 (75%)	NS
Age				
Median (yr)	65	60	69	NS
Sex				
% Female	52	29	100	.01

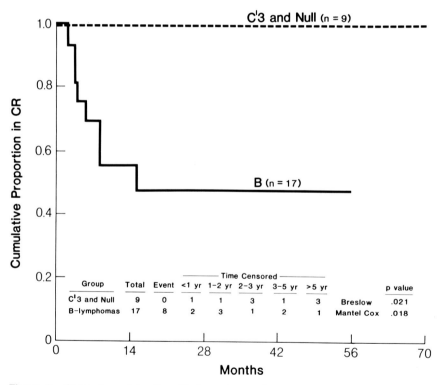

Figure 2. Comparison of duration of first complete remission (CR) of patients with diffuse large cell lymphomas (G and H of the International Working Formulation for Clinical Usage) according to immunologic groups.

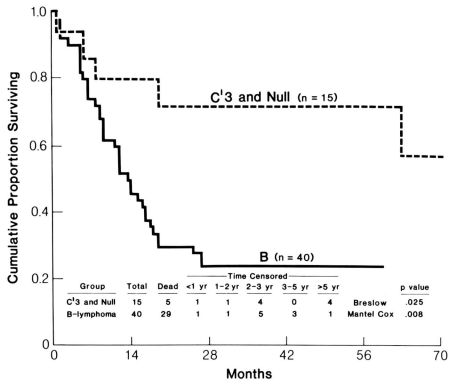

Figure 3. Comparison of survival of patients with diffuse large cell lymphomas according to immunologic groups.

did significantly worse. In contrast, survival curves according to histology (G versus H) and the presence or absence of C'3 receptors were essentially identical.

Monoclonal Antibody Phenotypes in Lymphoma

Tumor masses from a subset of 96 consecutive untreated patients were studied with the monoclonal antibody panel described earlier. Seventy-two cases were classified as having B lymphoma. Patients with B lymphoma ranged in age from 12 to 84 years (median 63). Forty-nine percent were female. By Ann Arbor criteria, 6 patients had stage I, 6 stage II, 15 stage III, and 44 stage IV disease. The results of phenotyping with various monoclonal antibodies by histologic classes for the B-lymphomas are shown in Table 3. All cases were negative for TdT, T3, T4, T8, T11, and OKM antigens. Almost all were HLA-DR positive, 82% were C'3 positive, and 75% were BA-1 positive. T101 was a good marker of small lymphocytic lymphoma; it was present in 62% of these cases and rarely found in other histologic groups. Follicular lymphomas were SIg positive, often CIg negative and were the predominant type of B lymphoma that expressed BA-3 (CALLA) antigen. In contrast, small lymphocytic (A) and diffuse large cell (G and H) lymphomas often had cells containing CIg and were almost always BA-3 negative. Only immuno-

Table 3. *Phenotypes of 72 B-Lymphomas**

Histology	No. pts	Percent positive cases						
		CIg only	C'3	Fc	BA-1	BA-2	BA-3	T101
A. Small lymphocytic	14	0	100	86	100	29	0	62
B. Follicular small cleaved cell	21	0	85	65	81	33	48	5
C. Follicular mixed small cleaved and large cell	7	0	100	50	57	29	29	0
D. Follicular large cell	6	0	80	50	67	50	17	0
E. Diffuse small cleaved cell	3	0	100	67	100	67	0	0
F. Diffuse mixed small and large cell	1	—	—	—	0	100	0	0
G. Diffuse large cell	13	0	60	50	54	69	8	8
H. Diffuse large cell immunoblastic	4	50	50	50	50	0	0	0
J. Small noncleaved cell	2	0	0	0	100	100	100	0
Other	1	0	0	0	100	100	0	0
Total			82	60	75	44	22	15

*100% HLA-DR positive except one case of H (malignant lymphoma, immunoblastic.)

Table 4. *Phenotypes of 12 T-Lymphomas**

Histology	No. pts	Number positive cases						
		T3	T6	TdT	HLA-DR	BA-2	BA-3	C'3
A. Small lymphocytic	2†	2	0	0	1	0	0	0
K. Mycosis fungoides	2‡	2	0	0	0	0	0	0
E. Diffuse small cleaved cell	1	1	0	0	0	0	0	0
F. Diffuse mixed	4	4	0	0	3	1	1	0
I. Lymphoblastic	3	1/2**	3	3	0	1	1	3

*100% E, T11 and T8 and/or T4 positive.
†One was 100% T4 positive, in the other, 85% of T cells were T8 positive.
‡Both had "helper" phenotypes with T4:T8 ratios of 9.4 and 7.5.
**One positive for T3 of two studied.

blastic lymphomas (H) demonstrated monotypic CIg (always heavy and light chain) in the absence of SIg. Both small noncleaved cell lymphomas (J) had the same phenotype: SIg positive, C'3 negative, BA-1 positive, BA-2 positive, BA-3 positive.

Twelve patients had T lymphoma; they ranged in age from 13 to 78 years (median 53). Ninety-two percent were male. By Ann Arbor classification, 1 patient had stage I, 1 had stage III, and 10 had stage IV disease. The results of phenotyping these T lymphomas with various monoclonal antibodies by histologic class are shown in Table 4. All cases were positive for E, T11, T8 and/or T4, and 90% were positive for T3.

From an immunologic standpoint, these T lymphomas appear to represent two groups, immature and mature. The immature lymphomas consist of the histologic group I-malignant lymphoma, lymphoblastic type and have a thymocyte phenotype (positive for TdT, T6, T8 and T4, often for C'3). There appear to be two mature types of T-lymphoma—monotypic and mixed. Each has a postthymic phenotype (negative for TdT, T6, C'3). One type appears to consist of a monotypic T cell proliferation consisting of helper (T4+) T cells or suppressor (T8+) T cells. This was seen in lymphomas of small lymphocytic type and mycosis fungoides. The second type appears to consist of a mixture of T4 and T8 T cells. These cases also often expressed HLA-DR (i.e., a phenotype of "activated" T lymphoctyes). Mixed T-cell proliferations were seen most commonly among F-malignant lymphoma, diffuse mixed large and small cell type.

Twelve patients were negative for SIg, CIg, and E; these included "null" and C'3 lymphomas. These patients tended to be older than B- or T-lymphoma patients ($P = .07$), ranging in age from 54 to 87 years (median 67). Fifty-eight percent were male. They had more limited disease than B- or T-lymphoma patients ($P = .03$): 4 had stage I, 5 had stage III, and only 3 had stage IV disease. Most cases were histologically classified as having large cell lymphomas (groups D and G).

The results of phenotyping these 6 "null" and 6 C'3 lymphomas with various monoclonal antibodies are shown in Table 5. All cases were HLA-DR positive and all were T marker and TdT negative; about one-third were BA-1 positive. Most important, all cases demonstrated at least one lymphocyte-associated marker.

Prognostic Utility of BA-1, BA-2, and BA-3 in B-Lymphomas (SIg+ or CIg+)

Immunologically, about 75% of lymphomas are B. Thus, it would be very useful if there were some way to divide these into clinically distinct groups using monoclonal antibodies. We have evaluated the potential of BA-1, BA-2 and BA-3 to define clinically useful groups in B lymphoma.

B lymphomas can be divided into 6 groups based on these three monoclonal antibodies (Table 6). Although these groups currently do not show statistically significant differences in age, sex, or stage, they differ significantly in histology ($P = .003$). Of considerable interest was the poor response to treatment, short remission duration (Figure 4), and short survival (Figure 5) of patients who were

Table 5. *Phenotypes of 12 "Null" and C'3-Lymphomas**

| | | | | BA-2 or | T-cell | | |
Histology	No. pts	C'3	BA-1	BA-3	markers	OKM	TdT
A. Small lymphocytic	1	0	0	0	0	0	0
B. Follicular small cleaved cell	1	1	1	0	0	0	0
D. Follicular large cell	3	2	0	1	0	0	0
G. Diffuse large cell	7	3	3	0	0	0	0

*All 12 were HLA-DR positive.

Table 6. *Histology and Clinical Features by Monoclonal (BA-1, BA-2, BA-3) Phenotype in 67 B-Lymphomas*

	+ − − (n = 26)	+ + − (n = 16)	− + − (n = 7)	+ + + (n = 7)	− − − (n = 6)	+ − + (n = 5)
Histology (no. cases)*						
A. Small lymphocytic	10	4	0	0	0	0
B. Follicular small cleaved cell	6	4	0	3	1	4
C. Follicular mixed small cleaved and large cell	3	0	0	1	2	0
D. Follicular large cell	2	1	2	0	0	1
E. Diffuse small cleaved cell	1	2	0	0	0	0
F. Diffuse mixed small and large cell	0	0	1	0	0	0
G. Diffuse large cell	2	4	4	1	2	0
H. Diffuse large cell immunoblastic	2	0	0	0	1	0
J. Small noncleaved cell	0	0	0	2	0	0
Other	0	1	0	0	0	0
Stage (no. cases)						
I,IIA	5	0	3	0	3	0
IIB	0	0	1	0	0	0
IIIA	4	3	0	1	1	0
IIIB	1	1	0	1	1	0
IVA	11	10	2	3	1	4
IVB	5	2	1	1	0	1
Complete remissions/ number treated	15/23	6/13	4/6	4/5	5/5	2/4
Age						
Median (yr)	64	63	52	49	61	63
Sex						
% Male	58	75	43	43	33	20

+ − − is BA-1⁺, BA-2⁻, BA-3⁻; + + − is BA-1⁺, BA-2⁺, BA-3⁻; − + − is BA-1⁻, BA-2⁺, BA-3⁻; + + + is BA-1⁺, BA-2⁺, BA-3⁺; − − − is BA-1⁻, BA-2⁻, BA-3⁻; + − + is BA-1⁺, BA-2⁻, BA-3⁺.
*Histology differed significantly among monoclonal groups ($P = .003$). None of the clinical features differed significantly.

BA-1 positive, BA-2 positive, and BA-3 negative. At the current time, remission duration and survival are very similar for all of the other groups. Individual consideration of the presence or absence of each marker was not as useful for predicting remission duration or survival, although patients with BA-2 negative lymphomas lived significantly longer than those with BA-2 positive lymphomas.

CONCLUSION

We have now studied lymphocyte markers in neoplastic cells from lymph nodes or other primary tumor masses in over 200 patients with newly diagnosed lymphoma. This study has a number of important features. First, only tumor masses

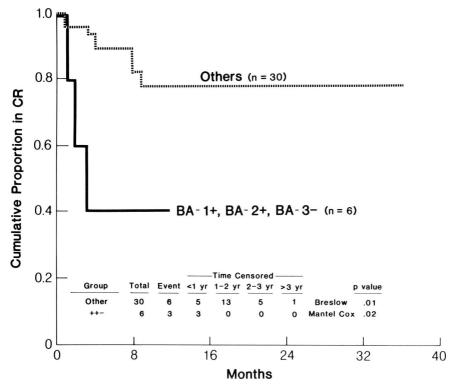

Group	Total	Event	<1 yr	1-2 yr	2-3 yr	>3 yr		p value
				Time Censored				
Other	30	6	5	13	5	1	Breslow	.01
++−	6	3	3	0	0	0	Mantel Cox	.02

Figure 4. Comparison of duration of first complete remission (CR) of patients with B lymphomas according to BA-1, BA-2, and BA-3 phenotype. Patients with lymphomas positive for BA-1 and BA-2 and negative for BA-3 (+ + −) have been compared to patients with other phenotypes (see text).

have been studied; many series include patients in whom neoplastic cells from only blood, bone marrow, or other body fluids have been studied. It has yet to be demonstrated that lymphocyte markers are identical, when studied simultaneously from different tissues; evaluation of many biologic properties, including morphology, suggest that they will not always be identical. Second, unlike most other large series, both cell suspensions and cryostat sections have been studied. We have reported the complementary nature of these two types of analysis for correctly phenotyping malignant lymphoma (Gajl-Peczalska et al. 1979). Finally, all patients have been studied at diagnosis; our sequential studies indicate that lymphocyte markers can differ at relapse. Even so, like all other studies, this one does not represent all newly diagnosed patients with malignant lymphoma seen at the University of Minnesota during this 10-year period; it includes only about one-half of the patients, i.e., those who had repeat peripheral lymph node biopsies taken or who required exploratory laparotomy for staging, diagnosis, or other problems. Moreover, as with most prior series, patients were not uniformly treated.

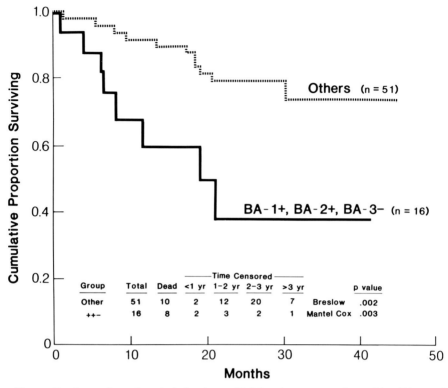

Figure 5. Comparison of survival of patients with B lymphomas according to BA-1, BA-2, and BA-3 phenotype (see legend Figure 4).

This study suggests that within histologic groups, lymphocyte markers (SIg, CIg, E, C′3) can add important prognostic information. Among patients with diffuse large cell lymphoma, patients with B lymphomas have significantly shorter remission durations and survivals. Similar results in smaller series have been reported (Warnke et al. 1980, Rudders et al. 1981). However, the number of patients is small and we cannot exclude the possibility that other prognostic factors, such as stage and tumor bulk, may explain the differences in response and survival among immunologic groups.

Most lymphomas, at least in adults, are B (SIg$^+$ or CIg$^+$). In our series, patients with B lymphoma had a median survival of about four years and about 35% are projected to live for more than six years. Clearly, it would be clinically useful to divide the B-lymphoma patients at diagnosis, if possible, into groups that would respond well to current treatments and those who would require new approaches. There are a number of B-cell monoclonal antibodies now available that could potentially subdivide the B-lymphomas into clinically useful groups. In this regard, we have explored the usefulness of three monoclonal antibodies, BA-1, BA-2, and BA-3, made at the University of Minnesota. More than 90% of B lymphomas mark with one of these monoclonal antibodies. They can be used to divide patients into six different groups, the most frequent of which is BA-1 positive, BA-2 negative, and BA-3 negative. When the six groups were evaluated for response to treatment and survival, one group (those patients with BA-1 positive, BA-2 positive, BA-3 negative lymphomas) had a somewhat lower remission rate than the other patients and significantly shorter remission durations and survival. This group represents 24% of the B-lymphoma patients.

Clearly, longer follow-up is required and more patients must be studied to confirm this preliminary observation. It will also be necessary to determine if the surface markers are an independent prognostic factor or whether the inferior survival of the BA-1 positive, BA-2 positive, BA-3 negative group is accounted for by some other prognostic factor. It is of potential therapeutic utility that the neoplastic cells of this poor prognosis group express the surface antigens recognized by the monoclonal antibodies BA-1 and BA-2, both of which are strongly cytotoxic in the presence of complement (LeBien et al. 1983). Thus, this may be a particularly good group in which to test the utility of autologous marrow transplantation early in the disease using monoclonal antibodies (plus complement or linked to ricin) to remove neoplastic cells ex vivo before reinfusion.

ACKNOWLEDGMENT

This investigation was supported in part by grant 17034, awarded by the National Cancer Institute, United States Department of Health and Human Services and the Coleman Leukemia Research Fund.

REFERENCES

Abramson CS, Kersey JH, LeBien TW. 1981. A monoclonal antibody (BA-1) reactive with cells of human B lymphocyte lineage. J Immunol 126:83–88.

Bloomfield CD, Gajl-Peczalska KJ. 1980. The clinical relevance of lymphocyte surface markers in leukemia and lymphoma. Curr Top Hematol 3:175–240.

Bloomfield CD, Gajl-Peczalska KJ, Frizzera G, Kersey JH, Goldman AI. 1979. Clinical utility of lymphocyte surface markers combined with the Lukes-Collins histologic classification in adult lymphoma. N Engl J Med 301:512–518.

Bloomfield CD, Kersey JH, Brunning RD, Gajl-Peczalska KJ. 1976. Prognostic significance of lymphocyte surface markers in adult non-Hodgkin's malignant lymphoma. Lancet ii:1330–1333.

Carbone PP, Kaplan HS, Musshoff K, Smithers DW, Tubiana M. 1971. Report of the committee on Hodgkin's disease staging classification. Cancer Res 31:1860–1861.

Gajl-Peczalska KJ, Bloomfield CD, Frizzera G, Kersey JH, LeBien TW. 1982. Diversity of phenotypes of non-Hodgkin's malignant lymphoma. *In* Vitetta E, ed., B and T Cell Tumors. Academic Press, New York, pp. 63–67.

Gajl-Peczalska KJ, Kersey JH, Bloomfield C, Frizzera G. 1979. The value of combined cell suspension and tissue frozen section studies in surface marker evaluation of non-Hodgkin's malignant lymphomas. (Abstract) Lab Invest 40:254.

Kersey JH, LeBien TW, Abramson CS, Newman R, Sutherland R, Greaves M. 1981. p24: A human leukemia-associated and lymphohemopoietic progenitor cell surface structure identified with monoclonal antibody. J Exp Med 153:726–731.

Kung PC, Goldstein G, Reinherz EL, Schlossman SF. 1979. Monoclonal antibodies defining distinctive human T-cell surface antigens. Science 206:347–349.

LeBien TW, Ash RC, Zanjani ED, Kersey JH. 1983. In vitro cytodestruction of leukemic cells in human bone marrow using a cocktail of monoclonal antibodies. *In* Neth R, Gallo RC, Greaves MF,

Moore MAS, Winkler K, eds. Haematology and Blood Transfusion, vol. 28, Modern Trends in Human Leukemia V. Springer-Verlag, Berlin, pp. 112–116.

LeBien TW, Boué DR, Bradley JG, Kersey JH. 1982. Antibody affinity may influence antigenic modulation of the common acute lymphoblastic leukemia antigen in vitro. J Immunol 129:2287–2292.

The Non-Hodgkin's Lymphoma Pathologic Classification Project. 1982. National Cancer Institute sponsored study of classification of non-Hodgkin's lymphomas. Cancer 49:2112–2135.

Reinherz EL, Schlossman SF. 1980. The differentiation and function of human T lymphocytes: A review. Cell 19:821–827.

Royston I, Majda JA, Baird SM, Meserve BL, Griffiths JC. 1980. Human T cell antigens defined by monoclonal antibodies: The 65,000-dalton antigen of T-cells (T65) is also found on chronic lymphocytic leukemia cells bearing surface immunoglobulin. J Immunol 125:725–731.

Rudders RA, Ahl ET, DeLellis RA. 1981. Surface marker and histopathologic correlation with long-term survival in advanced large-cell non-Hodgkin's lymphoma. Cancer 47:1329–1335.

Warnke R, Miller R, Grogan T, Pederson M, Dilley J, Levy R. 1980. Immunologic phenotype in 30 patients with diffuse large cell lymphoma. N Engl J Med 303:293–300.

UT M.D. Anderson Clinical Conference on Cancer,
Vol. 27, edited by R. J. Ford, L. M. Fuller, and
F. B. Hagemeister. Raven Press, New York © 1984.

Acquired Immunodeficiency Syndrome in the Development of Lymphoma

Benjamin Koziner, Carlos Urmacher,* R. S. K. Chaganti,† and
Bayard D. Clarkson

*Hematology/Lymphoma Service, Department of Medicine, *Department of Pathology and
†the Laboratory of Cancer Genetics and Cytogenetics, Memorial Sloan-Kettering
Cancer Center, New York, New York, 10021*

A steady increase in the incidence of disseminated Kaposi's sarcoma (KS), severe opportunistic infections (OI), and unexplained lymphadenopathy has been recently observed among sexually active homosexual men (Centers for Disease Control 1981, 1982a). Early in the course of this outbreak, it became clear that these patients were afflicted by a new variety of acquired immunodeficiency syndrome (AIDS) (Gottlieb et al. 1981, Siegal et al. 1981, Masur et al. 1981, Friedman-Kien et al. 1982, Urmacher et al. 1982). AIDS is defined by the Centers for Disease Control (CDC) as the appearance of KS (in patients under 60 years of age), life threatening OI, or both in patients with no known cause for immunosuppression. The term AIDS-related complex has recently been used to describe those patients who present with symptoms of lymphadenopathy, fever, or diarrhea, weight loss of 10% of total body weight, malaise, and immune abnormalities.

The unusual susceptibility to infectious agents such as *Pneumocystis carinii*, cytomegalovirus (CMV), herpes simplex, Epstein-Barr virus (EBV), *Mycobacterium tuberculosis* and *M. avium intracellulare, Candida, Cryptococcus* and other fungi, and parasitosis due to *Toxoplasma, Entamoeba histolytica* and *Giardia*, has been attributed to impaired cellular immunity. This immunodeficiency is reflected in the cutaneous anergy, lymphopenia, mostly at the expense of T-lymphocytes with decreased lymphocyte proliferative responses to antigens and mitogens, and defective natural killer cell activity. A characteristic finding in these patients has been the reversal of the ratio between the helper-inducer (OKT4+) and suppressor-cytotoxic (OKT8+) T-cell subsets because of a decrease in the proportion of helper-inducer T lymphocytes (Gottlieb et al. 1981, Koziner et al. 1982). Although the initial cases were exclusively among homosexual men and drug abusers, AIDS is now being reported among heterosexual men and women and their partners (Harris et al. 1983), children born of sexually promiscuous and drug addicted mothers (Oleske et al. 1983, Rubinstein et al. 1983), Haitians (Vieira et al. 1983, Pitchenik et al. 1983), hemophiliacs (Davis et al. 1983, Elliot et al. 1983, Poon et al. 1983), and transfusion recipients (Centers for Disease Control 1982c), which indicates a rapid spread of the epidemic to other sectors of the population and suggests an infectious etiology.

The United States and New York City statistics on AIDS cases, as obtained from the CDC on September 12, 1983 and from the most recent New York City Department of Public Health meeting, reveal that the total number of cases in the United States is 2290 and in New York City is 1058, which is about 40% of all cases reported. Approximately 75% of the new cases still appear in homosexual men and the mortality rate is 40%, a figure that has held for the past three years. One half of all known cases were reported in 1983. In the United States and in New York City, the median survival has been 17 months from diagnosis for patients with KS and 7 months for patients with OI. The Memorial Sloan-Kettering Cancer Center (MSKCC) statistics for AIDS cases seen since the start of the outbreak include 127 patients with KS, 35 patients with OI, and 4 patients who were homosexual drug users and presented with OI. The 166 AIDS cases seen at MSKCC represent 7%–8% of the United States total.

Recently, an increased incidence of secondary neoplasms including oral and rectal carcinomas (Lozada et al. 1982, Daling et al. 1982) and Burkitt's-like lymphoma has been noted in immunodeficient homosexual men (Centers for Disease Control 1982b). The development of malignant non-Hodgkin's lymphomas (NHL) has been observed, not only in AIDS patients but also in homosexual men without the syndrome but who have laboratory markers of immunodeficiency and epidemiologic backgrounds similar to patients with AIDS. More recently, a hemophiliac receiving factor VIII concentrate developed Burkitt's lymphoma (Gordon et al. 1983), raising concern about the possibility of this neoplasm occurring in other populations at risk.

The most common type of NHL seen in patients with AIDS at MSKCC is large cell lymphoma of the brain without involvement of other organs, while Burkitt's-like B-cell lymphomas are seen in homosexual patients who do not fit the strict definition of AIDS, which was formulated by the CDC. Because of its high incidence, we believe that B-cell NHL in homosexuals with the epidemiologic and immunologic backgrounds seen in AIDS should be included as part of the syndrome.

CASE MATERIAL

Burkitt's Lymphoma

The development of Burkitt's-like B-cell lymphoma in four homosexual men was initially reported from Arizona (Doll and List 1982) and California (Centers for Disease Control 1982b, Ziegler et al. 1982). We have reported two homosexual men (cases 1 and 2) who developed Burkitt's-like lymphoma and in whom the neoplastic cells showed chromosome translocations characteristically found in Burkitt's lymphoma (Chaganti et al. 1983, Chaganti 1983). Another patient (case 3) has been added to our series (Tables 1 and 2).

Table 1. *Clinical Characteristics of Male Homosexuals with Burkitt's Lymphoma*

Case	Age (yr)	Sites of involvement presentation/relapse				Therapy	Survival from diagnosis (months)
		LN	BM	CNS	Other		
New York (present series)							
1	39	+/+	+/+	−/+	−	L-17M	14
2	29	+/+	+/+	+/+	skin	L-17M High-dose Ara-C	5
3	37	+/	−/	−/	−	L-17M	5+
California (Ziegler et al. 1982)							
4	28	+/?	−/?	+/+	Orbit	CHOP	10
5	33	+/+	+/?	+/+	Mouth	Chemotherapy*	7
6	35	+/−	+/−	+/+	Mouth	Chemotherapy*	3
7	24	+/?	−/?	−/+	−	Chemotherapy*	7
Arizona (Doll and List 1982)							
8	24	+/−	−/−	−/−	Ileum	CHOP	24+

Chemotherapy*–not described.
LN–lymph node, BM–bone marrow, CNS–central nervous system CHOP–cyclophospha-mide, doxorubicin, vincristine, and prednisone.

Table 2. *Laboratory Findings in Male Homosexuals with Burkitt's Lymphoma*

Case	CMV	EBV-VCA	T4+/T8+ ratio	Phenotype	Tumor karyotype
New York (present series)					
1	1:16	1:640	0.9	Monoclonal κ	t(8;14)
2	1:16	1:640	1.0	IgM λ	t(8;22)
3	1:128	1:320	0.8	Monoclonal κ	t(8;14)
California (Ziegler et al. 1982)					
4	1:32	1:80	ND	ND	ND
5	1:32	1:320	ND	IgM-κ	ND
6	4:8	1:640	ND	IgM-κ	Normal
7	1:32	1:640	ND	IgM-κ	ND
Arizona (Doll and List 1982)					
8	ND	80	ND	ND	ND

ND–not done.
CMV–cytomegalovirus; EBV-VCA–Epstein-Barr virus-viral capsid antigen.

Case 1.

A 39-year-old sexually active homosexual man with a history of alcoholism, use of recreational drugs, and different sexually transmitted infections presented with a cutaneous genital lesion, which was consistent with KS, and a cervical mass and bone marrow involvement by Burkitt's-like cells that exhibited the t(8;14) translocation. EBV-viral capsid antigen (VCA) and CMV titers were 1:640, and cell surface marker analysis showed a predominance of monoclonal κ light chain-bearing cells. Despite treatment with MSKCC L17M protocol, recurrence in lymph nodes, bone marrow, and central nervous system (CNS) were documented. The patient died 14 months after presentation. The L17M induction and consolidation phases are depicted in Figures 1 and 2. The maintenance schedule included 2 sequences. The first sequence consisted of vincristine 2 mg/m² day 1 and 8 and prednisone 90 mg/m² q 12hr × 7 days, doxorubicin 20 mg/m² i.v. day 10–12 followed in 2 weeks by 6-mercaptopurine (6-MP) 90 mg/m² orally daily × 30 days, then methotrexate (MTX) 20 mg/m² orally × 30 days. Dactinomycin 600 μg/m² i.v. was given as a single dose one week after the conclusion of 6-MP and MTX. The second sequence was identical except that BCNU (bis-chloroethyl nitrosourea) 80 mg/m² i.v. and cyclophosphamide 800 mg/m² i.v. as single doses substituted for doxorubicin. The full course of treatment lasted approximately two years.

Case 2.

Another sexually active homosexual man, age 29, with a history of sexually related infections, presented with lymphadenopathy and CNS and bone marrow infiltration by small, noncleaved cell Burkitt's lymphoma (Figure 3). His chromosomal complement displayed the t(8;22) translocation. Therapy with MSKCC L17M protocol and high dose ARA-C (cytarabine) was only transiently effective and the patient died with generalized Burkitt's lymphoma, including CNS infiltration, five months after his initial presentation. EBV-VCA and CMV titers were 1:16. Cell surface marker analysis revealed a predominance of cells bearing monoclonal IgM-λ light chain.

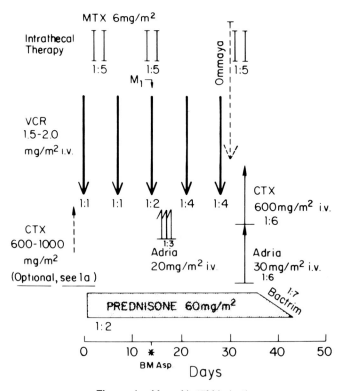

Figure 1. Map of L-17M induction.

CONSOLIDATION B

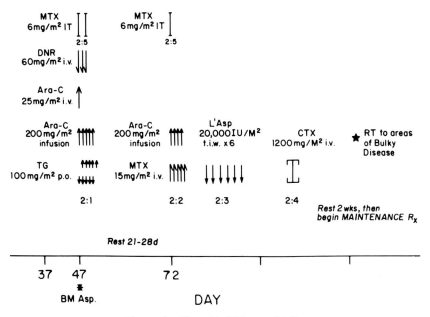

Figure 2. Map of L-17M consolidation.

Case 3.

This 37-year-old sexually active homosexual man presented at MSKCC with a one-month history of left axillary adenopathy. A biopsy was performed elsewhere and showed diffuse malignant lymphoma, small, noncleaved cell, Burkitt's type. Serological evaluation included *Toxoplasma* immunofluorescent antibody (IFA) total immunoglobulin 1:1024, IgM 1:4, and complement fixation (CF) 1:4. CMV complement-fixing antibody titer was 1:128 and EBV-VCA was 1:320. Staging work up included negative chest radiograph, abdominal computed tomographic (CT) scan, and bone marrow and spinal fluid aspiration for lymphomatous infiltration. Lymphangiogram, however, showed minimal enlargement of pelvic and para-aortic nodes and diffuse granular pattern. Surface markers analysis on lymphoid tissue from left axillary adenopathy showed a predominance of κ light-chain–bearing cells. Cytogenetic analysis on that specimen revealed a t(8;14) translocation. The patient remained alive and free of disease and was undergoing chemotherapy with MSKCC L17M protocol five months after his initial presentation.

Diffuse Histiocytic Lymphoma (DHL)

Case 4.

A 31-year-old man initially presented to MSKCC in October, 1982 with weight loss and malaise. He was an active homosexual with multiple partners, and he frequented bath houses. Workup showed a herpes simplex antibody titer of 1:32; CMV 1:64;

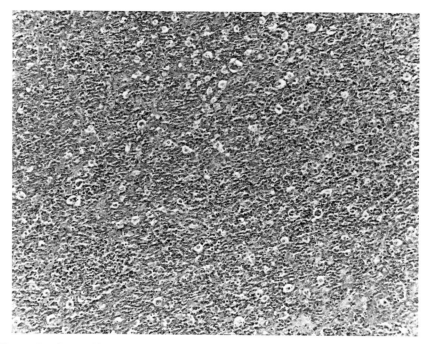

Figure 3. Case 2. Malignant lymphoma, small noncleaved cell, Burkitt's type. Hematoxylin and eosin stain. × 40.

Toxoplasma IFA (total immunoglobulin 1:16, IgM 1:4), complement fixing 1:2. Blood cultures grew *Staphylococcus aureus*. He was reevaluated in March, 1983 and had recurrence of *S. aureus* bacteremia. Because of persistent fever, he was readmitted to MSKCC in April, 1983. Physical examination showed left posterior cervical lymphadenopathy. Chest radiographic films revealed discrete round nodules in both lungs. Abdominal CT scan revealed massive enlargement of pelvic and para-aortic nodes. The spleen was enlarged. There was enlargement of the liver with a lucency noted on the anterior aspect of the dome of the right lobe. Barium enema did not show evidence of an intrinsic or extrinsic mass. Rectal examination and proctoscopy revealed a 1 × 1.5 cm hard nodule. Biopsy was obtained and showed malignant DHL, large cleaved-cell type. Bone marrow aspirate and biopsy results did not show evidence of lymphoma. Cerebrospinal fluid was negative for malignant cells. In May, 1983, the patient was started on the MSKCC NHL-7 protocol for stage IV DHL including cyclophosphamide, methyl GAG (methylglyoxal bis-guanylhydrazone), bleomycin, and prednisone alternated with doxorubicin, vincristine, and prednisone. The patient was free of disease and was undergoing chemotherapy six months after the diagnosis of DHL was made.

Lymphoplasmacytoid Lymphoma (LP Immunocytoma)

Case 5.

A 38-year-old homosexual man was first diagnosed as having KS in December, 1981. His medical history included multiple sexual contacts (over one thousand in the previous year) and venereal diseases. He also had a history of street-drug abuse. He was first admitted to MSKCC in March, 1982 for the treatment of KS with recombinant leukocyte A interferon, following a course of bovine transfer factor administered elsewhere. Serological evaluation included CMV by ELISA, IgG 1:512, IgM 1:16, and CMV complement-fixing antibody 1:64. *Toxoplasma* IFA total immunoglobulin was 1:16, IgM 1:4 and CF 1:2. EBV-VCA was 1:320. Immunoelectrophoresis revealed IgG 953 mg/dl, IgM 138 mg/dl, and IgA 280 mg/dl. No monoclonal paraprotein was found. He was readmitted to MSKCC for the final time in May, 1982 with increasing shortness of breath, new bilateral pulmonary infiltrates on chest radiographic examination, and hepatomegaly. Bronchoscopy revealed numerous erythematous lesions, but no organisms were identified when special stains were used. Bone marrow biopsy showed hypocellularity with adequate megakariocytes and megaloblastic changes. A liver biopsy revealed multiple periportal granulomas. Subsequently, cultures obtained from the lung, liver, and bone marrow were positive for *M avium intracellulare*. In late July, 1982 he began having hematemesis and died, approximately 20 months after the initial diagnosis of KS was made.

Postmortem findings included KS involving skin, lymph nodes, lungs, liver, spleen, duodenum, and tongue and diffuse lymphoplasmacytoid lymphoma (Figure 4A and B), involving multiple lymph node groups, lungs, stomach, spleen, and small and large bowel. Other conditions diagnosed at autopsy were disseminated *M avium intracellulare* and CMV infection, including chronic encephalitis that was due to CMV. *Candida albicans* was also recovered from lungs, adrenals, and lymph nodes.

Malignant Plasmacytoma

Case 6.

A 39-year-old bisexual man from St. Thomas, Virgin Islands presented to MSKCC, with a two-year history of hyperplastic lymphadenopathy, documented in repeated lymph node biopsies, and recurrent venereal infections. Several months prior to consultation, total protein was 10.9 g/dl and globulin was 7 g/dl. Although at that time a polyclonal increase in serum IgG of 4.3 g/dl with normal IgM and IgA was noted, serum immune electrophoresis at presentation at MSKCC showed a monoclonal IgG-κ paraprotein and urine immune electrophoresis revealed a significant amount of κ chain. Skeletal survey revealed no lesions and bone marrow aspiration and biopsy showed less than 5% mature plasma cells. Further laboratory testing revealed lymphopenia and a ratio of helper to suppressor T cells of 1.1:1 (normal 1.8 ± 0.8). Lymph node biopsy revealed follicular hyperplasia with fibrosis and plasmacytosis. Titer of EBV-VCA was 1:1280, CMV 1:8, and *Toxoplasma* 1:16.

Six months later the patient was readmitted because of severe back pain and a vesicular herpetic eruption at the level of L1-2 dermatome. Radiographic films of the thoracic spine revealed loss of the right pedicle of T2, myelogram showed 95% obstruction by a posterior epidural mass. Bone marrow aspirate and biopsy showed no diagnostic increase in plasma cells. Decompressive laminectomy revealed a soft tissue mass, which upon histological examination revealed a plasma cell tumor invading the bone. Immunoperoxidase stain showed that the cells contained intracytoplasmic IgG-κ immunoglobulin. Involved field radiotherapy was administered and the patient had not required further therapy in the 10 months following laminectomy. This case points out the potential for rapid progression from polyclonal to monoclonal B-cell proliferation and development of plasma cell tumor.

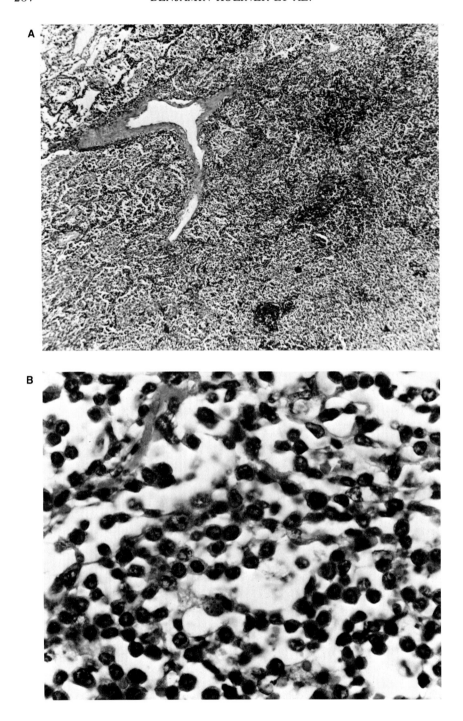

Figure 4. Case 5. **A.** Malignant lymphoma, lymphoplasmacytoid type in lung. Hematoxylin and eosin stain. × 200. **B.** × 500.

Acute Lymphoblastic Leukemia

Case 7.

A 33-year-old sexually active homosexual man with a recent diagnosis of pulmonary tuberculosis (TB) and KS presented to MSKCC complaining of fatigue, weight loss, fever to 39°C, and progressive skin lesions. Leukocyte count was 3,000/mm³ with 21% lymphocytes. High antibody titers to CMV and EBV-VCA were observed. OKT4+/ OKT8+ ratio was 1.7:1, although lymphocyte proliferative response to phytohemagglu- tinin stimulation was deficient. Bone marrow aspirate initially showed 3.5% blasts. However, an increased number of intermediate-size lymphocytes was observed. TdT (terminal deoxynucleotidyl transferase) determination using immunofluorescence showed 20% positive cells. A repeat bone marrow aspiration, taken 10 days later, showed 10.5% blasts and 25% TdT-positive cells. Flow cytometric analysis of the bone marrow aspirate showed a hyperdiploid clone (2.2 c). This abnormal clone represented 40% of the bone marrow cells. Biopsy of a cervical lymph node showed KS involving lymphoid and perinodal tissue. Although the significance of the elevated proportion of TdT- positive and aneuploid cells remains unexplained, it could be hypothesized that they represent evidence of early lymphoblastic neoplasia or, alternatively, reactive prolifer- ation with maturational arrest of lymphoid cells (Ciobanu et al. 1983).

Malignant Lymphomas of the Brain

Cases 8–10.

Malignant lymphomas that primarily involve the brain are being recognized more often in patients with AIDS (case records of the Massachusetts General Hospital 1983, Snider et al. 1983). Three patients in this series developed NHL with only brain involvement (Table 3). The primary cerebral lymphomas presented as space-occupying lesions and were histologically classified as large cell or DHL in two cases and lymphoplasmacytoid lymphoma in one case. Of the large-cell lymphomas one was noncleaved (Figure 5) and the other was cleaved-cell type. All lesions were unifocal. The infiltrates were associated with necrosis and, in addition, had characteristic vessel wall involvement. The diagnosis of brain lymphoma was made on postmortem examination in two cases; the other patient died one day after craniotomy because of massive hemorrhage into the operative site. This diagnosis can be extremely difficult to make in AIDS patients because of the variety of infectious processes that could produce a cerebral mass lesion, such as TB, fungi, and toxoplasmic encephalitis (Hauser et al. 1982). Increased aware- ness about the unusual incidence of brain lymphomas in AIDS patients could lead to earlier diagnosis and administration of effective therapy.

Finding Clonal Excess in AIDS Patients

The analysis of surface membrane light-chain clonal excess (CE) by means of flow cytometry was used to detect minimal B-cell disease in multiple tissues of AIDS patients. The analysis of CE is based on the early work of Ligler et al. (1980) who identified neoplastic B cells by an excess of cells bearing one light-chain type on the cell surface at discrete levels of fluorescence intensity, as measured on a fluorescence-activated cell sorter. CE was defined as the value obtained by applying the formula % κ^+ − % λ^+ cells/total number of light-chain–bearing cells for every

Table 3. *Clinical and Laboratory Characteristics of AIDS Patients with Brain Lymphomas*

Case	Age (yr)/ race	History	EBV-VCA titer	T4⁺/T8⁺ ratio	Brain lymphoma		Other postmortem findings	Survival (months)
					Location	Histology		
8	35/white	Criptosporidiosis *P. carinii* pneumonia	1:320	0.3	Right medial temporo-occipital	Lympho-plasmacytoid lymphoma	Anoxic encepha-lopathy Focal leucoen-cephalopathy Chronic encepha-litis	9
9	40/white	KS infiltrating skin and lymph nodes Interferon therapy	1:640	0.1	Right frontal cortex	DHL (large non-cleaved)	Massive postop-erative hemor-rhage in right frontal cortex Disseminated CMV infection	12
10	26/black	*P. carinii* pneumonia *Mycobacterium avium intracellu-lare*	1:320	0.2	Left frontal lobe	DHL (large cleaved)	CMV subacute encephalitis Disseminated CMV, *Candida albicans* and *Mycobacterium avium intracell-ulare*	18

EBV-VCA-Epstein-Barr virus-viral capsid antigen; KS-Kaposi's sarcoma; CMV-cytomegalovirus; DHL-diffuse histiocytic lymphoma.

10 channels of fluorescence intensity. The CE of normal lymph nodes and peripheral blood was between 0.4 and − 0.4 in all channels.

Figure 6 is a graphic example of a normal control blood sample and the resulting CE analysis. The upper figure is the flow cytometric frequency distributions of κ versus λ light-chain–bearing cells. Dissecting this curve by CE analysis yields the bottom figure. A value greater than zero indicates a majority of κ-bearing cells, a value less than zero indicates a majority of λ-bearing cells. In two homosexual men with extensive KS treated with interferon, atypical lymphocytes with plasmacytoid morphology were detected in the bone marrow; CE detected a predominance of κ (Figure 7) and λ light-chain–bearing cells, respectively. However, no evidence of lymphoma was detected on their postmortem examinations. These findings suggest that AIDS patients have the potential for developing B-cell monoclonal proliferations, which could eventually result in overt lymphomatous disease.

DISCUSSION

Homosexual men presently afflicted with AIDS appear to be at high risk of developing lymphoproliferative malignancies, similar to the patients with congenital (Gatti and Good 1971) or acquired immunodeficiencies (Penn 1970). Patients with the genetically induced immunodeficiencies ataxia telangiectasia (11.7%), Wiskott-Aldrich syndrome (15.4%), and IgM deficiency (10%) have greater risk for developing cancer, and more than 50% of the neoplasias they develop are lymphoreticular tumors (Spector et al. 1978b). The acquired immunodeficiencies include the immu-

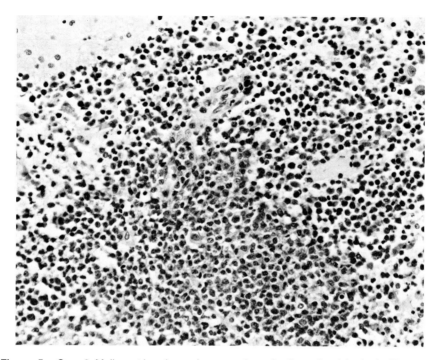

Figure 5. Case 9. Malignant lymphoma, large noncleaved cell type involving brain. Hematoxylin and eosin stain. × 200.

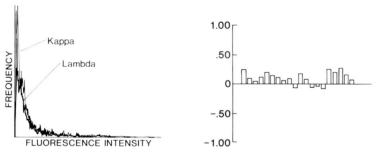

Figure 6. Clonal excess calculation of surface kappa and lambda light chain-bearing cells in a normal control.

nosuppression observed after organ transplantation (Penn 1979, 1981), which is similar to the congenital forms and has resulted in a cancer frequency 100-fold greater than the rate expected for the general population with a predominance of NHL. The average development of malignant lymphoma was noted approximately two years following organ homograft transplantation and predominantly afflicted a young patient population (mean age, 36 years) (Penn 1981). Another drug-induced immunodeficiency that has resulted in an increased incidence of secondary NHL is the one that follows the combined use of chemo- and radiotherapy for the treatment of Hodgkin's disease. Krikorian et al. (1979) from Stanford University

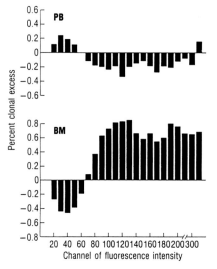

Figure 7. Clonal excess calculations in the peripheral blood and bone marrow from a patient with AIDS and KS. Overt κ light chain clonal excess was detected in the bone marrow from this patient. The peripheral blood did not exhibit clonal excess. PB-peripheral blood; BM-bone marrow.

have reported an incidence of secondary NHL of 4.4% at 10 years for the entire patient population treated with radiotherapy or chemotherapy and 15.2% for those treated with combined modality. Histologically, most of the secondary NHL reported have represented morphological variants (large cleaved, large noncleaved, and immunoblastic cell types) of activated B lymphocytes of follicular center origin (Lukes and Collins 1974, The Non-Hodgkin's Lymphoma Pathologic Classification Project 1982), which was previously encompassed in the DHL category of the Rappaport classification (Byrne 1977). The histologic subtype of systemic NHL reported in AIDS patients and found in three of our cases was small noncleaved-cell Burkitt's type (The Non-Hodgkins' Lymphoma Pathologic Classification Project 1982, Grogran et al. 1982) undifferentiated lymphoma, according to the Rappaport scheme (Byrne 1977). Clinically, the undifferentiated or Burkitt's-like lymphomas developing in homosexual men have usually shown an aggressive course with shortened survival rates and predilection for CNS infiltration. Two of our three patients died from progressive disease including CNS involvement despite intensive multidrug chemotherapy (L17M protocol).

Preneoplastic Potential of Lymphadenopathy in Homosexual Men and AIDS Patients

Lymphadenopathy may represent an early stage of AIDS, since it has preceded this syndrome in many cases and, in addition, could represent a preneoplastic stage to the development of malignant lymphomas (Centers for Disease Control 1982). The New York Hospital group has reported on the prognostic value of histopathology of generalized lymphadenopathy in homosexual men (Fernandez et al. 1983). Three different patterns were recognized: (1) follicular hyperplasia with focal coalescence of follicles, (2) follicular involution with small hypocellular germinal centers and paracortical hyperplasia, and (3) mixed pattern of follicular hyperplasia and involution in different portions of a lymph node, most likely representing a transitional stage between (1) and (2). Clinical correlation showed that the group with lymphoid follicular involution had the most severe T-cell dysfunction and neoplastic potential, since 5 patients each, out of a total of 17, developed NHL and KS. Brynes et al. (1983) observed follicular and paracortical hyperplasia in most lymph node specimens from 21 homosexual men. No disease progression was observed in this group at a median follow-up of 16 months. However, in three cases, an atypical pattern of lymphoid proliferation resembling angioimmunoblastic lymphadenopathy and peripheral T-cell lymphoma was observed, which correlated clinically with the rapid development of NHL or OI. Similar conclusions in regard to histopathologic patterns and clinical correlation were reported by Ioachim et al. from the Lenox Hill Hospital in New York City (1983). Furthermore, this group reported that in a patient in whom an NHL (diffuse, large, noncleaved-cell type) and lymphadenitis coexisted in the same node, the origin of the lymphoma could be traced to the hyperplastic germinal centers.

The inflammatory pattern observed in lymphoid tissue from homosexual men presenting with adenopathy resembles viral lymphadenitis. It seems pertinent to point out that electron microscopic examination of specimens from homosexual men with lymphadenopathy—some of them also afflicted with AIDS—have shown tubuloreticular structures (Zucker-Franklin 1983) and an unusual cytoplasmic structure termed vesicular rosette (Ewing et al. 1983), which suggests viral infection. Analysis of T-lymphocyte subsets in lymphoid tissue from homosexual men with lymphadenopathy or KS or both has shown the presence of numerous suppressor cells (OKT8[+]) in the follicular center and mantle regions, sites where, under normal conditions, suppressor T cells are rare (Modlin et al. 1983).

Pathogenetic Role of CMV in the Development of KS and Malignant Lymphomas

The striking association of aggressive and disseminated KS with the new outbreak of AIDS has brought new interest into the study of this neoplasia, which may potentially represent a model for a virus-associated human cancer (Safai and Good 1981). A high incidence of secondary cancers and, most particularly, lymphoreticular neoplasms has been observed in patients with the classical form of KS. In a retrospective study of 92 patients with KS seen at MSKCC from 1949 to 1975, a 30% incidence of second malignancies was observed with a 20-fold increase in the incidence of lymphoreticular neoplasms (Safai et al. 1980).

Giraldo and co-workers, in 1972, found herpes-type virus particles in tissue culture cell lines developed from African cases of KS. A serological association between CMV and KS in African, European (Giraldo et al. 1975), and North American patients (Giraldo et al. 1978) was subsequently established. CMV viral DNA sequences were detected in biopsy specimens from KS patients, and the expression of CMV-related antigens was seen in biopsy specimens and tissue cultures from KS patients (Giraldo et al. 1977, 1980). It is of interest that there is a close geographical association between KS (related to CMV) and Burkitt's lymphoma (associated with EBV) in equatorial Africa. Both EBV and CMV are lymphotropic and immunosuppressive DNA viruses that could be putatively oncogenic.

Antibodies to CMV can be detected in most homosexual men (94%), since the virus seems to be endemic and can be transmitted by semen, urine, and blood from infected individuals (Drew et al. 1981). Sexual promiscuity augments the probability of repeated exposure, which might lead to immunosuppression and secondary infection with other herpes viruses (Howard and Najarian 1974, Rinaldo et al. 1980). It has been proposed (Sonnabend et al. 1983) that AIDS might develop upon repeated exposure to CMV and allogeneic sperm, in highly promiscuous homosexual men. A hereditary predisposition (perhaps related to the HLA-DR5 locus) (Friedman-Kien et al. 1982) and the immunosuppressive effects of amyl nitrite (Goedert et al. 1982) could be contributing factors to the development of defective T-cell immunoregulation with eventual reactivation of herpes viruses such as EBV.

Pathogenetic Mechanisms for Lymphoma Development

Lymphoid oncogenesis in the background of genetic or acquired immunodeficiency could result from increased permissiveness for neoplastic growth due to deficient immune surveillance mechanisms (Ehrlich 1957, Thomas 1959, Burnet 1971). However, the disproportionately high incidence of malignant lymphomas over any other type of spontaneous tumor argues against this interpretation (Penn 1981). Alternatively, the immune deficiency may enhance lymphoid proliferation, malignant transformation, and clonal development. Several hypothetical mechanisms for this development have been postulated, such as chromosomal instability and marked sensitivity to chemical and physical agents with a defect in the DNA repair mechanisms similar to ataxia telangiectasia (Waldman et al. 1983), prolonged and repetitive antigenic stimulation, such as the one that occurs in allograft organ transplantation (Gleichman et al. 1975), and activation of endogenous viruses or infection with exogenous oncogenic viruses (Schwartz 1972, Hirsch et al. 1977).

Role of EBV in Lymphoma Development

Evidence for EBV being oncogenic is based on experimental animal models, such as the cotton top marmoset (Miller et al. 1977), and its relation to Burkitt's lymphoma and nasopharyngeal carcinoma in humans (Ziegler et al. 1977). EBV infection and malignant lymphoid proliferation of B-cell type have been seen in patients with severe combined immune deficiency who were treated with thymus transplantation, in immunosuppressed patients who had renal transplantation, in patients with X-linked lymphoproliferative syndrome, and, recently, in a patient who may have had an immunoregulation defect (Purtilo 1980, 1981, Hanto et al. 1981, Snydman et al. 1982). This viral infection may initially cause a polyclonal

B-cell response, which develops into a malignant proliferation because of a defect in suppressor T-cell response (Tosati et al. 1979).

In all the cases reported in this series, elevated EBV-VCA titers were observed, although Burkitt's lymphoma was reported in two homosexual patients without KS who had EBV titers of only 1:80. No marker studies were done in these patients, but the lymphomas were histologically typical (Doll and List 1982, Ziegler et al. 1982, case 1). Tumor cells in two of the four cases reported by Ziegler et al. (1982) contained EBV-associated nuclear antigen (EBNA) and one case contained both EBNA and CMV antigen. In a recent study (Lipscomb et al. 1983), all male homosexuals with lymphadenopathy were seropositive for EBV and three of five lymph node specimens from these individuals contained significant numbers of EBV-genome copies, suggesting on etiologic role. Moreover, a patient with small noncleaved (Burkitt's-like) lymphoma carried the EBV genome but lacked evidence of viral reactivation, which could have been indicated by the presence of antibodies to EBV-EA (early antigens).

Burkitt's Lymphoma as a Model for Lymphoma Development

Klein (1979) has postulated an hypothesis for the development of Burkitt's lymphoma resulting from EBV infection and initially involving the immortalization of cells that differentiate along the B-cell lineage and are able to continue division. During B-cell division, defective differentiation in preneoplastic polyclonal B cells persists under particular conditions of antigenic stimulation, such as endemic malaria in Africa. Emergence of a single clone with a chromosome marker, such as the t(8;14) translocation, might develop, and this cytogenetic change, which causes the activation of a c-*onc* gene, could provide the afflicted cell with a selective growth advantage to overcome host defenses, resulting in monoclonal development and neoplastic behavior.

Recent data showing that sites of chromosome breaks in specific translocations seen in Burkitt's lymphomas involve the positions of the determinants for immunoglobulin κ light chain (2p12 cen), μ heavy chain (14q32), and λ light chain (22q) (Kirsch et al. 1982, Malcolm et al. 1982, McBride et al. 1982) suggest that the sites of chromosomal translocation are associated with those of genes that are actively transcribing immunoglobulin determinants. Furthermore, as previously reported (Lenoir et al. 1982) and supported by our cases, a correspondence between site of translocation and respective immunoglobulin expression has been observed. The c-*myc* cellular oncogene recently has been localized on chromosome 8 at band q24, the site where a break occurs in the Burkitt's lymphoma translocation (Neel et al. 1982). Moreover, recent evidence demonstrates that c-*myc* becomes translocated to chromosome 14, in the t(8;14) translocation, in addition to undergoing transcriptional activation in Burkitt's lymphoma cells (Dalla Favera et al. 1982, Taub et al. 1982, Erikson et al. 1982). This event might result in functional activation of the c-*onc* gene and monoclonal proliferation with development of B-cell neoplasia.

Development of Brain Lymphomas: Its Relationship with EBV

Brain lymphomas are rare among the neoplasias afflicting the CNS, and it has been estimated that it represents the primary site of less than 2% of extranodal NHL (Schaumburg et al. 1972, Henry et al. 1974). Their increased occurrence in cases of IgA deficiency (Gregory and Hughes 1973), ataxia telangiectasia (Spector et al. 1978a), Wiscott-Aldrich syndrome (Model 1977), organ transplantation (Schaumburg et al. 1972, Schneck and Penn 1971, Lanza et al. 1983), and acquired immune suppression (Varadachari et al. 1978, Jellinger et al. 1979) has been noted, which indicates that there is a pathogenetic role of immunosuppression in some stage of lymphoma development or the peculiar location determination. The three cases reported in this series, in addition to those already published (case records of the Massachusetts General Hospital 1983, Snider et al. 1983) indicate that there are similar developmental mechanisms in patients with AIDS.

A hypothetical model for the development of brain lymphoma and its relationship to EBV infection could be found in the experiments reported by Nilsson et al. (1977). When normal diploid lymphoblastoid cell lines derived from EBV-infected B cells were injected subcutaneously into nude mice, rejection took place, but a brain tumor resulted from the intracerebral injection. However, when aneuploid lymphoblastoid cell lines, derived from Burkitt's tumors, were subcutaneously and intracerebrally injected into nude mice, tumors grew in both places. The postulated polyclonality of immunoblastic sarcomas seen after renal transplantation suggests that these tumors originated from diploid cells (Matas et al. 1976). Recent evidence based on the finding of the EBV genome on DNA preparations from a primary cerebellar lymphoma of an immunocompetent patient suggests an etiopathogenetic role for EBV in the development of lymphoma (Hochberg et al. 1983).

Oncogenicity of Retroviruses

Recently, type C RNA tumor viruses or retroviruses have been claimed to be oncogenic, not only in experimental animals but also in a significant proportion of naturally occurring leukemias and lymphomas in animals (Wong-Staal and Gallo 1982). A human T-cell leukemia virus (HTLV) was initially isolated from an established T-cell line from a patient thought to have a cutaneous T-cell lymphoma (Poiesz et al. 1980). Several neoplastic disorders of mature T cells, including the Japanese variety of adult T-cell leukemia (Robert-Guroff et al. 1982) and the T-cell lymphosarcoma cell leukemia of Caribbean blacks (Schupbach et al. 1983) as well as a recently characterized type of adult T-cell lymphoma in the United States (Bunn et al. 1983), have a strong seroepidemiological association with HTLV. Of particular interest, in light of the new outbreak of AIDS, has been the finding that 36% of a group of patients with AIDS had antibodies to cell membrane antigens associated with HTLV, whereas only 1.2% of asymptomatic homosexual controls reacted in that way (Gallo et al. 1983, Gelman et al. 1983, Marx 1983, Essex et al. 1983a). An increased incidence of this antibody to HTLV-membrane antigens has also been found in hemophiliacs (Essex et al. 1983b), another population at high risk to develop AIDS. However, evidence for the T-cell lineage of the malignant lymphomas and leukemias developing in patients with AIDS is lacking, so is their direct pathogenetic association with HTLV.

Concluding Remarks

The development of B-cell lymphoproliferative disorders represents an increasingly observed epiphenomenon in patients with AIDS and the AIDS-related complex. Pathogenetic mechanisms for neoplastic development appear to be similar to the ones previously proposed in patients with congenital and drug-induced immunodeficiencies, including the probable activation of endogenous viruses or infection with exogenous oncogenic viruses.

Although a variety of B-cell neoplasias have been observed, large cell lymphomas of the brain and systemic Burkitt's-like lymphomas are more frequent. Serologic and cytogenetic evidence suggests EBV involvement in the pathogenesis of these neoplasms. However, the causative agent of AIDS remains elusive, but current evidence points to a retrovirus as the most likely candidate. Considering the interest and commitment that AIDS research is generating, this most challenging human model for the study of immunodeficiency and secondary neoplastic development might provide useful information toward the understanding of tumorigenesis in general.

ACKNOWLEDGMENT

The authors wish to express their appreciation to Drs. Bijain Safai, Jonathan Gold, Susan Krown, David J. Straus, Roland Mertelsmann, and Sanford Kempin for allowing us to review material on their patients. We are most grateful to Nina Hotvedt for excellent editorial assistance.

This investigation was supported in part by grants CA-08748, CA-05826, and CA-34775 awarded by the National Cancer Institute, United States Department of Health and Human Services, The Cancer Research Institute, Inc., and the Zelda Weintraub Cancer Fund.

REFERENCES

Brynes RK, Chan WC, Spira TJ, Ewing EP, Chandler FW. 1983. Value of lymph node biopsy in unexplained lymphadenopathy in homosexual men. JAMA 250:1313–1317.

Bunn PA, Schecter GP, Jaffe E, Blayney D, Young RC, Matthews MJ, Blattner W, Broder S, Robert-Guroff M, Gallo RC. 1983. Clinical course of retrovirus-associated adult T-cell lymphoma in the United States. N Engl J Med 309:257–264.

Burnet FM. 1971. Immunological surveillance in neoplasia. Transplant Rev 7:3–25.

Byrne GE, Jr. 1977. Rappaport classification of non-Hodgkin's lymphoma: Histologic features and clinical significance. Cancer Treat Rep 61:935–944.

Case Records of the Massachusetts General Hospital. 1983. (Case 32-1983). N Engl J Med 309:359–369.

Centers for Disease Control. 1981. Kaposi's sarcoma and pneumocystis pneumonia among homosexual men - New York City and California. MMWR 30:305–308.

Centers for Disease Control. 1982a. Persistent, generalized lymphadenopathy among homosexual males. MMWR 31:249–251.

Centers for Disease Control. 1982b. Diffuse, undifferentiated non-Hodgkin's lymphoma among homosexual males - United States. MMWR 31:277–279.

Centers for Disease Control. 1982c. Possible transfusion-associated acquired immune deficiency syndrome (AIDS) - California. MMWR 31:652–654.

Chaganti RSK. 1983. Significance of chromosome change to hematopoietic neoplasms. Blood 62:515–524.

Chaganti RSK, Jhanwar SC, Koziner B, Arlin Z, Mertelsmann R, Clarkson BD. 1983. Specific translocations characterize Burkitt's-like lymphoma of homosexual men with the acquired immunodeficiency syndrome. Blood 61:1269–1271.

Ciobanu N, Andreeff M, Safai B, Koziner B, Mertelsmann R. 1983. Lymphoblastic neoplasia in a homosexual patient with Kaposi's sarcoma. Ann Intern Med 98:151–155.

Dalla Favera R, Bergni M, Erikson J, Patterson D, Gallo RC, Croce CM. 1982. Human c-myc oncogene is located on the region of chromosome 8 that is translocated in Burkitt's lymphoma cells. Proc Natl Acad Sci USA 79:7824–7827.

Daling JR, Weiss NS, Klopfenstein LL, Cochran LE, Wong HC, Daifuku R. 1982. Correlates of homosexual behavior and the incidence of anal cancer. JAMA 247:1988–1990.

Davis KC, Horsburgh CR, Hasiba U, Schocket AL, Kirkpatrick CH. 1983. Acquired immunodeficiency syndrome in a patient with hemophilia. Ann Intern Med 98:284–286.

Doll DC, List AF. 1982. Burkitt's lymphoma in a homosexual (Letter). Lancet 1:1026–1027.

Drew WL, Mintz L, Miner RC, Sands M, Ketterer B. 1981. Prevalence of cytomegalovirus infection in homosexual men. J Infect Dis 143:188–192.

Ehrlich P. 1957. Uber den jetzigen Stand der Karzinomforschung. *In* The Collected Papers of Paul Ehrlich, vol. 2. Pergamon Press, Oxford, p. 550.

Elliott JL, Hoppes WL, Platt MS, Thomas JG, Patel IP, Gansar A. 1983. The acquired immunodeficiency syndrome and Mycobacterium avium-intracellulare bacteremia in a patient with hemophilia. Ann Intern Med 98:290–293.

Erikson J, Ar-Rushud A, Drwinga HL, Nowell PC, Croce CM. 1982. Transcriptional activation of the translocated c-myc oncogene in Burkitt lymphoma. Proc Natl Acad Sci USA 80:820–824.

Essex M, McLane MF, Lee TH, Falk L, Howe CWS, Mullins JI. 1983a. Antibodies to cell membrane antigens associated with human T-cell leukemia virus in patients with AIDS. Science 220:859–862.

Essex M, McLane MF, Lee TH, Tachibana N, Mullins JI, Kreiss J, Kasper CK, Poon MC, Landay A, Stein SF, Francis DP, Cabradilla C, Lawrence DN, Evatt BL. 1983b. Antibodies to T-cell leukemia virus membrane antigens (HTLV-MA) in hemophiliacs. Science 121:1061–1063.

Ewing EP, Spira TJ, Chandler TW, Callaway CS, Brynes RK, Chan WC. 1983. Unusual cytoplasmic body in lymphoid cells of homosexual men with unexplained lymphadenopathy: A preliminary report. N Engl J Med 308:819–822.

Fernandez R, Mouradian J, Metroka C, Davis J. 1983. The prognostic value of histopathology in persistent generalized lymphadenopathy in homosexual men. N Engl J Med 309:186–187.

Friedman-Kien AE, Laubenstein LJ, Rubinstein P, Buimovici-Klein E, Marmor M, Stahl R, Spigland I, Kwang SK, Zolla-Pazner S. 1982. Disseminated Kaposi's sarcoma in homosexual men. Ann Intern Med 96:693–699.

Gallo RC, Sarin PS, Gelmann EP, Robert-Guroff M, Richardson E. 1983. Isolation of human T-cell leukemia virus in acquired immune deficiency syndrome (AIDS). Science 220:865–867.

Gatti RA, Good RA. 1971. Occurrence of malignancy in immunodeficiency diseases. A literature review. Cancer 28:89–98.

Gelmann EP, Popovic M, Blayney D, Masur H, Sidhu G, Stahl RE, Gallo RC. 1983. Proviral DNA of a retrovirus, human T-cell leukemia virus, in two patients with AIDS. Science 220:862–865.

Giraldo G, Beth E, Haguenau F. 1972. Herpes-type virus particles in tissue culture of Kaposi's sarcoma from different geographic regions. JNCI 49:1509–1526.

Giraldo G, Beth E, Hammerling U, Tarro G, Kourilski FM. 1977. Detection of early antigens in nuclei of cells infected with cytomegalovirus of herpes simplex virus type 1 and 2 by anti-complement immunofluorescence and use of a blocking assay to demonstrate their specificity. Int J Cancer 19:107–116.

Giraldo G, Beth E, Henle W, Henle G, Mike V, Safai B, Huraux JM, McHardy J, DeThe G. 1978. Antibody patterns to herpes viruses in Kaposi's sarcoma. II. Serologic association of American Kaposi's sarcoma with cytomegalovirus. Int J Cancer 22:126–131.

Giraldo G, Beth E, Hung ES. 1980. Kaposi's sarcoma and its relationship to cytomegalovirus (CMV). III. CMV, DNA and CMV early antigens in Kaposi's sarcoma. Int J Cancer 26:23–29.

Giraldo, G, Beth E, Kourilsky FM, Henle W, Henle G, Mike V, Huraux JM, Anderson MK, Gharbi MR, Kyalwazi SK, Puissant A. 1975. Antibody patterns of herpes viruses in Kaposi's sarcoma: serological association of European Kaposi's sarcoma with cytomegalovirus. Int J Cancer 15:839–848.

Gleichmann E, Gleichmann H, Schwartz RS, Weinblatt A, Armstrong MYK. 1975. Immunologic induction of malignant lymphoma: Identification of donor and host tumors in the graft-versus-host model. JNCI 54:107–116.

Goedert JJ, Wallen WC, Mann DL, Strong DM, Neuland CY, Greene MH, Murray C, Fraumeni JF, Blattner WA. 1982. Amyl nitrite may alter lymphocytes in homosexual men. Lancet 1:412–416.

Gordon EM, Berkowitz RJ, Strandjord SE, Kurczynski EM, Goldberg JS, Coccia PF. 1983. Burkitt lymphoma in a patient with classic hemophilia receiving factor VIII concentrates. J Pediatr 103:75–77.

Gottlieb MS, Schroff R, Schanker HM, Weisman JD, Fan PT, Wolf RA, Saxon A. 1981. Pneumocystis carinii pneumonia and mucosal candidiasis in previously healthy homosexual men: Evidence of a new acquired immunodeficiency. N Engl J Med 305:1425–1430.

Gregory MC, Hughes JT. 1973. Intracranial reticulum cell sarcoma associated with immunoglobulin A deficiency. J Neurol Neurosurg Psychiatry 36:769–776.

Grogran TW, Warnke RA, Kaplan HS. 1982. A comparative study of Burkitt's and non-Burkitt's "undifferentiated" malignant lymphoma: Immunologic cytochemical, ultrastructural, cytologic, histopathologic, clinical and cell culture features. Cancer 49:1817–1828.

Hanto DW, Frizzera G, Purtilo DT, Sakamoto K, Sullivan JL, Saemundsen AK, Klein G, Simmons RL, Najarian J. 1981. Clinical spectrum of lymphoproliferative disorders in renal transplant recipients and evidence for the role of Epstein-Barr virus. Cancer Res 41:4253–4261.

Harris C, Small CB, Klein RS, Friedland GH, Moll B, Emeson EE, Spigland I, Steigbigel NH. 1983. Immunodeficiency in female sexual partners of men with the acquired immunodeficiency syndrome. N Engl J Med 308:1181–1184.

Hauser WE, Luft BJ, Conley FK, Remington JS. 1982. Central nervous system toxoplasmosis in homosexual and heterosexual adults. N Engl J Med 307:498–499.

Henry JM, Heffner RR, Dillard SH, Earle KM, Davis RL. 1974. Primary malignant lymphomas of the central nervous system. Cancer 34:1293–1302.

Hirsch MS, Proffitt MR, Black PH. 1977. Autoimmunity, oncornaviruses, and lymphomagenesis. Contemp Top Immunobiol 6:209–227.

Hochberg FH, Miller G, Schooley RT, Hirsch MS, Feorino P, Henle E. 1983. Central-nervous system lymphoma related to Epstein-Barr virus. N Engl J Med 309:745–748.

Howard RJ, Najarian JS. 1974. Cytomegalovirus-induced immune suppression. II. Cell mediated immunity. Clin Exp Immunol 18:119–126.

Ioachim HL, Lerner CW, Tapper ML. 1983. Lymphadenopathies in homosexual men: Relationships with the acquired immune deficiency syndrome. JAMA 250:1306–1309.

Jellinger K, Kothbauer P, Weiss R, Sunder-Plassmann E. 1979. Primary malignant lymphoma of the CNS and polyneuropathy in a patient with necrotizing vasculitis treated with immunosuppression. J Neurol 220:259–268.

Kirsch IR, Morton CC, Nakahara K, Leder P. 1982. Human immunoglobulin heavy chain genes map to a region of translocations in malignant B lymphocytes. Science 216:301–303.

Klein G. 1979. Lymphoma development in mice and humans: diversity of initiation is followed by convergent cytogenetic evolution. Proc Natl Acad Sci USA 76:2442–2446.

Koziner B, Denny T, Myskowski D, Kris M, Safai B. 1982. Increased suppressor T-cell activity in male homosexuals with Kaposi's sarcoma. N Engl J Med 306:933–934.

Krikorian JG, Burke JS, Rosenberg SA, Kaplan HS. 1979. Occurrence of non-Hodgkin's lymphoma after therapy for Hodgkin's disease. N Engl J Med 300:452–458.

Lanza RR, Cooper DK, Cassidy MJD, Barnard CN. 1983. Malignant neoplasms occurring after cardiac transplantation. JAMA 249:1746–1748.

Lenoir GM, Preud'homme JL, Bernheim A, Berger R. 1982. Correlation between immunoglobulin light chain expression and variant translocation in Burkitt's lymphoma. Nature 298:474–476.

Ligler FS, Graham Smith R, Kettman JR, Hernandez JA, Himes JB, Vitteta ES, Uhr JW, Frenkel EP. 1980. Detection of tumor cells in the peripheral blood of non leukemic patients with B-cell lymphoma: analysis of "clonal excess." Blood 55:792–801.

Lipscomb H, Tatsumi E, Harada S, Yetz J, Davis J, Bechtold T, Volsky DJ, Kuzynski C, Purtilo D, Sonnabend JA, Wallace J, McLain K, Metroka C, Tubbs R. 1983. Epstein-Barr virus and chronic lymphadenomegaly in male homosexuals with acquired immunodeficiency syndrome. AIDS Research 1:59–82.

Louie S, Schwartz RS. 1978. Immunodeficiency and the pathogenesis of lymphoma and leukemia. Semin Hematol 15:117–138.

Lozada F, Silverman S, Conant M. 1982. New outbreak of oral tumors, malignancies and infectious diseases strikes young male homosexuals. Calif Dent J 10:39–42.

Lukes RJ, Collins RD. 1974. Immunologic characterization of human malignant lymphomas. Cancer 34:1488–1503.

Malcolm S, Barton P, Murphy C, Ferguson-Smith MA, Bently DL, Rabbits TH. 1982. Localization of human immunoglobulin kappa light chain variable region genes to the short arm of chromosome 2 by in situ hybridization. Proc Natl Acad Sci USA 79:4957–4968.

Marx JL. 1983. Human T-cell leukemia virus linked to AIDS. Science 220:806–809.

Masur H, Michelis MA, Greene JB, Onorato I, Vande Stowe RA, Holzman RS, Wormser G, Brettman L, Lange M, Murray HW, Cunningham-Rundles S. 1982. An outbreak of community acquired Pneumocystis carinii pneumonia: Initial manifestation of cellular immune dysfunction. N Engl J Med 305:1431–1438.

Matas AJ, Hertel BF, Rosai J, Simmons RL, Najarian JS. 1976. Post-transplant malignant lymphoma: Distinctive morphologic features related to its pathogenesis. Am J Med 61:716–720.

McBride OW, Swan D, Leder P, Hieter P, Hollis G. 1982. Chromosomal location of human immunoglobulin light chain constant region genes. Human Gene mapping 5 (1981): Fifth International Workshop on Human Gene Mapping. Cytogenet Cell Genet 32:297–298.

Miller G, Shope T, Coope D, Waters L, Pagano G, Bornkamm GW, Henle W. 1977. Lymphomas in cotton-top marmosets after inoculation with Epstein-Barr virus: Tumor incidence, histological spectrum, antibody responses, demonstration of viral DNA, and characterization of viruses. J Exp Med 145:948–967.

Model LM. 1977. Primary reticulum cell sarcoma of the brain in Wiskott-Aldrich syndrome: report of a case. Arch Neurol 34:633–635.

Modlin RL, Meyer PR, Hofman FM, Mehlmauer M, Levy NB, Lukes RJ, Parker JW, Ammann AJ, Conant MA, Rea TH, Taylor CR. 1983. T-lymphocyte subsets in lymph nodes from homosexual men. JAMA 250:1302–1305.

Neel BG, Jhanwar SC, Chaganti RSK, Hayward WS. 1982. Two human c-onc genes are located on the long arm of chromosome 8. Proc Natl Acad Sci USA 79:7842–7846.

Nilsson K, Giovanella BC, Stehlin JS, Klein G. 1977. Tumorigenicity of human hematopoietic cell lines in athymic nude mice. Int J Cancer 19:337–344.

Oleske J, Minnefor A, Cooper R, Thomas K, dela Cruz A, Ahdieh H, Guerro I, Joshi VV, Desposito F. 1983. Immune deficiency syndrome in children. JAMA 249:2345–2349.

Penn I. 1970. Malignant Tumors in Organ Transplant Recipients. Springer-Verlag, New York.

Penn I. 1979. Tumor incidence in human allograft recipients. Transplant Proc 9:1047–1051.

Penn I. 1981. Depressed immunity and the development of cancer. Clin Exp Immunol 46:459–474.

Pitchenik AE, Fischl MA, Dickinson GM, Becker DM, Fournier AM, O'Connell MT, Colton RM, Spira TJ. 1983. Opportunistic infections and Kaposi's sarcoma among Haitians: Evidence of a new acquired immunodeficiency state. Ann Intern Med 98:277–284.

Poiesz BJ, Ruscetti FW, Gazdar AF, Bunn PA, Minna JD, Gallo RC. 1980. Detection and isolation of type-C retrovirus particles from fresh and cultured lymphocytes of a patient with cutaneous T-cell lymphoma. Proc Natl Acad Sci USA 77:7415–7419.

Poon MC, Landay A, Prasthofer EF, Stagno S. 1983. Acquired immunodeficiency syndrome with Pneumocystis carinii pneumonia and mycobacterium avium-intracellulare infection in a previously healthy patient with classic hemophilia: Clinical, immunologic, and virologic findings. Ann Intern Med 98:287–290.

Purtilo DT. 1980. Epstein-Barr virus-induced oncogenesis in immune-deficient individuals. Lancet 1:300–303.

Purtilo DT. 1981. Immune deficiency predisposing to Epstein-Barr virus-induced lymphoproliferative disease: The X-linked lymphoproliferative syndrome as a model. Adv Cancer Res 34:279–312.

Rinaldo CR, Carney WP, Richter BS, Black PH, Hirsch MS. 1980. Mechanisms of immunosuppression in cytomegalovirus mononucleosis. J Infect Dis 141:488–495.

Robert-Guroff M, Nakao Y, Natake K, Ito Y, Sliski A, Gallo RC. 1982. Natural antibodies to the human retrovirus, HTLV, in a cluster of Japanese patients with adult T-cell leukemia. Science 215:975–978.

Rubinstein A, Sicklick M, Gupta A, Bernstein L, Klein N, Rubinstein E, Spigland I, Fruchter L, Litman N, Lee H, Hollander M. 1983. Acquired immunodeficiency with reversed T4/T8 ratios in infants born to promiscuous and drug-addicted mothers. JAMA 249:2350–2356.

Safai B, Good RA. 1981. Kaposi's sarcoma: A review and recent development. CA 31:2–12.

Safai B, Mike V, Giraldo B, Beth E, Good RA. 1980. Association of Kaposi's sarcoma with second malignancies, possible etiopathogenic implications. Cancer 45:1472–1479.

Schaumburg HH, Plank CR, Adams RD. 1972. The reticulum cell sarcoma-microglioma group of brain tumours: A consideration of their clinical features and therapy. Brain 95:199–212.

Schneck SA, Penn I. 1971. De-novo brain tumors in renal-transplant recipients. Lancet 1:983–986.

Schupbach J, Kalyanaraman VS, Sarngadharan MG, Blattner, WA, Gallo RC. 1983. Antibodies against three purified proteins of the human type C retrovirus, human T-cell leukemia-lymphoma patients and healthy blacks from the Caribbean. Cancer Res 43:886–891.

Schwartz RS. 1972. Immunoregulation, oncogenic viruses and malignant lymphomas. Lancet 1:1266–1269.

Siegal FP, Lopez C, Hammer GS, Brown AE, Kornfeld SJ, Gold I, Hassett J, Hirschman SZ, Cunningham-Rundles C, Adelsberg BR, Parham DM, Siegal M, Cunningham-Rundles S, Armstrong D. 1981. Severe acquired immunodeficiency in male homosexuals, manifested by chronic perianal ulcerative herpes simplex lesions. N Engl J Med 305:1439–1444.

Snider WD, Simpson DM, Aronyk KE, Nielsen SL. 1983. Primary lymphoma of the nervous system associated with acquired immuno-deficiency syndrome. N Engl J Med 308:45.

Snydman DR, Rudder RA, Daoust P, Sullivan JL, Evans AS. 1982. Infectious mononucleosis in an adult progressing to fatal immunoblastic lymphoma. Ann Intern Med 96:737–742.

Sonnabend J, Witkin SS, Purtilo DT. 1983. Acquired immunodeficiency syndrome, opportunistic infections and malignancies in male homosexuals, a hypothesis of etiologic factors in pathogenesis. JAMA 249:2370–2374.

Spector BD, Perry GS, Good RA, Kersey JJ. 1978b. Immunodeficiency disease and malignancy. *In* Twomey GG, Good RA, eds., Immunopathology of Lymphoreticular Neoplasms. New York, Plenum Press, pp. 815–823.

Spector BD, Perry GS, Kersey JH. 1978a. Genetically determined immunodeficiency disease (GDID) and malignancy: Report from the immunodeficiency cancer registry. Clin Immunol Immunopathol 11:12–19.

Taub R, Kirsch I, Morton C, Lenoir G, Swan D, Tronick S, Aaronson S, Leder P. 1982. Translocation of the c-myc gene into the immunoglobulin heavy chain locus in human Burkitt's lymphoma and murine plasmacytoma cells. Proc Natl Acad Sci USA 79:7837–7841.

The Non-Hodgkin's Lymphoma Pathologic Classification Project. 1982. National Cancer Institute sponsored study of the classifications of non-Hodgkin's lymphomas. Summary and description of a working formulation for clinical usage. Cancer 49:2112–2125.

Thomas L. 1959. Discussion of Medawar PB. Reaction to homologous tissue antigens in relation to hypersensitivity. *In* Lawrence HS, ed., Cellular and Humoral Aspects of the Hypersensitive States. Paul Hoeber, New York, pp. 529–533.

Tosati G, McGrath I, Koski EI, Doodley N, Blaesc M. 1979. Activation of suppressor T-cells during Epstein-Barr virus induced infectious mononucleosis. N Engl J Med 301:1133–1137.

Urmacher C, Myskowski P, Ochoa M, Kris M, Safai B. 1982. Outbreak of Kaposi's sarcoma with cytomegalovirus infection in young homosexual men. Am J Med 72:569–575.

Varadachari C, Palutke M, Climiem ARW, Weise RW, Chason JL. 1978. Immunoblastic sarcoma (histocytic lymphoma) of the brain with B cell markers: case report. J Neurosurg 49:887–892.

Vieira J, Frank E, Spira TJ, Landsman SH. 1983. Acquired immune deficiency in Haitians: Opportunistic infections in previously healthy Haitian immigrants. N Engl J Med 308:125–129.

Waldmann TA, moderator. 1983. Ataxia telangiectasia: A multi system hereditary disease with immunodeficiency, impaired organ maturation, X-ray hypersensitivity and a high incidence of neoplasia. Ann Intern Med 99:367–379.

Wong-Staal F, Gallo RC. 1982. Retroviruses and leukemia. In Gunz F, Henderson E, eds., Leukemia. Grune and Stratton, New York, pp. 329–358.

Ziegler JL, Magrath IT, Gerber P, Levine PH. 1977. Epstein-Barr virus and human malignancy. Ann Intern Med 86:323–326.

Ziegler JL, Miner RC, Rosenbaum E, Lennette ET, Shillitoe E, Casavant C, Drew WL, Mintz L, Gershow J, Greenspan J, Beckstead J, Yamamoto K. 1982. Outbreak of Burkitt's-like lymphoma in homosexual men. Lancet 2:631–633.

Zucker-Franklin D. 1983. "Looking" for the cause of AIDS. N Engl J Med 308:837–838.

Therapy of Non-Hodgkin's Lymphoma

UT M.D. Anderson Clinical Conference on Cancer,
Vol. 27, edited by R. J. Ford, L. M. Fuller, and
F. B. Hagemeister. Raven Press, New York © 1984.

Management of Patients with Nodular Lymphoma

Peter McLaughlin, William S. Velasquez, Roger W. Rodgers,
Hagop Kantarjian, J. J. Butler,* and Lillian M. Fuller†

*Department of Hematology, *Department of Pathology, and †Department of Radiotherapy,
The University of Texas M. D. Anderson Hospital and Tumor Institute at Houston,
Houston, Texas 77030*

Patients with nodular (follicular) lymphoma make up almost one half of all cases of non-Hodgkin's lymphoma in the Western world. This is generally an older group of patients, with a median age at diagnosis of about 50 years. In contrast to the preponderance of males for most types of non-Hodgkin's lymphomas, there is a slight female preponderance for the nodular lymphomas. While it is clear that the nodular lymphomas are B-cell diseases, little is known about predisposing or etiologic factors. Recently, a consistent chromosome translocation t(14;18) has been described in some cases of nodular and other lymphomas of B-cell origin (Yunis et al. 1982).

Numerous classification schemes exist for the non-Hodgkin's lymphomas. Table 1 illustrates the modified Rappaport scheme that will be used in this chapter (modified by substituting "large cell" for the semantically incorrect term "histiocytic") and its relationship to the recent National Cancer Institute sponsored Working Formulation (Non-Hodgkin's Lymphoma Pathologic Classification Project 1982).

The treatment approach to patients with nodular lymphoma is controversial. While nodular lymphomas are often called "favorable" diseases, they remain among the few categories of lymphoma for which there is no substantial chance of cure. Patients respond to multiple therapies, yet they almost inevitably relapse at a fairly constant rate, about 10%–15% yearly (Rosenberg 1979). This therapeutic impasse has led to a somewhat nihilistic attitude about therapy for these diseases, an attitude that it hardly matters when therapy is given or what therapy is chosen. In this chapter we propose to challenge some of those attitudes, to indicate that there are patients with potentially curable disease, and to argue that it can be very important to make timely and correct treatment decisions for these patients.

STAGES I AND II NODULAR LYMPHOMA

Until recently, most published data on patients with stages I and II nodular lymphoma consisted of fairly short follow-up of small groups of patients with

Table 1. *Nodular Lymphoma: Histologic Synonyms*

Modified Rappaport*	Working Formulation†
Nodular poorly differentiated lymphocytic	Follicular, small cleaved
Nodular mixed	Follicular, mixed
Nodular large cell ("histiocytic")	Follicular, large cell

*Rappaport (1966).
†The Non-Hodgkin's Lymphoma Pathologic Classification Project (1982).

Table 2. *Nodular Lymphoma Stages I and II: Patient Characteristics*

% with:	Low grade		Intermediate grade
	NPDL (n = 49)	NML (n = 16)	NLCL (n = 17)
Constitutional symptoms	8	19	24
Extranodal sites	16	19	41
HGB <12 g/dl	9	7	29
LDH >225 U/L	4	27	33

NPDL–nodular poorly differentiated lymphocytic lymphoma; NML–nodular mixed lymphoma, NLCL–nodular large cell lymphoma; HGB-hemoglobin; LDH–lactic dehydrogenase.

nonuniformly staged disease. One exception was Fuller's large series in which she reported a 65% five-year survival rate but a pattern of continual relapse up to five years (Fuller et al. 1975). More recently, two large series have been reported with median follow-up approaching ten years (Bush and Gospodarowicz 1982, Paryani et al. 1983). Both of these series demonstrated a pattern of rare relapse beyond five years, i.e., a plateau of the relapse-free survival curve that suggests cure. In both of these series, the treatment was radiotherapy alone, and the potentially cured fraction was approximately 50%.

The role of chemotherapy is uncertain and largely unexplored in patients with stages I and II disease. Monfardini et al. (1980) concluded that there was no significant benefit from adjuvant chemotherapy with COP (cyclophosphamide, vincristine, and prednisone), but they did show a trend for better survival with chemotherapy (93% versus 62% at five years, $P = .10$), which is noteworthy in their small group of 26 patients.

At UT M. D. Anderson Hospital, we have recently analyzed our results with 83 patients with stages I and II nodular lymphoma seen between 1974–1981. This series included 49 patients with poorly differentiated lymphocytic (NPDL) cell type, 16 with mixed (NML), 17 with large cell or histiocytic (NLCL), and 1 with nodular lymphoma, cell type uncertain (Table 2). Treatment strategies varied during the period of this review, partly in accord with increased appreciation of risk factors, which included large cell histology, involvement of extranodal sites, and the presence of constitutional symptoms (Bush et al. 1977). A comparable fraction of NPDL and NML patients received radiotherapy alone, while a disproportionate number of NLCL patients also received chemotherapy.

The overall survival and relapse-free survival curves are illustrated in Figure 1. A plateau in relapse-free survival at 50% appears beyond four years. As with the data of Bush and Paryani, we also expect that relapses will be rare beyond this four- to five-year period.

In this group of patients with stages I and II disease, we identified several pretreatment factors of possible prognostic importance. Patients with extranodal disease had significantly worse survival rates than those with nodal presentations (66% versus 75% at five years, $P = .03$). Those with elevated serum lactic dehydrogenase (LDH) had worse survival rates than those with normal LDH (31% versus 83%, $P = .07$). Patients who had bulky abdominal disease had shorter relapse-free survival periods than those who did not (38% versus 63%, $P = .06$).

Moreover, we assessed the impact of therapy. To date, there has been no significant difference in survival rates between those receiving radiotherapy only and

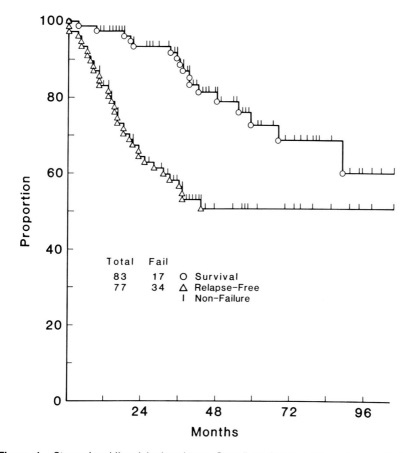

Figure 1. Stages I and II nodular lymphoma. Overall survival and relapse-free survival rates.

those receiving chemotherapy with or without radiation. But, the relapse-free survival rate (68% at five years) for patients receiving chemotherapy is significantly better than the corresponding figure for those receiving radiation alone (47%). This advantage applies if the analysis is restricted to patients with low grade cell types only (Figure 2) or if NLCL patients are included. While these data need prolonged follow-up and confirmation, it appears that the inclusion of chemotherapy with radiotherapy at least delays, and may prevent, relapse in some patients with stages I and II nodular lymphoma. Thus, chemotherapy may increase the fraction of patients with stages I and II disease who can be cured (McLaughlin et al. 1984).

NODULAR LARGE CELL LYMPHOMA

NLCL is a more aggressive disease than NPDL or NML, with a median survival in most series of approximately three years (Osborne et al. 1980, Glick et al. 1982,

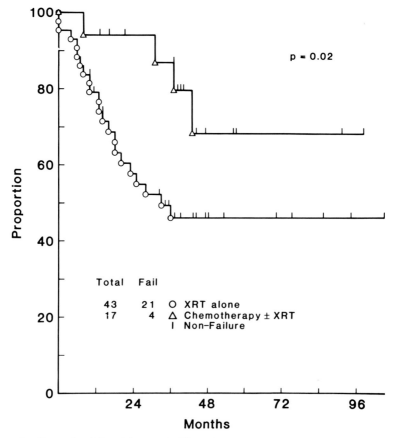

Figure 2. Stages I and II nodular poorly differentiated lymphocytic and mixed lymphoma. Relapse-free survival rates by treatment.

Jones et al. 1973, Anderson et al. 1982). It has been categorized in the Working Formulation as an intermediate grade lymphoma, and intensive chemotherapy has been widely advocated for its treatment. Improved treatment results and potential cures have been described following more intensive therapy (Osborne et al. 1980, Glick et al. 1982, McLaughlin et al. 1983).

We recently analyzed our experience with 62 patients with NLCL at UT M. D. Anderson Hospital. About 25% of our cases presented with stages I and II disease, in contrast to other reports that suggest that most NLCL patients have advanced stage disease. As noted previously (Table 2), our patients with stages I and II disease had a fairly high incidence of constitutional symptoms, extranodal sites of involvement, and elevation of serum LDH. Despite these adverse features, the survival and relapse-free survival rates of our stages I and II NLCL patients were similar to the outcome with NPDL and NML. This may have been partly because a higher percentage of the NLCL patients received chemotherapy in conjunction with radiotherapy. The pattern of relapse in stages I and II NLCL patients suggests that chemotherapy has an impact; of those treated with radiotherapy only, five of six have relapsed, whereas only two of eight patients who received chemotherapy plus radiotherapy have relapsed. Our current treatment approach for stages I and II NLCL is CHOP-Bleo (cyclophosphamide, doxorubicin, vincristine, prednisone, and bleomycin; Rodriguez et al. 1977) plus radiotherapy.

The survival and relapse-free survival rates of our stage III NLCL patients is quite similar to those patients with stage IV disease, despite the inclusion of radiotherapy in the treatment of the majority of stage III patients. Further analysis of our patients with stages III and IV disease identified a number of adverse prognostic factors, including the presence of bulky abdominal disease, mediastinal disease, thrombocytosis, and elevated serum LDH. The importance of thrombo-cytosis was unexpected. We did note that it correlated with bulky abdominal disease, but in a multivariate analysis, thrombocytosis remained a highly significant adverse factor.

Analysis of treatment variables for stages III and IV NLCL revealed two factors of major importance. The first was complete remission; patients achieving complete remission had significantly longer survival than those with partial or no response (76% versus 7% at five years, $P < .01$). The second important treatment variable was intensive therapy, defined as the administration of a minimum of six cycles of a doxorubicin-including regimen (CHOP-Bleo). Patients who received such inten-sive therapy showed a trend for improved survival than those receiving less intensive therapy (63% versus 40% at five years, $P = .1$).

While these results indicate that intensive chemotherapy has improved treatment results in NLCL, it must be emphasized that the prognosis for advanced NLCL remains worse than that of NPDL and NML. Treatment breakthroughs are needed. The emphasis on intensive chemotherapy in the treatment of NLCL, however, appears to be an important positive step.

STAGES III AND IV NPDL AND NML

For the majority of nodular lymphoma patients, those with stages III and IV NPDL and NML, there is no currently available treatment that appears to be curative. This fact underlies much of the controversy that exists about the choice of primary treatment for these patients. Comparisons of primary treatment are extremely difficult since it is not only the primary therapy but also the timing, choice, and effectiveness of rescue therapy that ultimately affect survival. Initial treatment approaches range from single alkylating agents to combination chemotherapy and from radiotherapy alone to combined modality therapy. In addition, deferral of initial therapy is a widely publicized consideration for selected asymptomatic patients (Portlock and Rosenberg 1979, Portlock 1982, DeVita and Hubbard 1982).

We do not advise deferring therapy for patients with advanced stage indolent lymphomas. Ultimately, therapy is inevitable for these patients, and the risks of delaying treatment outweigh the benefits. The first risk of deferring therapy is the fact that without treatment, the disease can progress. While these are not generally rapidly progressive diseases, they can be difficult to follow. The bone marrow and retroperitoneum are areas that are difficult to evaluate clinically and they can become extensively involved without symptoms. More extensive disease means worse prospects for disease control with therapy (Cabanillas et al. 1979, Stein et al. 1979, Rodgers et al. 1983, Flippin et al. 1983).

The next disadvantage to deferring therapy is the possibility of histologic transformation. The irony of this concern is that proponents of deferral speculate that transformation may carry with it the curative potential of the higher grade lymphoma (DeVita and Hubbard 1982). This is an intriguing theory, and certainly a better understanding of the biologic basis of transformation would be a tremendous advance in our knowledge about lymphoma. But, withholding therapy for this reason is a plan that could clinically backfire. All available data on transformed nodular lymphoma show dismal treatment results and survival data (Cullen et al. 1979, Armitage et al. 1981, Ostrow et al. 1981), analogous to the experience with Richter's syndrome in chronic lymphocytic leukemia. For the fraction who do survive, it will still take years to tell if they retain the potential for late relapse of the original nodular lymphoma.

Another point against deferring therapy is that no survival advantage has been demonstrated, despite its recommendation for selected favorable patients who might well be expected to do better than unselected treated patients. The available data indicate that the group with deferred therapy had about the same survival rate, or perhaps a little worse, than treated patients, which is an unsatisfactory result for a selected favorable group of patients.

Even more controversial than the timing of therapy is the choice of primary therapy. Three major areas of debate are the importance of complete remission, the comparison of single alkylators with combination chemotherapy, and the role of radiotherapy in advanced stage indolent lymphoma.

THE IMPORTANCE OF COMPLETE REMISSION

While complete remission is just one milestone in the course of a chronic disease, it is an important goal of primary therapy. Among our patients with stage IV disease, those achieving complete remission had a five-year survival rate of 77% compared to only 27% for those failing to achieve remission ($P < .01$) (Rodgers et al. 1983). Numerous other studies have demonstrated a similar survival advantage for patients achieving remission (Schein et al. 1974, Anderson et al. 1977, Lister et al. 1978, Cabanillas et al. 1979, Diggs et al. 1981). This goal of complete remission provides one useful guideline in choosing initial therapy.

SINGLE AGENTS OR COMBINATIONS?

There are numerous reports of combination chemotherapy for patients with nodular lymphoma, which generally show a 50%–80% complete remission rate (Anderson et al. 1977, Cabanillas et al. 1979, Diggs et al. 1981, Jones et al. 1983, Rodgers et al. 1983). The range of published complete remission rates with single alkylating agents is broader, 30%–70% (Luce et al. 1971, Jones et al. 1972, Portlock et al. 1976). Thus, combinations appear to give somewhat higher remission rates, although there is considerable overlap of reported results. Protracted courses of alkylators are required to give remission rates that are comparable to the results with combination regimens. In several controlled trials there was a consistent trend for higher complete remission rates with combination chemotherapy than with single agents (Hoogstraten et al. 1969, Kennedy et al. 1978, Hoppe et al. 1981, Lister et al. 1978). But the small size of these trials has left the issue statistically unsettled, with only Hoogstraten's and Kennedy's reports showing significantly higher remission rates with combinations.

The well-accepted rapidity of response with combinations is a clear advantage, especially in pressing clinical situations. Conversely, protracted courses of oral alkylating agents may increase the potential for long-term toxicity, including second malignancies. Thus, while controversy persists, most evidence suggests that combination chemotherapy is superior.

The optimum combination regimen for patients with nodular lymphoma has not been clearly established. Treatment results at UT M. D. Anderson Hospital suggest that the CHOP regimen is superior to COP in terms of complete remission rates (Cabanillas et al. 1979). However, data from the Southwest Oncology Group show comparable complete remission, relapse-free, and overall survival data with COP-Bleo (COP plus bleomycin) or CHOP. Trials at the National Cancer Institute show similar complete remission rates for three regimens COP, C-MOPP (cyclophosphamide, mechlorethamine, vincristine, prednisone, and procarbazine), and BACOP (bleomycin, doxorubicin, cyclophosphamide, vincristine, and prednisone; Anderson et al. 1977). These and other data do not allow the selection of one best chemotherapeutic regimen. At UT M. D. Anderson Hospital, we currently recommend CHOP-Bleo as one of the most consistently effective regimens for NPDL and NML.

THE IMPACT OF RADIOTHERAPY

While radiotherapy is effective for patients with stages I and II disease, less data are available about radiotherapy in advanced disease (Glatstein et al. 1976, Cox et al. 1981). Cox's trial of radiotherapy only for patients with stage III nodular lymphoma showed strikingly good results, a 97% complete remission rate, 78% five-year survival, and 61% five-year disease-free survival. These results compare favorably with most published treatment trials for these diseases.

At UT M. D. Anderson Hospital, we have treated patients with stage III disease using combined modality treatment, alternating CHOP-Bleo with sequential radiotherapy to the involved fields (Flippin et al. 1983). This series was expanded to include 75 patients with a median follow-up of 51 months. The overall complete remission rate was 88%, with a five-year survival rate of 80% and relapse-free survival of 52% (McLaughlin et al. 1982).

The survival analysis by cell type shows a significantly worse survival for stage III NLCL than for NPDL and mixed histology (Figure 3). While the median survival rate in our series for NLCL is no better than that generally reported in the literature, the five-year survival for NPDL of 88% and NML of 89% are well above the 50%–75% five-year data generally reported for advanced stage indolent lymphomas.

Unfortunately, the relapse-free survival curves do show a continuous pattern of late relapse for NPDL and NML (Figure 4). However, our five-year relapse-free survival rates of 58% for NPDL and 62% for NML also appear to be an improvement on most published data, which generally suggest a median relapse-free survival of about two to three years. Thus, we feel that this combined modality treatment approach is one of the most effective currently available programs for stage III NPDL and NML. Our results, in conjunction with the results of Glatstein and Cox, demonstrate that radiotherapy can indeed play an important role in the therapy of some patients with advanced nodular lymphomas.

THE PROBLEM OF RELAPSE

Even after intensive induction therapy, however, most patients with advanced stage nodular lymphomas suffer relapse. Prolonged maintenance chemotherapy has delayed, but not prevented, progression of disease; no survival benefit has been shown.

Immunotherapy has been used and results have been encouraging in a limited number of trials of patients with nodular lymphoma. *Bacillus Calmete-Guerin* treatment has been associated with a trend for prolonged survival in two trials and has prolonged the disease-free survival in another small trial at UT M. D. Anderson Hospital (Cabanillas et al. 1979, Hoerni et al. 1981, Jones et al. 1983).

The interferons are another form of biologic therapy that have shown activity in patients with nodular lymphomas (Louie et al. 1981, Gutterman et al. 1980). These encouraging results and the suitability of interferon for long-term administration have led us to incorporate maintenance therapy with leukocyte interferon into our

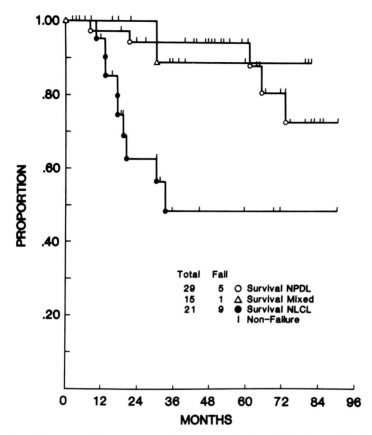

Figure 3. Stage III nodular lymphoma. Survival rates by histologic subtype. Statistical comparison showed: NPDL versus large cell, $P < .01$; mixed versus large cell, $P = .03$.

treatment plan for patients with advanced stage NPDL and NML who achieve complete remission.

CONCLUSION

There is evidence that a fraction of patients with nodular lymphoma may be curable, namely, those with stages I and II disease of all cell types and possibly those with all stages of NLCL. For all patients, the achievement of complete remission correlates with longer survival and should be a goal of initial therapy.

The choice of initial chemotherapy remains controversial, but available evidence suggests that combination chemotherapy probably yields higher complete remission rates than single alkylators and that combinations certainly result in earlier response.

Radiotherapy is also an effective modality even in some patients with advanced (stage III) disease, and it can be effectively integrated with chemotherapy in the treatment of these patients. However, new treatment approaches are needed to deal

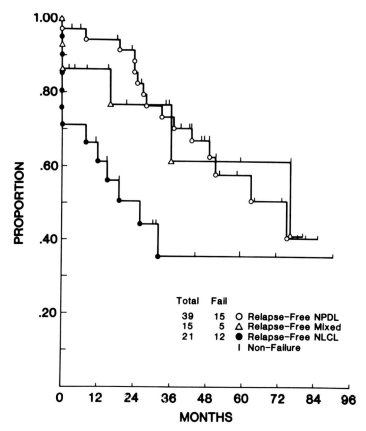

Figure 4. Stage III nodular lymphoma. Relapse-free survival rates by histologic subtype. Statistical comparison showed: NPDL versus large cell, $P < .01$; mixed versus large cell, $P = .1$.

with the continuing problem of relapse in patients with advanced stage nodular lymphoma.

REFERENCES

Anderson T, Bender RA, Fisher RI, DeVita VT, Chabner BA, Berard CW, Norton L, Young RC. 1977. Combination chemotherapy in non-Hodgkin's lymphoma: Results of long-term followup. Cancer Treat Rep 61:1057–1066.

Anderson T, DeVita VT, Simon RM, Berard CW, Canellos GP, Garvin AJ, Young RC. 1982. Malignant lymphoma: II. Prognostic factors and response to treatment of 473 patients at the National Cancer Institute. Cancer 50:2708–2721.

Armitage JO, Dick FR, Corder MP. 1981. Diffuse histiocytic lymphoma after histologic conversion: A poor prognostic variant. Cancer Treat Rep 65:413–418.

Bush RS, Gospodarowicz M, Sturgeon J, Alison R. 1977. Radiation therapy of localized non-Hodgkin's lymphoma. Cancer Treat Rep 61:1129–1136.

Bush RS, Gospodarowicz M. 1982. The place of radiation therapy in the management of localized non-Hodgkin's lymphoma. *In* Rosenberg SA and Kaplan HS, eds., Malignant Lymphomas: Etiology, Immunology, Pathology, Treatment. Academic Press, New York, pp. 485–502.

Cabanillas F, Smith T, Bodey GP, Gutterman JU, and Freireich EJ. 1979. Nodular malignant lymphomas: Factors affecting complete response rate and survival. Cancer 44:1983–1989.

Cox JD, Komaki R, Kun LE, Wilson JF, Greenberg M. 1981. Stage III Nodular lymphoreticular tumors (non-Hodgkin's Lymphoma): Results of central lymphatic irradiation. Cancer 47:2247–2252.

Cullen MH, Lister TA, Brearley RL, Shand WS, Stansfeld AG. 1979. Histological transformation of non-Hodgkin's lymphoma: A prospective study. Cancer 44:645–651.

Diggs CH, Wiernik PH, Ostrow SS. 1981. Nodular lymphoma: Prolongation of survival by complete remission. Cancer Clinical Trials 4:107–114.

DeVita VT, Hubbard SH. 1982. The curative potential of chemotherapy in the treatment of Hodgkin's disease and non-Hodgkin's lymphomas. *In* Rosenberg SA and Kaplan HS, eds., Malignant Lymphomas: Etiology, Immunology, Pathology, Treatment. Academic Press, New York, pp. 379–416.

Flippin T, McLaughlin P, Conrad FG, Fuller LM, Velasquez WS, Butler JJ, Shullenberger CC. 1983. Stage III nodular lymphomas: Preliminary results of a combined chemotherapy/radiotherapy program. Cancer 51:987–993.

Fuller LM, Banker RL, Butler JJ, Gamble JF, Sullivan MP. 1975. The natural history of non-Hodgkin's lymphomata stages I and II. Br J Cancer 31 (Suppl II):270–285.

Glatstein E, Fuks Z, Goffinet DR, Kaplan HS. 1976. Non-Hodgkin's lymphomas of stage III extent. Is total lymphoid irradiation appropriate treatment? Cancer 37:2806–2812.

Glick JH, McFadden E, Costello W, Ezdinli E, Berard CW, Bennett JM. 1982. Nodular histiocytic lymphoma: Factors influencing prognosis and implications for aggressive chemotherapy. Cancer 49:840–845.

Gutterman J, Blumenschein GR, Alexanian R, Yap HY, Buzdar AU, Cabanillas F, Hortobagyi GN, Hersh EM, Rasmussen SL, Harmon M, Kramer M, Pestka S. 1980. Leukocyte interferon-induced tumor regression in human metastatic breast cancer, multiple myeloma, and malignant lymphoma. Ann Intern Med 93:399–406.

Hoerni B, Durand M, Eghbali H, Hoerni-Simon G, Lagarde C. 1981. Adjuvant BCG-therapy of non-Hodgkin's malignant lymphomas. *In* Salmon SE and Jones SE, eds., Adjuvant Therapy of Cancer III. Grune and Stratton, New York, pp. 99–106.

Hoogstraten B, Owens AH, Lenhard RE, Glidewell OJ, Leone LA, Olson KB, Harley JB, Townsend SR, Miller SP, Spurr CL. 1969. Combination chemotherapy in lymphosarcoma and reticulum cell sarcoma. Blood 33:370–378.

Hoppe RT, Kushlan P, Kaplan HS, Rosenberg SA, Brown BW. 1981. The treatment of advanced stage favorable histology non-Hodgkin's lymphoma: A preliminary report of a randomized trial comparing single agent chemotherapy, combination chemotherapy, and whole body irradiation. Blood 58:592–598.

Jones SE, Fuks Z, Bull M, Kadin ME, Dorfman RF, Kaplan HA, Rosenberg SA, Kim H. 1973. Non-Hodgkin's lymphomas: IV. Clinicopathologic correlation in 405 cases. Cancer 31:806–823.

Jones SE, Grozea PN, Metz EN, Haut A, Stephens RL, Morrison FS, Talley R, Butler JJ, Byrne GE, Hartsock R, Dixon D, Salmon SS. 1983. Improved complete remission rates and survival for patients with large cell lymphoma treated with chemoimmunotherapy. A Southwest Oncology Group Study. Cancer 51:1083–1090.

Jones SE, Rosenberg SA, Kaplan HS, Kadin ME, Dorfman RF. 1972. Non-Hodgkin's lymphomas: II. Single agent chemotherapy. Cancer 30:31–38.

Kennedy BJ, Bloomfield CD, Kiang DT, Vosika G, Peterson BA, Theologides A. 1978. Combination versus successive single agent chemotherapy in lymphocytic lymphoma. Cancer 41:23–28.

Lister TA, Cullen MH, Beard MEJ, Brearley RL, Whitehouse JMA, Wrigley PFM, Stansfeld AG, Sutcliffe SBJ, Malpas JS, Crowther D. 1978. Comparison of combined and single-agent chemotherapy in non-Hodgkin's lymphoma of favourable histological type. Br Med J 1:533–537.

Louie AC, Gallagher JG, Sikora K, Levy R, Rosenberg SA, Merigan TC. 1981. Follow-up observations on the effect of human leukocyte interferon in non-Hodgkin's lymphoma. Blood 58:712–718.

Luce JK, Gamble JF, Wilson HE, Monto RW, Isaacs BL, Palmer RL, Coltman CA Jr., Hewlett JS, Gehan EA, Frei E III. 1971. Combined cyclophosphamide, vincristine, and prednisone therapy of malignant lymphoma. Cancer 28:306–317.

McLaughlin P, Kantarjian H, Fuller LM, Smith T, Osborne B, Velasquez W, Cabanillas F. 1983. Nodular large cell lymphoma-A review of 62 cases. (Abstract) Proceedings of the American Society of Clinical Oncology 2:222.

McLaughlin P, Fuller LM, Butler JJ, Sullivan JA. 1984. Stage I–II nodular (follicular) lymphoma. (Abstract) Proceedings of the American Society of Clinical Oncology 3:249.

McLaughlin P, Fuller LM, Conrad FG, Butler JJ, Velasquez WS, Hagemeister FB, Shullenberger CC. 1982. Stage III nodular lymphoma: Results of combined modality therapy. (Abstract) Proceedings of the 13th International Cancer Congress, p. 412.

Monfardini S, Banfi A, Bonadonna G, Rilke G, Milani F, Valagussa P, Lattuada A. 1980. Improved five year survival after combined radiotherapy-chemotherapy for stage I-II non-Hodgkin's lymphoma. Int J Radiat Oncol Biol Phys 6:125–134.

Non-Hodgkin's Lymphoma Pathologic Classification Project. 1982. National Cancer Institute sponsored study of classifications of non-Hodgkin's lymphomas. Summary and description of a Working Formulation for clinical usage. Cancer 49:2112–2135.

Osborne CK, Norton L, Young RC, Garvin AJ, Simon RM, Berard CW, Hubbard S, DeVita VT. 1980. Nodular histiocytic lymphoma: An aggressive nodular lymphoma with potential for prolonged disease-free survival. Blood 56:98–103.

Ostrow SS, Diggs CH, Sutherland JC, Gustafson J, Wiernik PH. 1981. Nodular poorly differentiated lymphocytic lymphoma: Changes in histology and survival. Cancer Treat Rep 65:929–933.

Paryani S, Hoppe R, Cox R, Colby T, Rosenberg S, Kaplan H. 1983. Follicular non-Hodgkin's lymphomas, stage I and II. (Abstract) Proceedings of the American Society of Clinical Oncology 2:220.

Portlock CS, Rosenberg SA, Glatstein E, Kaplan HS. 1976. Treatment of advanced non-Hodgkin's lymphomas with favorable histologies: Preliminary results of a prospective trial. Blood 47:747–756.

Portlock CS, Rosenberg SA. 1979. No initial therapy for stage III and IV non-Hodgkin's lymphomas of favorable histologic types. Ann Intern Med 90:10–13.

Portlock CS. 1982. Deferral of initial therapy for advanced indolent lymphomas. Cancer Treat Rep 66:417–419.

Rappaport H. 1966. Tumors of the hematopoietic system. *In* Atlas of Tumor Pathology. Section III, Fascicle 8. Armed Forces Institute of Pathology, Washington, D.C., pp. 97–161.

Rodgers RW, McLaughlin P, Sullivan JA, Favors A, Butler JJ, Gresik M, Conrad FG. 1983. Prognostic factors in stage IV nodular lymphoma. (Abstract) Proceedings of the American Society of Clinical Oncology 2:217.

Rodriquez V, Cabanillas F, Burgess MA, McKelvey EM, Valdivieso M, Bodey GP, Freireich EJ. 1977. Combination chemotherapy ("CHOP-Bleo") in advanced (non-Hodgkin) malignant lymphoma. Blood 49:325–333.

Rosenberg SA. 1979. Current concepts in cancer: Non-Hodgkin's lymphoma–selection of treatment on the basis of histologic type. N Engl J Med 301:924–928.

Schein PS, Chabner BA, Canellos GP, Young RC, Berard C, DeVita VT. 1974. Potential for prolonged disease-free survival following combination chemotherapy of non-Hodgkin's lymphoma. Blood 43:181–189.

Stein RS, Cousar J, Flexner JM, Graber SE, McKee LC, Krantz S, Collins RD. 1979. Malignant lymphomas of follicular center cell origin in man. III. Prognostic features. Cancer 44:2236–2243.

Yunis JJ, Oken MM, Kaplan ME, Ensrud KM, Howe R, Theologides A. 1982. Distinctive chromosomal abnormalities in histologic subtypes of non-Hodgkin's lymphoma. N Engl J Med 307:1231–1236.

UT M. D. Anderson Clinical Conference on Cancer,
Vol. 27, edited by R. J. Ford, L. M. Fuller, and
F. B. Hagemeister. Raven Press, New York © 1984.

Treatment of Pediatric Patients with Stages I and II Lymphoma

Margaret P. Sullivan and Irma Ramirez

Department of Pediatrics, The University of Texas M. D. Anderson Hospital at Houston, Houston, Texas 77030

For some time, the favorability of stages I and II presentations of the non-Hodgkin's lymphomata (NHL) of childhood was obscured by the relative infrequency of their occurrences. Such limited disease has been found in 24 of 99 (22%) eligible and evaluable patients in the Pediatric Oncology Group (POG) study of LSA_2-L_2 therapy (Sullivan et al. unpublished data). Localized disease occurred in 60 of 211 (22%) patients on the Children's Cancer Study Group comparative evaluation of treatment results using LSA_2-L_2 and COMP (cyclophosphamide, vincristine, methotrexate, and prednisone) (Anderson et al. 1983). In the POG study cited, the ratio of stage I:II patients was 9:15 or 1:1.6.

Wollner's first report of LSA_2-L_2 therapy versus historical controls or "nonprotocol" patients with NHL in 1976 showed 100% survival for the 10 stages I and II patients given LSA_2-L_2 therapy versus 40% survival for 10 stages I and II control patients (Wollner et al. 1976). The proportion of stages I and II patients on this LSA_2-L_2 study was 10 of 43 (23%). LSA_2-L_2 patients received 10 chemotherapeutic agents and radiotherapy; the nonprotocol group had been treated initially with nitrogen mustard derivatives and radiotherapy, with or without maintenance regimens of single chemotherapeutic agents.

In a subsequent report of these patients, reduction in the dose of irradiation from "curative" doses to 2000 rad was suggested to accommodate the intensity of chemotherapy and the number, as well as the volumes, of the treatment fields that might be employed in more advanced disease (Wollner et al. 1979). Further study of the impact of radiotherapy on the outcome of LSA_2-L_2 therapy shows no effect on survival, but radiotherapy was again strongly recommended as a means of preventing local recurrences (Jereb et al. 1981).

In the Children's Cancer Study Group, comparison of LSA_2-L_2 and COMP therapies, two-year disease-free survival rates for patients with localized disease were 84% and 89% for the regimens, respectively (Anderson et al. 1983). In this study, both regimens employed radiotherapy. In the POG study of LSA_2-L_2 therapy, irradiation was required only for those patients with residual disease following the completion of induction therapy (Sullivan et al. 1984). All POG stage I patients and 10 of the 15 (67%) stage II patients were disease free two years after entering the study.

Less-intensive lymphoma therapy, in the form of an antileukemic regimen designated APO (doxorubicin, prednisone, and vincristine), was developed at the Dana-Farber Cancer Institute, Children's Hospital Medical Center (Boston) and produced greater than an 80% two-year survival rate in children with NHL, regardless of disease stage (Weinstein and Link 1979). Patients with diffuse undifferentiated histology of the Burkitt's-type lymphoma responded poorly to APO and have not been given this type of therapy since December 1975.

Less-intensive short-term chemotherapy with involved-field radiotherapy, 2000 rad, has been employed by Murphy and co-workers at the St. Jude Children's Research Hospital since 1982; 85.7% disease-free survival was achieved by 28 stages I and II patients (Murphy et al. 1983). Relapse occurred in only four patients with diffuse undifferentiated histology.

At the UT M. D. Anderson Hospital, LSA_2-L_2 therapy, with modifications, has been given to pediatric patients with NHL from the time of Wollner's first presentation of LSA_2-L_2 results in 1974. As our institutional field trial showed poor results among patients with Burkitt's lymphoma, this group was given a specially devised regimen employing cyclophosphamide (Cytoxan®) and methotrexate in high doses. The outcome of therapy for UT M. D. Anderson Hospital stages I and II patients is herewith examined with respect to survival, histology, the contribution of radiotherapy, and the length of treatment, in an effort to identify important elements of therapy.

MATERIALS AND METHODS

Demographic Characteristics

Thirty children with NHL, stages I and II, have been treated at the UT M. D. Anderson Hospital since Novemeber, 1974. The male to female ratio was 3:1 (Table 1). The ratio was slightly higher in stage II disease. Ages of the patients ranged from $2^6/12$ years to $16^3/12$ years. The number of whites greatly exceeded blacks, 28:2. It is of some interest that 19 children had Spanish surnames; of these, 17 were from families speaking Spanish as their language of preference.

Table 1. *Sex and Age at Diagnosis of 30 Patients with NHL of Childhood, Murphy Stages I and II UT M. D. Anderson Hospital*

Stage	Sex (M:F)	Age range (yrs)	Median age (yr)
I N = 16	12:4	4 2/12–14 6/12	8 2/12
II N = 14	11:3	2 6/12–16 3/12	6 9/12

Disease Characteristics

The histologic subtype of disease is shown, with respect to stage, in Table 2. The paucity of lymphoblastic disease is of importance. Large-cell and diffuse undifferentiated histologies were observed in equal numbers of patients and, together, constituted 87% of the study group. Of those with undifferentiated histology, the number with Burkitt's-type lymphoma was approximately twice that of the non-Burkitt's type. Primary sites of involvement are shown in Table 3. The preponderance of cases originating in the small bowel, 12 of 30, or 40%, is of importance. These tumors were all said to have been removed completely and showed no evidence of recurrence when treatment was initiated; second surgical explorations were not done prior to the initiation of treatment.

Therapeutic Assignments

The various treatments given our stages I and II study populations are correlated with disease stage in Table 4. Four children were included in the UT M. D. Anderson Hospital field trial of LSA_2-L_2 therapy that was activated in November, 1974. With these patients, every effort was made to give therapy as described by Wollner in her publications and in telephone conversations. As all four Burkitt's

Table 2. *Histologic Subtypes of 30 Patients with NHL of Childhood, Murphy Stages I and II UT M. D. Anderson Hospital*

Histologic type	Stage I no. patients	Stage II no. patients	Total no. (%)
Lymphoblastic	1	0	1(3.3)
Large cell	6	7	13(43.3)
Undifferentiated, Burkitt's	4	5	9(30)
Undifferentiated, non-Burkitt's	4	0	4(13.3)
Unclassified	1	2	3(10)
Total	16	14	30(100)

Table 3. *Primary Sites of Disease of 30 Patients with NHL of Childhood, Murphy Stages I and II UT M. D. Anderson Hospital*

Site	Stage I	Stage II	Total
Distal ileum, cecum, appendix	4	8	12
Peripheral nodes	7	2	9
Eyelids, orbit	2	1	3
Facial bones (jaw)	2	0	2
Oro- and nasopharynx	2	0	2
Testicle	1	0	1
Long bones (tibia)	1	0	1
Total	19	11	30

Table 4. Therapeutic Programs and Treatment Results of 30 Patients with NHL of Childhood, Murphy Stages I and II UT M. D. Anderson Hospital–November 1974–July 1983

Treatment	Patients		Given radiotherapy	Relapses/ deaths	Survival
	Stage I	Stage II			
Radiotherapy only	1	0	1	0	1
LSA$_2$-L$_2$ field trial	1	3	4	2*/1	3
POG 7615	4	2	3	1†/1	5
Second generation	6	3	0	0	9
T-cell modification (T-3-A)	1	0	0	0	1
High cyclophosphamide High methotrexate	3	6	0	0	9
Total	16	14	8	3/2	28

*One responded to radiotherapy.
†Relapse in radiotherapy treatment field.

lymphoma patients in the field trial relapsed, individuals in this histologic category were no longer considered eligible for treatment with LSA$_2$-L$_2$-derived regimens.

Beginning in September, 1976, modified LSA$_2$-L$_2$ therapy was given to six stages I and II patients treated in accordance with the Southwest Oncology Group (later POG) protocol study 7615 (Sullivan et al. unpublished data). As irradiation interfered with ongoing chemotherapy in the field trial, radiotherapy was recommended only for postinduction residual disease in the group study. A futher modification was the requirement for an absolute granulocytic count of 1000/μL for continuation of therapy. From the activation time of this study, the ineligible stages I and II patients with Burkitt's lymphoma (N = 9) were entered on a new institutional study employing high doses of Cytoxan® and methotrexate with coordinated intrathecal therapy consisting of methotrexate, cytosine arabinoside, and hydrocortisone (Ramirez 1979). Treatment for advanced stages of the disease is completed in 54 weeks; patients with stages I and II disease now complete therapy in 36 weeks.

With the closure of POG 7615 to patient entries in August, 1979, an institutional "second generation" LSA$_2$-L$_2$ protocol was activated. Therapeutic modifications included intensification of intrathecal central nervous system prophylaxis, intensification of cytosine arabinoside therapy during consolidation, and the deletion of thioguanine from the consolidation phase of treatment. Six stage I and three stage II patients received second generation LSA$_2$-L$_2$ therapy. Stage I patients had received an even more altered LSA$_2$-L$_2$ regimen that was devised for patients with T-cell disease. Treatment time has now been reduced from two years from complete remission date to one year or to the completion of three treatment cycles, whichever comes first.

A single stage I patient, given radiotherapy only, fell within the study time span and perforce is included in the data base.

RESULTS

Survival

Three of the 30 patients have relapsed. As indicated in Table 4, one responded to radiotherapy; the two other patients have died. Twenty-eight of 30 (90%) survive (Figure 1). One patient with disease died following the recurrence of tumor at the primary site, which had been irradiated. A second patient died of diffuse large-cell lymphoma of the bowel complicated by acute pancreatitis and diabetes, occurring as toxic side effects of L-asparaginase therapy. During the long period in which therapy was withheld from this patient, because of side effects, a single nodule developed in the liver and was resected. Consent for further therapy was withdrawn when new disease manifestations became apparent. Both patients who died had large-cell disease; one had recurrent peripheral nodal disease and the other had primary disease of the bowel. The significance of these findings, however, cannot be determined because of the small number of patients in each diagnostic

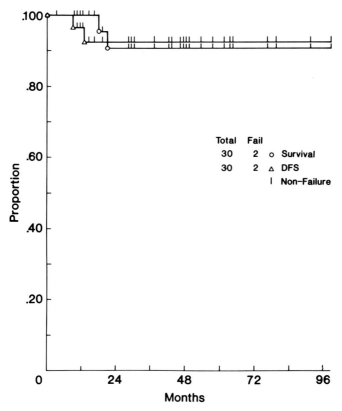

Figure 1. Survival and disease-free survival of children with stages I and II non-Hodgkin's lymphoma. UT M. D. Anderson Hospital and Tumor Institute 1974–1983.

category. The presenting site of the disease does not appear to have been an important determinant of outcome in our group.

Contribution of Radiotherapy

Table 3 shows the number of patients receiving radiotherapy and the outcome of treatment. One child relapsed in a previously irradiated peripheral nodal mass, and a second child who had Burkitt's lymphoma with nodal relapse responded to radiotherapy. None of the 18 children given second generation LSA_2-L_2 or high Cytoxan®-high methotrexate therapy received radiotherapy; with chemotherapy only, all survive. These data contribute to the feeling that the role of radiotherapy in NHL of childhood needs to be redefined.

Length of Treatment

Relapse in large cell and diffuse undifferentiated lymphoma of childhood characteristically occurs eight months from diagnosis or earlier (Sullivan et al. unpublished data). The experience to date with the high Cytoxan®-high methotrexate protocol indicates that 54 weeks is adequate time for therapy for diffuse undifferentiated disease. Through the randomization process, the POG is determining the effectiveness of 36 weeks of therapy in advanced disease; in our institutional study, this question is addressed for stages I and II patients. The follow-up period has been too short for definitive statements, but there have been no adverse consequences to date.

CONCLUSIONS

The data presented together with those previously published indicate a very favorable prognosis for children with stages I and II non-Hodgkin's lymphoma who are treated with multiagent chemotherapy, with or without radiotherapy. The inclusion of Cytoxan® in the treatment of undifferentiated lymphoma, Burkitt's type, appears essential to the success of the regimen. Radiotherapy is not required for successful treatment. Treatment for Burkitt's lymphoma may be terminated at 54 weeks without jeopardizing the response. Thirty-six week treatment schedules are being conducted, but time on study is not sufficient for reporting. Short-term second generation LSA_2-L_2 therapy also appears adequate, but this conclusion also requires further follow-up.

ACKNOWLEDGMENT

This study was supported in part by grant CA-03713 from the National Institutes of Health, United States Department of Health and Human Services.

REFERENCES

Anderson JR, Wilson JF, Jenkin DT, Meadows AT, Kersey J, Chilcote RR, Coccia P, Exelby P, Kushner J, Siegel S, Hammond D. 1983. Childhood non-Hodgkin's lymphoma: The results of a randomized therapeutic trial comparing a 4-drug regimen (COMP) with a 10-drug regimen (LSA$_2$-L$_2$). N Engl J Med 308:559–565.

Jereb B, Wollner N, Kosloff C, Exelby P. 1981. The role of local radiation in the treatment of non-Hodgkin's lymphoma in children. Med Pediatr Oncol 9:157–166.

Murphy SB, Husto HO, Rivera G, Berard CW. 1983. End results of treating children with localized non-Hodgkin's lymphomas with a combined modality approach of lessened intensity. Journal of Clinical Oncology 1:326–330.

Ramirez I, Sullivan MP, Wang Y-M, Martin RG, Butler JJ. 1979. Effective therapy for Burkitt's lymphoma: High dose cyclophosphamide-high dose methotrexate with coordinated intrathecal therapy: Plasma and cerebrospinal fluid methotrexate levels. Cancer Chemother Pharmacol 3:103–109.

Sullivan MP, Boyett J, Pullen J, Doering EJ, Trueworthy R, Huizdala E, Ruymann F. 1984. Pediatric Oncology Group experience with modified LSA$_2$-L$_2$ therapy in 107 children with non-Hodgkin's lymphoma (Burkitt's lymphoma excluded). Cancer (In press).

Weinstein HJ, Link MP. 1979. Non-Hodgkin's lymphoma in childhood. Clin Haematol 8:699–716.

Wollner N, Burchenal JH, Lieberman PH, Exelby P, D'Angio G, Murphy ML. 1976. Non-Hodgkin's lymphoma in children: A comparative study of two modalities of therapy. Cancer 37:123–134.

Wollner N, Exelby PP, Lieberman PH. 1979. Non-Hodgkin's lymphoma in children: A progress report on the original patients treated with the LSA$_2$-L$_2$ protocol. Cancer 44:1990–1999.

UT M. D. Anderson Clinical Conference on Cancer,
Vol. 27, edited by R. J. Ford, L. M. Fuller, and
F. B. Hagemeister. Raven Press, New York © 1984.

B-Cell Small Noncleaved Undifferentiated Lymphoma in Adults

Alexandra M. Levine, Zdena Pavlova,* John W. Parker,* Annlia
Paganini-Hill,† Darleen R. Powars,‡ Robert J. Lukes,*
and Donald I. Feinstein

*Departments of Medicine, *Pathology, †Family and Preventative Medicine, and
‡Pediatrics, University of Southern California School of Medicine, and the Los Angeles
County-University of Southern California Medical Center, Los Angeles, California 90033*

BACKGROUND

Burkitt's lymphoma was first described in 1958 by Dennis Burkitt who noted a peculiar type of tumor, oriented about the jaw, in children living in Uganda. An extremely rapid rate of tumor growth was noted in these cases, with small nodules growing to extreme proportions sometimes within a matter of days. After single agent cyclophosphamide therapy, approximately 85% of the patients experienced complete resolution of disease, although two-thirds of them subsequently relapsed, usually within two to three months. The tumor was later found to be endemic, not only in Uganda but also throughout the malaria belt of equatorial Africa. In these regions, an association between the Epstein-Barr virus (EBV) and the development of lymphoma was found. de-The and colleagues (1978) studied 42,000 children in Uganda, obtaining serum to analyze for exposure to and infection with the EBV. He returned to this region, to ascertain which of the children had developed Burkitt's lymphoma in the interval. Those children who did develop Burkitt's lymphoma were found to have significantly higher antibody titers to the viral capsid antigen (VCA) of EBV, when compared to those children who remained well. Further, by DNA hybridization studies, EBV genomic material was found within tumor cell DNA from Burkitt's lymphoma cases occurring in the endemic regions.

A morphologically identical tumor has been described in the United States and in other nonendemic areas of the world. Although identical under the microscope, these cases differ clinically, in that no apparent relationship exists between the tumor and the EBV. Further, the anatomic orientation of the disease is different; the majority of tumors occur in the abdomen, as opposed to the jaw. Affected individuals in the nonendemic regions are somewhat older than those described in Africa. The African and nonendemic cases are similar in that both are potentially curable in children. In both variants, a specific chromosomal translocation t(8;14) has been described.

Aside from the classic Burkitt's tumor, another morphologic variant has been described in nonendemic regions, termed non-Burkitt's, or Burkitt's-like. Burkitt's lymphoma was first pathologically classified within the undifferentiated category of Rappaport (1966). With an appreciation that the tumor is of B cell or follicular center cell (FCC) derivation, Lukes and Collins (1974) chose to classify it descriptively under the designation of small noncleaved FCC lymphoma. Within this group, two subtypes were described, the Burkitt's type and the non-Burkitt's variant. A similar categorization has been suggested by the Non-Hodgkin's Lymphoma Pathology Classification Project (1982), in which, under the designation of high grade tumors, the small noncleaved lymphoma could be further classified as Burkitt's variant if the tumor met the morphologic criteria for this subtype as published by the World Health Organization.

The accurate pathologic designation of a small noncleaved FCC tumor into the Burkitt's or non-Burkitt's variants may, at times, be difficult. Moreover, such a distinction may not be necessary, if, in fact, these entities are clinically and biologically similar. In an attempt to define the clinicopathologic features of Burkitt's versus non-Burkitt's subtypes in the United States, we studied the precise clinical and pathologic characteristics in 42 patients with small noncleaved FCC lymphoma, from whom biopsy material was collected for multiparameter studies. Twenty-five patients with the Burkitt's variant and 17 with the non-Burkitt's subtype were reviewed.

MATERIALS AND METHODS

For inclusion in the study, a morphologic diagnosis of small noncleaved FCC lymphoma was required. Additionally, we required that pretreatment diagnostic material be available, as well as adequate fresh pathologic tissues for multiparameter immunologic studies.

All cases interpreted and coded as small noncleaved FCC lymphoma at Los Angeles County-University of Southern California (USC) Medical Center, and the Southern California Lymphoma Group between January, 1974 and January, 1980 were pathologically reviewed and subclassified into Burkitt's or non-Burkitt's variants by two of us (ZP, RJL). Clinical charts were reviewed in all cases, independent of pathologic review. When the clinical and pathologic reviews were complete, the data were collated; all cases were assigned specific diagnoses as to the pathologic subtype, and the clinical characteristics of Burkitt's versus non-Burkitt's variants were compared.

Detailed cellular morphology was assessed on tissue that was fixed in Zenker's solution, and B-5 fixative or formalin, or both, embedded in paraffin, sectioned at 4 to 6 μm intervals and stained with hematoxylin and eosin and methyl green pyronin.

All immunologic marker studies were performed on pretreatment diagnostic material. Spontaneous sheep erythrocyte rosette formation, cell surface immunoglobulin studies, and the immunoperoxidase method for detecting intracytoplasmic immunoglobulin were all performed as described.

RESULTS

Histopathologic Findings

Of the 42 cases in this study, 25 fulfilled the morphologic criteria for Burkitt's lymphoma, as defined by the World Health Organization. The remaining 17 cases were considered to be non-Burkitt's. The non-Burkitt's variant exhibited greater variation in the size and shape of the nucleus, and the nucleoli were more prominent than in the Burkitt's type. In addition, a greater amount of cytoplasm and more variability in the degree of amphophilia were seen in the non-Burkitt's cases.

Immunoglobulin Marker Studies

Multiparameter immunologic studies confirmed the B-cell nature of small noncleaved FCC lymphoma. Using both cell surface markers and the immunoperoxidase technique, 20 of 24 (83%) Burkitt's and 13 of 16 (81%) non-Burkitt's cases proved to be monoclonal (Levine et al. 1983).

Age and Sex

Of the 25 Burkitt's patients, 18 were male and 7 were female. The median age of the Burkitt's group was 31 years (2.5–93 years). In the non-Burkitt's category, 9 of 17 were male, and 8 were female. The median age for the group was 56 years (8–79 years) (Levine et al. 1983).

Method of Presentation

The initial method of presentation in the two variants was quite distinct. Eighteen of 25 Burkitt's patients (72%) first sought medical attention because of disease in extranodal sites, compared to 5 of 17 (30%) in the non-Burkitt's group ($P = .02$) (Levine et al. 1983). Of the 18 Burkitt's patients who presented with extranodal disease, 15 were first seen because of disease in the gastrointestinal (GI) tract. Eight of these were initially hospitalized with ileocecal intussusception related to tumor. Other sites of GI involvement in the Burkitt's group included the stomach in one, stomach and duodenum in two, duodenum in one, jejunum in one, rectum in one, and massive retroperitoneal tumor bilaterally involving all areas of GI tract from diaphragm to sacrum in one patient. Aside from the GI tract, other sites of extranodal presentation in the Burkitt's group included the uterus in one patient, central nervous system in one, and a subcutaneous mass lesion in one.

In the non-Burkitt's group, five patients initially presented with extranodal disease, including the stomach in two, cecum in one, ileum and cecum in one, and breast in one patient. The difference in GI involvement between the two variants was significant ($P < .05$).

Initial Staging

Full staging evaluation of the patients revealed advanced stage of disease in the majority of both variants. Using the Ann Arbor system, stage III or IV disease was detected at diagnosis in 20 of 25 (80%) Burkitt's patients and 14 of 17 (82%) non-Burkitt's cases. Using the distinct staging system for Burkitt's lymphoma proposed by Ziegler (1981) there were three Burkitt's patients with stage A, one with AR, eight with B, five with C, and eight with D disease. In the non-Burkitt's group, 1 patient had stage A, 11 had B, 2 had C, and 3 had D disease. Systemic B symptoms were seen in 10 of 25 (40%) Burkitt's patients and 4 of 17 (24%) non-Burkitt's cases (Levine et al. 1983).

In spite of widespread disease in both variants and in spite of extensive abdominal disease in many of the Burkitt's patients, there was remarkable sparing of the bone marrow. At diagnosis, only 1 of 22 (4.5%) Burkitt's patients had involvement of the bone marrow, compared to 6 of 16 (37.5%) non-Burkitt's cases. This difference was significant ($P<.05$). Frank leukemic involvement at diagnosis was observed in two non-Burkitt's patients and in no case of the Burkitt's variant.

Response to Therapy

The results of therapeutic intervention were almost identical in the two variants (Levine et al. 1983). A total of 14 patients with stage II, III, or IV disease received either BACOP (bleomycin, doxorubicin, cyclophosphamide, vincristine, and prednisone) or CHOP (cyclophosphamide, doxorubicin, vincristine, and prednisone). This resulted in a 57% complete remission rate in both Burkitt's and non-Burkitt's cases. The COP (cyclophosphamide, vincristine, and prednisone) or COPP (COP plus procarbazine) regimens were used in seven Burkitt's patients and five non-Burkitt's cases. No response to these regimens was documented in 71% of Burkitt's and 80% of non-Burkitt's cases. The COM (cyclophosphamide, vincristine, and methotrexate) regimen was administered to two Burkitt's patients, resulting in complete response in one and no response in one. Similar results were obtained on the two Burkitt's patients who were treated with the POMP (prednisone, vincristine, methotrexate, and mercaptopurine) regimen.

A total of seven Burkitt's patients with disseminated disease attained complete remission. Five of these remain alive without evidence of disease, from 21 to more than 74 months after diagnosis; four are children.

A total of six patients with advanced disease in the non-Burkitt's category attained complete remission. Three of these patients were alive, without evidence of disease, from 32 to 48 months after diagnosis. A fourth complete responder, the only child in this category, was lost to follow-up at 6 months.

Stage I disease was found in only four patients in the entire small noncleaved group. All four received radiotherapy as the sole modality, resulting in long-term disease-free survival in the three Burkitt's patients and no response in the one patient who had non-Burkitt's variant.

Survival

The overall survival in the two variants was similar and short. Median survival in the Burkitt's group was 10.5 months, compared to 7.7 months in the non-

Burkitt's group (Levine et al. 1983). Nine patients in this study were less than 18 years of age (seven Burkitt's and two non-Burkitt's). Complete remission was attained in five of these (four Burkitt's, one non-Burkitt's). The median survival of the pediatric group was in excess of 74 months.

SMALL NONCLEAVED FCC LYMPHOMA IN HOMOSEXUAL MALES

From January, 1982 through October, 1983, 17 homosexual males with malignant B-cell lymphomas were seen at Los Angeles County-USC Medical Center. Six of these patients had small noncleaved FCC lymphoma, including four with the non-Burkitt's and two with the Burkitt's variant. Four of these six patients presented with stage IV disease, including involvement of the bone and kidney in one, small bowel in one, bone marrow and central nervous system in one, and lung in one. Three patients gave histories of multiple recreational drug abuse; one patient had a history of persistent, generalized lymphadenopathy. The ratio of helper to suppressor T-lymphocytes in the peripheral blood was reversed in five. One patient died at 3 months, and the other five were alive, on chemotherapy, from 1 to 15 months from initial diagnosis. The clinical and pathologic characteristics of these cases are fully consistent with what has been described by Levine et al. (1984) in homosexual males; the lymphomas that develop in these individuals are aggressive, B-lymphocyte diseases, which are often extranodal in presentation and associated with the immunologic abnormalities that have been described in the acquired immunodeficiency syndrome.

CONCLUSIONS

The current study has demonstrated that the morphologic separation between the Burkitt's and non-Burkitt's variants of small noncleaved FCC lymphoma is fairly easy to make in the majority of cases. The B-cell nature of this tumor has been confirmed by the demonstration of surface or intracytoplasmic immunoglobulin in the majority of both variants. Clinical distinctions between the subtypes have been noted; Burkitt's patients tend to present at an earlier age. Additionally, the anatomic orientation of the disease appears different. The Burkitt's tumor presents initially in the abdomen and GI tract, with relative sparing of the bone marrow, which is in contradistinction to the non-Burkitt's cases. Both variants may be seen in homosexual males with immunologic abnormalities similar to those described in the acquired immunodeficiency syndrome. In spite of short survival, common to both types, we believe that significant biologic differences between the variants that may be of potential value to the clinician have been demonstrated.

ACKNOWLEDGMENT

This investigation was supported in part by grant CA 19449, awarded by the National Cancer Institute and the Lowell M. Hill, Paul K. Wesler, Mark Clair, and Martin Ward Lymphoma Research Funds.

REFERENCES

Burkitt D. 1958. A sarcoma involving the jaws in African children. Br J Surg 46:218–223.

de-The G, Geser A, Day NE, Tukei PM, William EH, Beri DP, Smith PG, Dean AG, Bornkamm GW, Feorino P, Henle W. 1978. Epidemiological evidence for causal relationship between Epstein-Barr virus and Burkitt's lymphoma from Ugandan prospective study. Nature 274:756–761.

Levine AM, Meyer PR, Begandy MK, Parker JW, Taylor CR, Irwin L, Lukes RJ. 1984. Development of B cell lymphoma in homosexual men: Clinical and immunologic findings. Ann Intern Med 100:7–13.

Levine AM, Pavlova Z, Pockros AW, Parker JW, Teitelbaum AH, Paganini-Hill A, Powars DR, Lukes RJ, Feinstein DI. 1983. Small noncleaved follicular center cell (FCC) lymphoma: Burkitt and Non-Burkitt variants in the United States. I. Clinical Features. Cancer 52:1073–1079.

Lukes RJ, Collins RD. 1974. Immunologic characterization of human malignant lymphomas. Cancer 34:1488–1503.

Non-Hodgkin's Lymphoma Pathology Classification Project. 1982. National Cancer Institute sponsored study of classification of non-Hodgkin's lymphomas: Summary and description of a working formulation for clinical usage. Cancer 49:2112–2135.

Rappaport H. 1966. Tumors of the hematopoietic system. *In* Atlas of Tumor Pathology. Section III, Fascicle 8. Armed Forces Institute of Pathology, Washington, D.C., pp. 97–161.

Ziegler JL. 1981. Burkitt's lymphoma. N Engl J Med 305:735–745.

UT M.D. Anderson Clinical Conference on Cancer,
Vol. 27, edited by R. J. Ford, L. M. Fuller, and
F. B. Hagemeister. Raven Press, New York © 1984.

T-Cell Convoluted/Lymphoblastic Undifferentiated Lymphoma in Adults

Alexandra M. Levine, Paul R. Meyer,* Robert J. Lukes,* and
Donald I. Feinstein

*Division of Hematology, Department of Medicine, and the *Division of Hematopathology,
Department of Pathology, Los Angeles County-University of Southern California Medical
Center, Los Angeles, California 90033*

BACKGROUND

Lymphoblastic lymphoma, also known as convoluted T-cell lymphoma, has been recognized as a distinct clinicopathologic entity for less than a decade. The unique clinical and pathologic characteristics of the disease could not be appreciated in the past, since early cases were classified within the spectra of acute lymphocytic leukemia of childhood and diffuse, poorly differentiated lymphocytic (DPDL) lymphoma of the Rappaport system (Barcos and Lukes 1975, Nathwani et al. 1976).

The classic natural history of this disease may serve to clarify earlier misconceptions. The vast majority of cases are of T-lymphocyte origin, often derived from the mid-thymocyte stage of T-cell differentiation. Presumably, then, it first begins in the thymus, presenting clinically as a mediastinal mass (DPDL lymphoma of Rappaport; Sternberg's sarcoma). From the mediastinum, the disease spreads rapidly and predictably to involve the bone marrow and thereafter, the peripheral blood, such that a picture resembling acute lymphocytic leukemia may become apparent. The distinctive morphologic appearance of this tumor was described by Barcos and Lukes (1975) who noted an irregular and convoluted nuclear outline with primitive nuclear chromatin and inconspicuous nucleoli. Since the malignant cells formed rosettes with sheep erythrocytes and were, presumably, T lymphocytes, the authors descriptively characterized the entity as "convoluted T-cell lymphoma." Later, noting that a minority of cases had nonconvoluted nuclear outlines, Rappaport termed the illness "lymphoblastic lymphoma."

The relationship between convoluted/lymphoblastic lymphoma and T-cell acute lymphocytic leukemia (T-ALL) remains somewhat controversial. Using monoclonal antibodies to characterize the malignant cells from 51 children with T-ALL (50 had greater than 85% replacement of marrow by T lymphoblasts and one had 55% replacement) and 17 children with convoluted/lymphoblastic lymphoma (none had marrow involvement), Roper et al. (1983) found significant overlap between the cases. Of the T-ALL group, approximately one-third had markers of early thymocyte origin (OKT/9$^+$ or OKT/10$^+$), one-third had markers of mid-thymocyte (OKT/6$^+$ or both OKT/4$^+$ and OKT/8$^+$), and one-third had markers of mature T lymphocyte (OKT/3$^+$). None of the convoluted/lymphoblastic cases had markers of early thymocyte derivation, whereas approximately one-half were mid-thymic, and one-half were mature T lymphocytic. Aside from the remarkable overlap in phenotypic expression between the two entities, clinical overlap was noted as well, with no difference in any clinical parameter reported, except marrow and blood involvement in the T-ALL patients.

CLINICAL CHARACTERISTICS

The clinical characteristics of convoluted/lymphoblastic lymphoma, as it occurs in the adult population, have been reported by Rosen et al. (1978) and Nathwani et al. (1976). Additional series reported from various institutions have been remarkably consistent with regard to the clinical characteristics of this disease. The majority of patients are either older children or young adults in the second or third decades of life. The range in age may be great, however, and patients 70 to 80 years old have also been described. The disease is one of male preponderance, as high as 75% of patients described.

The most common presentation in adults is mediastinal mass, occurring in 75% of the cases described by Rosen et al. (1978). In the majority of these patients, initial symptoms were directly attributable to compression of the trachea or esophagus or to pericardial or pleural disease. This tumor is locally invasive within the mediastinum, and it is quite common for affected patients to present with symptoms of an emergent nature, including superior vena caval syndrome, pericarditis, severe dyspnea, or other compromise of vital intrathoracic structures.

Aside from mediastinal disease, adult patients may first seek medical attention with symptoms and signs related to bone marrow infiltration and overt leukemia. Of the 12 patients reported by Rosen et al. (1978), approximately 40% presented with frank leukemia, while an additional 20% had marrow involvement, although an overt leukemic picture was absent at diagnosis. The peripheral white blood cell count in these patients may be extremely high, with counts in excess of 200,000/μl. Interestingly, the hemoglobin and platelet counts, although depressed, may be higher than one would expect from the degree of hyperleukocytosis.

Aside from prominent mediastinal and marrow involvement, one third of the patients reported by Rosen et al. (1978) had central nervous system (CNS) involvement some time during the course of illness. Symptoms and signs related to CNS involvement may include headache, cranial nerve palsy, increased intracranial pressure, or mass lesion in the cerebrum. Involvement of the CNS may, at times, be asymptomatic and diagnosis might only be made at the time of the spinal tap for administration of prophylactic intrathecal chemotherapy.

Clinically, the disease appears to be fairly consistent in its presentation. Most adult patients present either with mediastinal masses, leukemic marrow infiltration, or both. Depending on the presentation, the case may be characterized as a lymphoma or a leukemia. Mediastinal involvement is frequently associated with medical emergencies, and occasionally, the situation in these patients is so critical that adequate tissue for diagnosis cannot be procured until the clinical status is stabilized by pericardiocentesis, radiotherapy, or other such measures. The CNS becomes involved in a significant number of cases, especially those with diffuse marrow infiltration. Because the tumor disseminates so predictably and rapidly, routine staging procedures are of no use in devising therapeutic plans for treating individual patients. These patients must be considered to have widely disseminated disease at diagnosis and must be treated accordingly. In the series reported by Rosen et al. (1978), patients were treated with combinations of radiation therapy, as well as cyclophosphamide, vincristine, prednisone, doxorubicin, and bleomycin. The initial response in these patients was very dramatic. Rapid tumor regression led, in some instances, to metabolic complications of tumor lysis. However, even though these patients responded rapidly they also relapsed rapidly, and overall median survival in most reported series has been in the range of one year.

THERAPEUTIC CONSIDERATIONS

Because of the proclivity for bone marrow and CNS involvement in this disease, patients with convoluted/lymphoblastic lymphoma should be treated with systemic therapy, probably similar to that employed for childhood leukemia and lymphoma, with the early inclusion of prophylactic CNS therapy. Several such therapeutic approaches have recently been reported, and results from these initial trials indicate a significant change in the overall prognosis of these patients.

Weinstein et al. (1983) recently updated the results of the APO regimen (doxorubicin, prednisone, and vincristine) administered to 21 pediatric patients whose median age was 13 years (range 2.5 to 22 years). Treatment continued for two years, consisting of a modified ALL regimen, including doxorubicin, preventative cranial irradiation, and intrathecal methotrexate. Complete remission was attained in 20 patients, although 3 required mediastinal irradiation in order to achieve complete remission. With median follow-up of six years, the actuarial method of Kaplan and Meier showed an estimate of disease-free survival at three years of 58%. Six of the 20 complete responders have relapsed, including three with CNS disease and two with testicular disease. Patients with bone marrow involvement (T-ALL) were excluded from this series.

Coleman et al. (1981) recently reported results of a one-year treatment protocol administered to 13 adult patients with lymphoblastic lymphoma and a fourteenth patient who was considered to have T-ALL. A modified CHOP (cyclophosphamide, doxorubicin, vincristine, prednisone) induction regimen was employed and was followed by consolidation and CNS prophylaxis, which consisted of L-asparaginase, high-dose systemic methotrexate, and intrathecal methotrexate. Maintenance phase consisted of daily mercaptopurine and weekly methotrexate, patterned after maintenance for childhood ALL, and continued for one year. At three years, the actuarial survival rate was 61% for the group and a relapse-free survival rate of 56%. Although high-dose methotrexate was administered in these patients, relapse of disease in the CNS occurred in 3 of 13, causing the investigators to modify their regimen to include earlier prophylaxis to the CNS and to include radiotherapy to this site.

At the University of Southern California, Levine et al. (1983) reported on 15 adult patients with convoluted/lymphoblastic lymphoma who were treated with an aggressive regimen, modified from the LSA_2-L_2 protocol used for childhood lymphoma developed by Wollner et al. (1976,1979). The treatment schema consisted of an induction phase, including cyclophosphamide, vincristine, prednisone, and doxorubicin and 2,000 rad to the mediastinum, as well as intrathecal methotrexate, given as early as day one of therapy. The consolidation phase included cytosine arabinoside, 6-thioguanine, L-asparaginase, and CCNU (chloroethyl cyclohexyl nitrosourea), along with cranial irradiation and further intrathecal methotrexate. The maintenance phase consisted of cyclical chemotherapy and intrathecal methotrexate, continuing for a total of three years. The median age in the group was 25 years (range 16–73 years). There were eight males and seven females. At diagnosis, nine patients had mediastinal involvement, and nine had bone marrow involvement. Five of these (one-third of the entire group) demonstrated malignant cells in the peripheral blood (median white blood cell count of 121,000/μl) and would have been classified as having T-ALL by some investigators. Complete clinical response was attained in 11 patients (73%), including 4 of the 5 patients with leukemic presentations. Three patients achieved partial response (Levine et al. 1983). With median follow-up of 24 months (range 7 to more than 85 months), the median survival for the group was 27.9 months, while median survival for complete responders was 41.8 months, and median relapse-free survival for complete responders was 37.3 months. Relapse of disease has occurred in five complete responders, including two of the four completely responding patients with initial leukemic pictures. Sites of relapse included CNS in one (who had refused cranial irradiation), CNS and bone marrow in two, and nodal sites in one. The bone marrow was the site in one patient who presented with overt leukemia and relapsed at 42 months, 6 months after cessation of all therapy. Of the five patients who had frank leukemia at diagnosis, only one remains alive at more than 16 months from diagnosis. Two patients relapsed and subsequently died (17 and 46 months from diagnosis). One patient died of *Candida tropicalis* meningitis 11 months after diagnosis and had no evidence of lymphoma at autopsy. This patient experienced intracerebral hemorrhage at the time of diagnosis, requiring emergency neurosurgery and ventriculostomy. At that time, her peripheral white blood cell count was 368,000/μl. One patient never achieved complete remission and died 14 months after diagnosis.

At the University of Southern California, the current therapeutic protocol for patients with convoluted/lymphoblastic lymphoma and T-ALL includes high dose cytosine arabinoside, vincristine, prednisone, and L-asparaginase, given in the induction phase. It is followed by cranial irradiation and intrathecal cytosine arabinoside, as continued CNS prophylaxis. The consolidation phase consists of CHOP with continued intrathecal cytosine arabinoside. The maintenance phase consists of 6 mercaptopurine and oral, weekly methotrexate, which is given for a total treatment period of two years.

In patients who are refractory to the newer regimens, several therapeutic options may still be available. Russell et al. (1981) have described the successful use of 2' deoxycoformycin in four patients with resistant T-ALL. Antithymocyte globulin was reported to be effective in inducing a partial remission in one patient (Wong et al. 1982). O'Leary et al. (1983) and Kaizer et al. (1982) reported the successful use of bone marrow transplantation, when performed at the time of complete remission status, in a few refractory patients.

In summary, convoluted/lymphoblastic lymphoma is a very distinct clinicopathologic entity. Its diagnosis implies widely disseminated disease, in spite of apparent localization. The prognosis has been quite poor with conventional therapeutic approaches. The median survival has been in the range of one year. With aggressive therapeutic regimens, similar to those used in childhood lymphoma and leukemia, and with early institution of prophylactic therapy to the CNS, long-term, disease-free survival may be expected in the majority of patients. Prior classifications place this disease into the category of diffuse poorly differentiated lymphocytic lymphoma, diffuse undifferentiated lymphoma, or acute lymphocytic leukemia and therefore, would not alert the clinician to the distinctive natural history, course, or response to therapy.

ACKNOWLEDGMENT

This investigation was supported in part by grant CA 14674, PO1 CA 19449-01, and TO 1 CA 05205; GM 06905 (USPHS), awarded by the National Cancer Institute and the Lowell M. Hill Leukemia Research Fund.

REFERENCES

Barcos MQP, Lukes RJ. 1975. Malignant lymphoma of convoluted lymphocytes. A new entity of possible T-cell type. *In* Sinks LF, Godden JO, eds., Conflicts in Childhood Cancer, vol. 4. Allan R. Liss, Inc., New York, pp. 147–178.

Coleman CN, Cohen JR, Rosenberg SA. 1981. Adult lymphoblastic lymphoma—results of a pilot therapy protocol. Blood 57:679–684.

Kaizer H, Levy R, Cote JP, Johnson RJ, Fuller D, Santos GW. 1982. Autologous bone marrow transplantation in lymphoblastic lymphoma and T-ALL. Blood 60:169a.

Levine AM, Forman SJ, Meyer PR, Koehler SC, Liebman H, Paganini-Hill A, Pockros A, Lukes RJ, Feinstein DI. 1983. Successful therapy of convoluted T-lymphoblastic lymphoma in the adult. Blood 61:92–98.

Levine AM, Koehler S, Meyer PR, Forman SJ, Feinstein DI. 1983. Successful therapy of convoluted lymphocytic lymphoma (lymphoblastic lymphoma) in adults: A pilot study. Blood 57:679.

Nathwani BN, Kim H, Rappaport H. 1976. Malignant lymphoma, lymphoblastic. Cancer 38:964–983.

O'Leary M, Ramsay NKC, Nesbit ME, Hurd D, Woods WG, Krivit W, Kim TH, McGlave P, Kersey J. 1983. Bone marrow transplantation for non-Hodgkin's lymphoma in children and young adults. A pilot study. Am J Med 74:497–501.

Roper M, Crist WM, Metzgar R, Ragab AH, Smith S, Starling K, Pullen J, Leventhal B, Bartolucci AA, Cooper MD. 1983. Monoclonal antibody characterization of surface antigens in childhood T-cell lymphoid malignancies. Blood 61:830–837.

Rosen PJ, Feinstein DI, Pattengale PK, Tindle BH, Williams AH, Cain MJ, Bonorris JB, Parker JW, Lukes RJ. 1978. Convoluted lymphocytic lymphoma in adults: A clinicopathologic entity. Ann Intern Med 89:319–324.

Russell NH, Prentice HG, Lee N, Piga A, Ganeshaguru K, Smyth JF, Hoffbrand AV. 1981. Studies on the biochemical sequelae of therapy in Thy-ALL with adenosine deaminase inhibitor 2′deoxycoformycin. Br J Haematol 49:1–9.

Weinstein HJ, Cassady JR, Levey R. 1983. Long-term results of the APO Protocol (Vincristine, Doxorubicin (Adriamycin) and Prednisone) for treatment of mediastinal lymphoblastic lymphoma. J Clin Oncol 1:537–541.

Wollner N, Burchenal JH, Lieberman PH, Exelby P, D'Angio G, Murphy ML. 1976. Non-Hodgkin's lymphoma in children: A comparative study of two modalities of therapy. Cancer 37:123–134.

Wollner N, Burchenal JH, Lieberman PH, Exelby P, D'Angio G, Murphy ML. 1979. Non-Hodgkin's lymphoma in children: A progress report on the original patients treated with the LSA$_2$-L$_2$ protocol. Cancer 44:1990–1999.

Wong KK, Sweet DL, Variakogis D. 1982. The treatment of lymphoblastic lymphoma with anti-thymocyte globulin. Cancer 50:57.

UT M.D. Anderson Clinical Conference on Cancer,
Vol. 27, edited by R. J. Ford, L. M. Fuller, and
F. B. Hagemeister. Raven Press, New York © 1984.

Initial Chemotherapy for Clinically Staged Localized Non-Hodgkin's Lymphomas of Unfavorable Histology

Thomas P. Miller and Stephen E. Jones

Section of Hematology/Oncology, Department of Medicine, and the Cancer Center at the University of Arizona, and the Veterans Administration Hospital, Tucson, Arizona 85724

The strategy for the initial treatment of patients with localized diffuse non-Hodgkin's lymphoma of unfavorable histology is controversial (Miller and Jones 1980). Traditionally, patients with stages I and II disease have received initial treatment with radiotherapy (RT) alone with modest success (Chen et al. 1979, Jones et al. 1973). Carefully selecting patients by means of vigorous staging techniques, including laparotomy, has improved the results of RT for a small group of patients with very localized (stage I) disease (Levitt et al. 1980, Sweet et al. 1981). Adjuvant chemotherapy (ChT) has been used in an attempt to improve upon the results of RT alone and has had mixed results (Bonadonna et al. 1979, Glatstein et al. 1977, Landberg et al. 1979). Less than satisfactory results with adjuvant ChT are probably related to the delay in initiating systemic treatment for a disease with a known propensity for early hematogenous spread and to the use of relatively ineffective ChT regimens (Miller and Jones 1980).

In 1979, we reported our early results of treatment for localized diffuse lymphomas using initial doxorubicin-containing drug combinations (Miller and Jones 1979). The strategy of using combination ChT as initial therapy resulted in continuous disease-free survival for 21 of 22 patients during a median follow-up time of 27 months. Cabanillas et al. (1980) have obtained comparable results in a series of 30 patients. In this chapter we are updating our experience, which now includes 49 patients with localized lymphoma and a median follow-up time of 41 months.

PATIENTS AND METHODS

Between November, 1971 and November, 1983, 49 patients were treated for localized non-Hodgkin's lymphoma with initial ChT. Analysis of the data is available through July 1, 1983.

The original biopsy material was classified according to the new Working Formulation (Non-Hodgkin's Pathologic Classification Project 1982) and showed the following histologic distribution: 47 patients had diffuse large cell lymphoma, and

2 patients had follicular large cell lymphoma. In all patients, disease was clinically staged and classified according to the criteria of the Ann Arbor symposium. The clinical evaluation included a physical examination, complete blood counts and chemistries, chest radiographs, and bone marrow biopsies and aspirate. Lymphangiograms were performed on all patients prior to 1977. Since 1977, patients received either a lymphangiogram, computed tomographic (CT) scan, or ultrasonic examination of the abdomen and pelvis. Radionuclide scans of the liver and spleen or bone were performed if symptoms or serum enzymes suggested disease involvement. Laparotomies were performed on 13 patients in order to establish the histologic diagnosis. Surgery did not include significant tumor resection or thorough pathologic staging in most patients.

All patients received intensive initial induction therapy with combination ChT. Thirty patients received ChT as the only therapy, and 19 patients received combination ChT and RT. In this nonrandomized pilot study, patients were assigned treatment with ChT alone or ChT and RT on the basis of bone marrow reserve and tumor response to initial ChT. Patients who required reduction in the dose rate of ChT (usually older than 65 years) or failed to achieve a complete response (CR) after three courses of initial ChT were treated with ChT and RT. Forty-eight of 49 patients received ChT with the doxorubicin-containing drug regimen CHOP (cyclophosphamide, doxorubicin, vincristine, and prednisone) (McKelvey et al. 1976). The ChT was repeated every 21 days. A single patient received combination ChT without doxorubicin because of preexisting heart disease. Patients treated with ChT alone received between 6 and 11 courses of CHOP. Patients treated with both ChT and RT received between two and eight courses of CHOP. These patients were treated with involved field RT with a minimum dose of 3,600 rad (range 3,600–6,000 rad). Patients were not excluded from treatment on the basis of age or surgical risk.

At the completion of therapy, disease in all patients was restaged with particular attention to reassessing initially involved sites. Patients were classified as having achieved CR when there was no objective evidence of residual tumor or subjective symptoms of persistent disease. Following restaging no additional therapy was administered.

Survival was measured from the time of diagnosis until the date of last contact or death. Relapse-free survival (RFS) was measured from the completion of all therapy until the time of relapse or last contact. The actuarial method of Kaplan and Meier (1958) was used to plot survival and RFS curves. Comparisons were made using Gehan's modification (1965) of the Wilcoxon two-tailed test.

RESULTS

The clinical characteristics and results of treatment of these 49 patients are summarized in Table 1. Thirty-one patients (63%) had stage II disease. Potentially adverse prognostic features, including B symptoms, extranodal disease, gastrointestinal tract involvement, bulky disease, and age greater than 65 years, were

Table 1. *Clinical Features and Results of Treatment of 49 Patients with Localized Lymphoma*

Clinical feature	Chemotherapy alone		Chemotherapy and radiotherapy	
	No. patients	No. relapses	No. patients	No. relapses
Male/female	15/15	2/4	11/8	1/1
Stage I	6	1	3	0
Stage IE	5	1	4	0
Stage II	11	3	2	1
Stage IIE	8	1	10	0
B symptoms	1	1	2	0
Gastrointestinal involvement	4	0	2	1
Disease above/below diaphragm	18/12	3/3	14/5	1/1
Bulky disease*	7	1	8	1
Older than 65 years	7	1	7	1

*Bulky disease = mass 7 cm in greatest diameter.

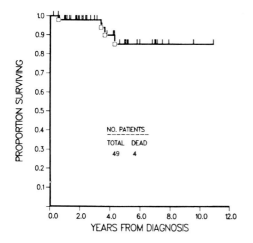

Figure 1. Actuarial survival for 49 patients with localized non-Hodgkin's lymphoma from the time of diagnosis.

common in this group (Table 1). For 30 patients treated with ChT alone, the median age was 57 (range 24–85) years, and for 19 patients treated with ChT and RT was 61 (range 25–86) years.

Forty-eight of 49 patients achieved complete response. One patient with stage IIE disease involving the mesentary and spleen achieved a partial response while receiving CHOP ChT but developed progressive disease while receiving involved field RT. Actuarial survival and RFS are indicated in Figures 1 and 2. One patient is currently receiving therapy. Forty-five patients (92%) were alive with a median follow-up time of 41 months (range 3–131). Forty-one patients (84%) remained continuously free of disease with a median follow-up time from completing therapy of 34 months. Survival and RFS at two years are not statistically different after

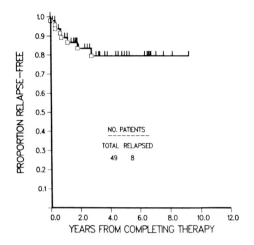

Figure 2. Actuarial relapse-free survival of 49 patients with localized non-Hodgkin's lymphoma from the time of completing therapy.

Table 2. *Survival and Relapse-Free Survival (RFS) of 49 Patients with Localized Lymphoma*

Clinical feature	No. patients	Survival (%)*	P value	RFS (%)*	P value
All	49	96	—	86	—
Chemotherapy alone	30	96		76	
Chemotherapy + radiotherapy	19	95	>0.96	92	>0.07
Stage I	18	100	0.21	77	0.92
Stage II	31	94		84	
Extranodal disease present	27	96		88	
Extranodal disease absent	22	94	0.59	77	0.35
Bulky disease present	25	93	0.51	86	0.82
Bulky disease absent	34	97		84	
Older than 65 years	14	100	0.30	82	0.73
Younger than 65 years	35	94		84	

*Actuarial survival and RFS measured at 2 years.

comparing the following variables: 1) type of treatment, 2) stage, 3) extranodal disease, 4) bulky disease, and 5) age (Table 2).

Eight patients failed treatment. Six of 30 patients (20%) failed treatment with ChT alone. These patients have suffered recurrence at distant as well as at initially involved sites. Two of 19 patients (11%) failed treatment with initial ChT followed by involved field RT. Both of these patients suffered recurrence within the previously irradiated field. Only 2 of 14 patients (14%) who were older than 65 years at the time of diagnosis have relapsed. This older group of 14 patients has, in general, received less intensive initial ChT with CHOP. Patients relapsing after initial treatment have been retreated with either ChT or RT. Five of eight patients achieved second complete remissions. Four patients were alive and remained disease free from the time of their second treatment (6 +, 14 +, 35 +, and 36 + months).

The toxicity and side effects of treatment were generally mild and manageable. Leukopenia was moderate but uncomplicated by serious infection. Nausea, vomiting, and hair loss were common but did not interrupt therapy. No cardiotoxicity resulting from doxorubicin has been observed.

DISCUSSION

The results of this study indicate that initial systemic ChT with doxorubicin-containing regimen is an effective treatment strategy for patients with clinically apparent localized lymphomas of unfavorable histology. Furthermore, treatment with effective initial ChT obviates the need for extensive surgical staging. We have included two patients with minimally nodular large cell lymphomas in this series, based on reports that this variant probably has the same potential for cure (Osborne et al. 1979, Jones et al. 1973).

Traditionally, patients with localized large cell lymphomas have been treated with RT alone, and 45%–50% of patients remain free of disease two years after treatment (Jones et al. 1973, Chen et al. 1979). The failure of RT alone probably relates to several clinical features of the disease. First, the large cell lymphomas are a high growth fraction tumor with a propensity for early and unpredictable hematogenous spread. This feature is clinically appreciated in the fact that approximately 10% of patients with clinically localized large cell lymphomas will have detectable intraabdominal disease at laparotomy (Goffinet et al. 1977) and in the observation that as many as 20% of patients treated with initial RT will develop new disease outside of the RT ports while receiving RT (Bajetta et al. 1983). Second, there is no clear-cut dose-response relationship of the non-Hodgkin's lymphomas to RT (Fuks and Kaplan 1973).

Results with RT can be improved by careful selection of patients. Aggressive surgical staging, including laparotomy, has improved the results of treatment with radiation alone, presumably by eliminating those patients with occult intraabdominal disease from analysis (Sweet et al. 1981, Glatstein et al. 1977). If, after staging laparotomy, patients are further selected to include only those with stage I disease, the results of RT alone will be quite good, and greater than 90% of these patients will remain free of disease (Sweet et al. 1981, Levitt 1980). Unfortunately, such rigorous selection results in treatment of only a very small proportion of patients who have stage I disease. Surgical staging is generally restricted to patients younger than 65 years, but diffuse large cell lymphomas are common in older patients. In this series, 14 of 49 patients (29%) were older than 65 years and would have been excluded from most RT series that used laparotomy to select patients.

Analysis of initial sites of relapse of the eight patients failing to respond to treatment with initial ChT does not help to identify a single weakness in treatment strategy. Two patients first treated with CHOP followed by involved field RT, initially relapsed at distant sites outside the radiation treatment ports. Four of six relapsing patients who were treated with ChT alone initially developed new disease outside the RT ports. In these patients, it seems unlikely that RT to the initial sites

Table 3. *Treatment of Stage II Lymphoma of Unfavorable Histology Series Using Aggressive Initial Chemotherapy*

Author	Treatment	Complete response (%)	Disease-free survival %
Miller, Jones, current series	CHOP ± RT	30/31 (97)	84
Cabanillas et al. 1980	CHOP	19/22 (86)	79
Skarin et al. 1983*	M-BACOD	13/15 (87)	80
Fisher et al. 1983	ProMACE/MOPP	14/17 (82)	+
Bajetta et al. 1983	BACOP + RT	62/64 (97)	81

*Includes two patients with stage IE disease
+ Not available.
M-BACOD-methotrexate, bleomycin, doxorubicin, cyclophosphamide, vincristine, and decadron; ProMace/MOPP-cyclophosphamide, doxorubicin, etoposide, and methotrexate plus mechlorethamine, vincristine, procarbazine, and prednisone; BACOP-bleomycin, doxorubicin, cyclophosphamide, vincristine, and prednisone.

of disease involvement would have prevented relapse of an apparently systemic disease. Two of six relapsing patients who were treated with ChT alone initially relapsed at the first site of disease involvement. Additional RT might have prevented these failures.

Recently, several series have been reported using ChT of proven curative potential as initial therapy for patients with localized lymphomas (Table 3). These series demonstrate remarkably consistent results. The complete response rates vary from 82%–87% among three series using ChT alone and approach 100% in series using combined ChT and RT. In addition, the percentage of patients remaining free of disease varies within exceptionally small limits (79%–84%) among the four series where disease-free survival is reported.

Initial treatment for localized diffuse large cell lymphoma with ChT regimens of proven curative potential in advanced disease is a successful treatment strategy and obviates the need for extensive surgical staging. However, surgical staging and treatment with RT alone appears to be an equally effective treatment alternative for the unusual patient with documented stage I or IE disease (Sweet et al. 1981, Levitt et al. 1980). The side effects and toxicities, including potential delayed complications of aggressive ChT, must be weighed and compared to the risks and morbidity of surgical staging, with its necessary delay in initiating treatment, in determining the best approach to patients with stage I disease. Patients with stage II disease, whether surgically or clinically determined, appear to benefit from initial ChT, with or without additional RT, compared to previous studies using initial RT. The optimal amount of initial systemic chemotherapy that is effective for the majority of patients remains to be defined. Prognostic factors that would predict drug and RT resistance in a minority of patients have to be identified.

ACKNOWLEDGMENT

This investigation was supported in part by grant CA 17094 awarded by the National Cancer Institute, United States Department of Health and Human Services.

REFERENCES

Bajetta E, Buzzoni R, Lattuada A, Valagussa P, Bonadonna G. 1983. Combined chemotherapy (CVP vs BACOP)—radiotherapy in PS I-II diffuse non-Hodgkin's lymphomas. (Abstract) Proceedings of the American Society of Clinical Oncology 2:223.

Bonadonna G, Lattuada A, Monfardini S, Milani F, Banfi A. 1979. Combined radiotherapy-chemotherapy in localized non-Hodgkin's lymphomas: 5-year results of a randomized study. *In* Jones SE, Salmon SE, eds., Adjuvant Therapy of Cancer II. Grune & Stratton, New York, pp. 145–153.

Cabanillas F, Bodey GP, Freireich EJ. 1980. Management with chemotherapy only of stage I and II malignant lymphoma of aggressive histologic types. Cancer 46:2356–2359.

Chen MG, Prosnitz LR, Gonzales-Serva A, Fischer DB. 1979. Results of radiotherapy in control of Stage I and II non-Hodgkin's Lymphoma. Cancer 43:1245–1254.

Fisher RI, DeVita VT, Hubbard SM, Longo DL, Wesley R, Chabner BA, Young RC. 1983. Diffuse aggressive lymphomas: Increased survival after alternating flexible sequences of ProMACE and MOPP chemotherapy. Ann Intern Med 98:304–309.

Fuks Z, Kaplan HS. 1973. Recurrence rates following therapy of nodular and diffuse malignant lymphomas. Radiology 108:675–684.

Glatstein E, Portlock C, Rosenberg SA, Kaplan HS. 1977. Combined modality treatment in the malignant lymphomas. *In* Salmon SE, Jones SE, eds., Adjuvant Therapy of Cancer. North Holland, New York, pp. 545–548.

Gehan EA. 1965. A generalized Wilcoxon test for comparing arbitrarily singly-censored samples. Biometrika 52:203–223.

Goffinet DR, Warnke R, Dunnick NR, Castellino R, Glatstein E, Nelsen TS, Dorfman RF, Rosenberg SA, Kaplan HS. 1977. Clinical and surgical (laparotomy) evaluation of patients with non-Hodgkin's lymphoma. Cancer Treat Rep 61:981–992.

Jones SE, Fuks Z, Kaplan HS, Rosenberg SA. 1973. Non-Hodgkin's lymphomas V. Results of radiotherapy. Cancer 32:682–691.

Kaplan EL, Meier P. 1958. Nonparametric estimation for incomplete observations. Journal of the American Statistical Association 53:457–481.

Landberg TG, Hakansson LG, Moller TR, Mattsson WKI, Landys KE, Johansson BG, Killander DCF, Molin BF, Westing PF, Lennet PH, Dahl OG. 1979. CVP-remission-maintenance in Stage I or II non-Hodgkin's lymphomas. Preliminary results of a randomized study. Cancer 44:831–838.

Levitt SH, Bloomfield CD, Frizzera G, Lee CKK. 1980. Curative radiotherapy for localized diffuse histiocytic lymphoma. Cancer Treat Rep 64:175–177.

McKelvey EM, Gottlieb JA, Wilson HE, Haut A, Talley RW, Stephens R, Lane M, Gamble JF, Jones SE, Grozea PN, Gutterman J, Coltman C, Moon TE. 1976. Hydroxyldaunomycin (adriamycin) combination chemotherapy in malignant lymphoma. Cancer 38:1484–1493.

Miller TP, Jones SE. 1980. Is there a role for radiotherapy in localized diffuse lymphomas? Cancer Chemother Pharmacol 4:67–70.

Miller TP, Jones SE. 1979. Chemotherapy of localized histiocytic lymphoma. Lancet 1:358–360.

Non-Hodgkin's Lymphoma Pathologic Classification Project. 1982. National Cancer Institute sponsored study of classifications of non-Hodgkin's lymphomas: Summary and description of a working formulation for clinical usage. Cancer 49:2112–2135.

Osborne CK, Merrill JM, Garvin AS, DeVita VT, Young RC. 1979. Nodular histiocytic lymphoma. An aggressive nodular lymphoma with potential for long term survival. (Abstract) Proceedings of the American Society of Clinical Oncology 20:442.

Skarin AT, Canellos GP, Rosenthal DS, Case DC, MacIntyre JM, Pinkus GS, Moloney WC, Frei E. 1983. Improved prognosis of diffuse histiocytic and undifferentiated lymphoma by use of high dose methotrexate alternating with standard agents (M-BACOD). Journal of Clinical Oncology 1:91–98.

Sweet DL, Kinzie J, Gaeke ME, Golomb HM, Ferguson DL, Ultmann JE. 1981. Survival of patients with localized diffuse histiocytic lymphoma. Blood 58:1218–1223.

UT M.D. Anderson Clinical Conference on Cancer,
Vol. 27, edited by R. J. Ford, L. M. Fuller, and
F. B. Hagemeister. Raven Press, New York © 1984.

Extranodal Lymphomas of the Stomach and Head and Neck

Lillian M. Fuller, Moshe H. Maor, Joseph S. Kong,
K. Thomas Robbins,* Mark C. Vlasak,† and
William S. Velasquez‡

*Departments of Clinical Radiotherapy and ‡Hematology, The University of Texas M. D.
Anderson Hospital and Tumor Institute at Houston, Houston, Texas 77030; *Department
of Otolaryngology Head and Neck Surgery, The University of Texas Medical School
at Houston, Houston, Texas 77030; and †Scott and White Memorial Hospital,
Temple, Texas 76501*

For more than three decades, our approach to the management of extranodal presentations of non-Hodgkin's lymphomas, stages IE and IIE, has included intensive radiotherapy for permanent control of the primary disease. This consistency of treatment has allowed us to compare differences in results according to histopathology, sequential staging, and combined modality treatment programs.

Early in the 1970s, we reported that radiotherapy results for localized extranodal presentations of diffuse lymphomas were related to both the clinical presentation and the status of adjacent lymph nodes (Fuller et al. 1975). In this study, the disease in approximately one half of the patients was staged by lymphangiography. For stage IE upper torso presentations, the majority of which originated in the head and neck region, the five-year survival figure was 52%; for stage IIE disease it was only 15%. For patients with lower torso presentations, it was generally not possible to distinguish between stage IE and IIE disease. However, the combined result for the two stages was only 30% (Figure 1). Most of these patients with stages IE and IIE disease had diffuse large cell lymphomas. A further analysis, by disease site, of response to radiotherapy demonstrated that the incidence of local control was also related to the location of the disease. Upper torso disease could generally be eradicated with intensive radiotherapy. However, the possibility of eliminating lower torso disease was dependent on the extensiveness of the involvement. Large abdominal masses were seldom controlled.

These results and the introduction of staging laparotomy in 1970 stimulated us to determine whether more precise staging, including laparotomy, could identify patients with truly localized upper torso disease who could be cured with regional radiotherapy. Because of our poor experience in controlling abdominal disease with radiotherapy alone we devised a combined modality program for lower torso presentations. The choice of combination chemotherapy was based on our experience

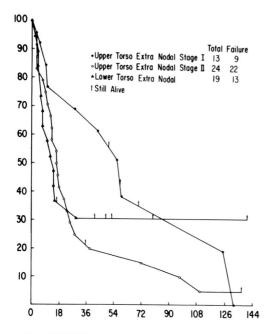

Figure 1. Survival curves for extranodal stage I versus stage II upper torso presentations and for the combined group of stage I and stage II lower torso presentations of diffuse histiocytic lymphomata. (Reproduced from Fuller et al. 1975, with permission of The Macmillan Press Ltd.)

(Within figure)

	Total	Failure
•Upper Torso Extra Nodal Stage I	13	9
∘Upper Torso Extra Nodal Stage II	24	22
▲Lower Torso Extra Nodal	19	13
↑ Still Alive		

with CHOP-Bleo (cyclophosphamide, doxorubicin, vincristine, prednisone, and bleomycin) in generalized disease (Rodriguez et al. 1977). Our plan was to give sequentially, four cycles of CHOP-Bleo, localized radiotherapy, another four cycles of CHOP-Bleo, and finally, four cycles of COP (cyclophosphamide, vincristine, and prednisone). Results of our combined modality program were gratifying. The five-year disease-free survival rate for patients with extranodal abdominal disease was 80% (Lester et al. 1982).

LAPAROTOMY-STAGED IE AND IIE UPPER TORSO DISEASE PRESENTATIONS

In most patients with extranodal upper torso presentations, the disease originated in the head and neck region. Despite a negative staging laparotomy, results in terms of both survival and disease-free survival were related again to the stage or status of adjacent lymph node regions. For 10 patients with stage IE head and neck disease who were treated with involved field (IF) radiotherapy only, the disease-free survival rate was 100%. The corresponding figure for stage IIE disease was only 60%. Also, the disease-free figure for patients with disease limited to the cervical nodes (eight stage I disease and one stage II disease patients) was only 39% (Lester et al. 1982).

Since these results were based on only 27 patients with head and neck disease, it was not possible to draw definite conclusions from these data. Moreover, in the majority of non-Hodgkin's lymphoma patients, who are generally elderly, laparotomy is impractical for staging the extent of this disease. In a retrospective review, we found that the mean age of 138 patients with stage IE and stage IIE Waldeyer's ring disease was 57 years. Also, approximately one half of these patients were outside of the 60 to 65 year age limit for elective staging laparotomy. Further, our yield of positive abdominal findings was relatively low, less than 20% for stages IE and IIE extranodal diffuse large cell lymphomas of the upper torso (Heifetz et al. 1980).

There is very little information on the relative incidence of localized extranodal to nodal presentations of diffuse lymphomas after sequential staging, exclusive of staging laparotomy. In our experience over the past 10 years, approximately 43% of all patients with localized disease had extranodal involvement (Table 1). More than one half of these patients presented with extranodal disease in the head and neck region, and Waldeyer's ring was the most common site (Table 2).

Currently, most patients with localized presentations of diffuse large cell lymphomas, including those with stage IE disease, are treated on our combined modality program. To determine to what extent combined modality treatment has improved results over radiotherapy alone, we initiated a retrospective review for all extranodal sites. This review included patients who were admitted to UT M.D. Anderson Hospital between 1947 and 1981. Eligibility for this study was determined by

Table 1. *Non-Hodgkin's Lymphomas: Incidence of Extranodal Stages IE-IIE and Nodal Stages I-II Disease Presentations 1974–1984*

Extranodal cases	226	
Head and neck	122	54%
Stomach	40	18%
Bone	16	
Reproductive		
Female	14	
Male	14	
Skin/soft tissues	6	28%
Breast	5	
Central nervous system	2	
Miscellaneous	7	
Nodal cases	229	
Total	525	

Table 2. *Extranodal Head and Neck Sites Stages IE and IIE Non-Hodgkin's Lymphomas— 1974–1984*

	Patients	Stage IE	Stage IIE
Waldeyer's ring	76	26	50
Paranasal sinuses	24	20	4
Thyroid	18	6	12
Miscellaneous	4	4	—
Total	122	56	66

whether sufficient pathologic material could be obtained for review and reclassification. Because of recent reports of surgical results for gastric lymphomas we decided to begin by reviewing our results for lymphomas of the stomach. Since then we have analyzed our results for the paranasal sinuses and for Waldeyer's ring. Currently, we are in the process of reviewing our results for the more unusual presentations.

GASTRIC LYMPHOMAS

Long-term survival figures ranging from 50% to 75% have been reported for gastric lymphomas following resection, with or without radiotherapy (Fleming et al. 1982, Brooks and Enterline 1983, Gospodarowicz et al. 1983). However, results for unresectable disease, which account for approximately one third of most series (Fleming et al. 1982, Connors and Wise 1974), have been uniformly poor. Also, the incidence of postoperative deaths has been on the order of 10% to 18% (Weingrad et al. 1982, Naqvi et al. 1969). Regardless of treatment, our five-year survival rate for 79 patients with Ann Arbor stage IE and IIE disease, for whom sufficient material was available for review and reclassification, has been 56% (Figure 2). Results for 35 patients with stage IE disease were 76% as compared with 42% for 44 patients with stage IIE disease. Although resectability influenced results, our best survival rate of 100% was obtained in patients who were treated during the past 10 years with combination chemotherapy and radiotherapy, with or without primary resection (Maor et al. 1984).

Traditionally, gastrectomy has been advocated as the first therapeutic step for patients with primary lymphoma of the stomach. The following are claimed to be advantages for this approach: a large specimen for histologic interpretation as compared with fragments obtained at endoscopic examination; immediate relief of

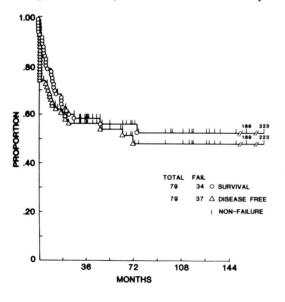

Figure 2. Survival and disease-free survival in patients with gastric lymphomas. (Reproduced from Maor et al. 1984, with permission of *Cancer*).

symptoms; more accurate staging; and a significant survival for patients treated with surgery alone. Also, the specter of perforation or hemorrhage during chemotherapy or radiotherapy has been cited as an additional reason to use surgery as the initial treatment (Hande et al. 1978). These reasons for favoring primary laparotomy and gastrectomy need to be reevaluated in the light of developments in medical technology and treatment during the past 20 years; the most important of these are the fiberscope, lymphangiography, computerized tomography (CT), megavoltage irradiation, and combination chemotherapy.

Treatment

During our earlier experience, gastrectomy was performed whenever possible as the first definitive step in the treatment of stomach malignancies, regardless of the eventual diagnosis. Forty-two patients had gastrectomy for lymphoma. In another 24, the disease was unresectable at laparotomy. Of the total group of 66 patients who had laparotomy, gastrectomy was generally feasible in those with stage IE lesions. However, in approximately half of the patients with stage IIE involvement, the diseased stomach could not be resected. Regardless of whether gastrectomy was feasible, the majority of these patients were treated with radiotherapy. A few received chemotherapy only or in combination with radiotherapy. Chemotherapy consisted of single agents, COP, and later, CHOP-Bleo. In seven of these patients who were treated with chemotherapy and radiotherapy, the chemotherapy was CHOP-Bleo. During the later years when the flexible fiberscope was available and the technique of endoscopic biopsy was perfected, 13 patients had endoscopic biopsy as their only surgical procedure (Table 3). Six of these patients were treated on our CHOP-Bleo and radiotherapy protocol.

In undertaking a retrospective review, we had three primary goals. One was to ascertain the feasibility and accuracy of endoscopic biopsies. A second was to determine our past results for patients who had gastrectomy and those who did not. The third was to determine, on the basis of information from both endoscopy and results of treatment, whether we would continue to advocate no further surgery in patients with positive endoscopic biopsy reports, in favor of treatment with combination chemotherapy and radiotherapy alone.

Table 3. *Surgical Procedures in Relation to Stage*

| Patients | Laparotomy | | Endoscopy and biopsy only |
	Gastrectomy	Unresectable	
Stage IE 35	21	4	10
Stage IIE 44	21	20	3
Total 79	42	24	13

Endoscopic Biopsies

Although advocates of surgery for lymphoma of the stomach continue to contend that endoscopic biopsies are unreliable or nondiagnostic (Brooks and Enterline 1983, Fleming et al. 1982), since 1974, our overall rate of obtaining a positive biopsy specimen using the flexible fiberscope has been 91%. This improvement over our past experience of approximately 50% has been due not only to better equipment but also to experience gained in obtaining adequate representative material and in interpreting the histopathologic findings (Nelson and Lanza 1974, Rosch et al. 1971, Hertzer and Hoerr 1976). However, nondiagnostic biopsy reports should not be accepted as a benign condition. The vast majority of lymphomas of the stomach are of the diffuse large cell variety. These can usually be diagnosed from endoscopic biopsy specimens. However, specimens are seldom adequate to diagnose lymphomas that are composed of small lymphocytes because this type of infiltrate can also occur in benign conditions (Evans et al. 1978). Usually, a laparotomy is required to obtain sufficient material to establish the diagnosis.

Treatment Results

The major differences in the results of the various treatments centered on whether the disease was resectable and on whether the treatment contained CHOP-Bleo chemotherapy (Table 4). Prior to the introduction of CHOP-Bleo, the best five-year survival figure of 66% was obtained in 12 patients who had gastrectomy only for very limited disease. However, the survival figure dropped to 52% for patients with more extensive disease who were treated with gastrectomy and radiotherapy. Nine patients who received CHOP-Bleo after gastrectomy, with or without radiotherapy, are surviving.

Results for unresectable disease were generally poor. In the immediate postoperative period, two patients died. The five-year survival rate for 15 patients who received radiotherapy after laparotomy was only 20%. Also, four patients who

Table 4. *Correlation of Five-Year Survival Figures with Treatment*

| | Primary treatment | | |
| | | Only | |
Additional treatment	Gastrectomy	Laparotomy	Endoscopy and biopsy
None	66%	0/2*	—
Radiotherapy	52%	20%	50%
CHOP-Bleo	55%	0/4	1/1
CHOP-Bleo and radiotherapy	4/4	3/3	6/6

*Postoperative deaths.
CHOP-Bleo—cyclophosphamide, doxorubicin, vincristine, prednisone, and bleomycin.

received only CHOP-Bleo died. By contrast, three patients who received CHOP-Bleo and radiotherapy are alive.

Thirteen patients whose diseases were diagnosed by means of endoscopic biopsy results without laparotomy were dependent on the treatment. All six patients who were treated with CHOP-Bleo and radiotherapy are surviving and are free of disease.

Conclusions

Several facts that are pertinent to current management of gastric lymphomas have emerged from this retrospective review. The first is that it is possible, with the flexible fiberscope, to establish the diagnosis through endoscopic biopsies in most patients. The second is that most patients can be treated successfully with CHOP-Bleo and radiotherapy without having preliminary gastric resection. In our patients, there were no major treatment complications, such as life-threatening hemorrhage or perforation, that have been cited as reasons for preliminary gastrectomy (Hande et al. 1978).

There are a number of reasons why an empirical gastrectomy should not be performed as the first step in the management of known gastric lymphoma. One is that lymphomas of the stomach generally occur in an elderly population. The reported postoperative mortality rate has ranged between 10% and 18%. Also, there is a significant incidence of prolonged morbidity after either a subtotal or particularly, a total resection of the stomach. By contrast, there has been very little morbidity following treatment with CHOP-Bleo and radiotherapy.

The major reason for not recommending a gastrectomy as the first therapeutic step is that in approximately one third of most surgical series the disease was unresectable. While it has been argued that laparotomy was important for establishing the extent of disease for radiotherapeutic fields, this line of reasoning is not really valid. The same information can be obtained from noninvasive procedures including gastrointestinal series, CT scans, and lymphangiography, in addition to endoscopy. Also, except for the Princess Margaret Hospital survival figures of 75% for gastrectomy and total abdominal irradiation (Gospodarowicz et al. 1983), reported survival figures for gastrectomy with or without radiotherapy have been in the order of 50% to 60%. These results are not acceptable by today's standards.

In a minority of patients, laparotomy is needed to establish the diagnosis. In such cases, gastrectomy is usually done to insure adequate material for analyses and for debulking. Gastrectomy is also indicated in the rare situation when disease has failed to respond to initial chemotherapy. Subsequent to reporting our results in which we had 100% survival for 13 patients who were treated with CHOP-Bleo and radiotherapy with or without preliminary gastrectomy, we have had a single failure during preliminary chemotherapy. This was discovered after two cycles of CHOP-Bleo, and the patient had a gastrectomy. In treating patients with combination chemotherapy and radiotherapy, follow-up endoscopic examinations are extremely important. If there is evidence of progressive disease or if the response is unsatisfactory, treatment should be changed to include immediate gastrectomy.

Radiotherapy alone has been inadequate as the only treatment for gastric lymphomas. In our experience, this has also been true of CHOP-Bleo. All five patients who were treated with CHOP-Bleo after laparotomy for inoperable disease died of lymphoma. However, there may be a role for chemotherapy alone as adjunctive treatment after adequate resection in patients whose disease was confined to the stomach. In our series, five patients who had CHOP-Bleo after gastrectomy are surviving. However, the percentage of patients who would fall in this category is small and, in our opinion, does not justify laparotomy and gastrectomy for all patients with gastric lymphomas.

HEAD AND NECK

The clinical behavior of extranodal lymphomas originating in the head and neck is remarkably similar to that of their carcinomatous counterparts. For carcinomas, it can be well correlated with the location and extent of the primary disease and the status of the neck by using the TNM_{AJCC} staging system (American Joint Committee on Cancer 1983).

It is well known that extranodal lymphomas of the head and neck can present as localized disease, which can be cured with radiotherapy alone. In the past, our overall survival figure for stages IE and IIE disease was 47% (Wong et al. 1975). While local control was excellent, there was a significant incidence of relapse in distant sites. This was particularly true for stage IIE presentations, but was also significant for stage IE disease. To determine whether the size of the extranodal disease and the status of the neck are related to the incidence of distant relapses, we have reanalyzed our results using the TNM_{AJCC} system as well as the modified Ann Arbor system for the various primary sites (Mill et al. 1980).

The majority of extranodal head and neck lymphomas present in Waldeyer's ring or the nasal cavity and paranasal sinuses. However, lymphomas originating in Waldeyer's ring represent a heterogenous group as compared with lymphomas of the nasal cavity and paranasal sinuses.

Nasal Cavity and Paranasal Sinus Presentations

The data on 38 patients with Ann Arbor-staged IE and IIE lymphomas of the nasal cavity and paranasal sinuses were analyzed after pathologic review and reclassification. The pathologic breakdown was diffuse large cell, 35; diffuse poorly differentiated lymphocytic, 2; and diffuse mixed, 1 (Fuller et al. 1984).

The radiologic reports and available paranasal sinus films and tomograms (25 patients), operative reports, surgical pathology reports, and clinical notes were used collectively to stage the extranodal disease according to the TNM_{AJCC} system for 33 patients with disease involving the maxillary antrum. In five patients whose tumors appeared to originate in the nasal cavity; the extent of involvement was arbitrarily staged as follows: T_1, disease confined to the nasal cavity; T_2, minimal extension to the anterior ethmoids; T_3, extension to the orbit; and T_4, direct extension through the cribriform plate to the anterior cranial fossa. The final breakdown was as follows: T_1 or T_2 disease, 13 patients and T_3 or T_4 disease, 25 patients. Among 15 patients with T_4 disease 3 had bilateral antral disease and 6 had disease extension into the nasopharynx. All of the patients with T_1 and T_2 disease belonged to the Ann Arbor stage IE group. All five patients who presented with disease in the neck (Ann Arbor stage IIE) had T_3 or T_4 disease. Regardless of the TNM staging, 70% of these patients were treated definitively with radiotherapy. The others were treated with CHOP-Bleo or COP and radiotherapy.

Treatment Results

Permanent local control of the extranodal and nodal disease was achieved in 36 patients. One patient had progressive disease during radiotherapy and one patient had a marginal relapse in the hard palate, five years following treatment with radiotherapy alone.

The overall survival and disease-free survival figures for the 38 patients was 56% and 46%, respectively. The corresponding results for patients with stage IE disease were 67% and 55%. No patient with stage IIE disease survived five years.

Patients with disease staged by means of lymphangiography had a somewhat better five-year survival than patients who did not have lymphangiogram. However, the difference between 69% for patients with lymphangiogram-staged disease and 40% for those with disease not staged by lymphangiography was not statistically significant.

When results for treatment with radiotherapy alone were analyzed according to the TNM_{AJCC} system, differences in disease-free survival rates were statistically significant. These were 89% for T_1 and T_2 lesions as compared with 25% for T_3 and T_4 disease ($P = .003$) (Figure 3). However, survival and disease-free survival

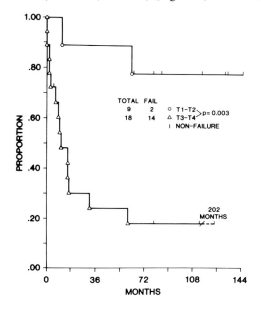

Figure 3. Comparison of disease-free survivals for patients staged as T_1-T_2 versus T_3-T_4 treated with radiotherapy only. (Reproduced from Kong et al. 1984, with permission of *Am J Clin Oncol.*)

for T_3 and T_4 disease patients who had no cervical adenopathy were somewhat better.

When the results were analyzed according to whether patients were treated with combination chemotherapy and radiotherapy or with radiotherapy alone, the disease-free survival rate was better for patients who were treated on the combined program (Figure 4). However, the difference of 63% for patients who were treated with CHOP-Bleo and radiotherapy was not statistically different from that of 53% for patients with lymphangiogram-staged disease or 39% for those with disease not staged by lymphangiogram and who were treated with radiotherapy only. The fact that there was no detectable significant difference between results for the two groups may have been because of the small numbers of patients in each group. The percentage of T_1 and T_2 patients whose disease relapsed after radiotherapy alone was considerably less than that observed in the T_3 and T_4 disease group (Table 5). Of the 13 patients with T_1 and T_2 disease, 10 received radiotherapy only and of these 10, 8 remained free of disease from 62 to 144 months. Of the three who received combination chemotherapy and radiotherapy, two are alive (Table 5). By contrast, of the 20 T_3 and T_4 disease patients with no cervical adenopathy (stage IE), 14 were treated with radiotherapy alone. Of these 14 patients, only 5 are free of disease. Six patients were treated with CHOP-Bleo and radiotherapy and of these, four are alive. All five T_3 and T_4 disease patients, whose diseases

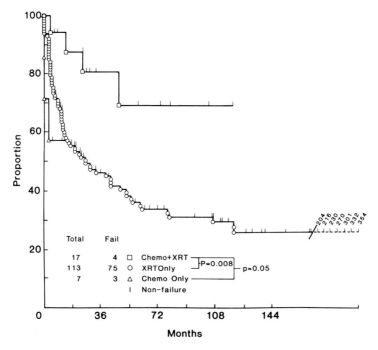

Figure 4. Comparative disease-free survival by treatment for all sites of Waldeyer's ring. (Reproduced from Kong et al. 1984, with permission of *Am J Clin Oncol.*)

Table 5. *Response to Treatment*

TNM$_{AJCC}$	Treatment		NED	Relapsed (DOD)	Complication
T$_1$-T$_2$-N$_0$	XRT	10	8	2* (2)	
	CHOP-Bleo + XRT	2	2		
	COP + XRT	1		1 (1)	
T$_3$-T$_4$-N$_0$	XRT	14	5	9 (7)	
	CHOP-Bleo + XRT	6	4	1	1†
T$_3$-T$_4$-N$_+$	XRT	5		5 (5)	
Total		38	19	18 (15)	1

*Marginal relapse at five years in one patient.
†Patient died of hemorrhage due to thrombocytopenia during chemotherapy.
NED–no evidence of disease; DOD–dead of disease; N$_0$–no diseased neck nodes; N$_+$–positive neck nodes; XRT–radiotherapy; CHOP-Bleo–cyclophosphamide, doxorubicin, vincristine, prednisone, and bleomycin; COP–cyclophosphamide, vincristine, and prednisone.

were staged as IIE and who were treated with radiotherapy only are dead. In summary, although the numbers are small, it would appear that radiotherapy alone is sufficient treatment for patients with T$_1$ and T$_2$ disease. However, for T$_3$ and T$_4$ disease patients, aggressive combination chemotherapy and radiotherapy is needed.

Waldeyer's Ring

Of all the non-Hodgkin's lymphoma extranodal presenting sites, Waldeyer's ring is the most common. At the time the Ann Arbor system of staging was developed, it was primarily for Hodgkin's disease, and Waldeyer's ring was considered "like a lymph node" for staging purposes. Later, when the concept of extranodal "E" disease was introduced, the definition of Waldeyer's ring was not addressed. However, since Waldeyer's ring is an extranodal site, our policy has been to designate disease localized to Waldeyer's ring as stage IE and as IIE when the neck nodes are also involved.

Among 137 patients with involvement of Waldeyer's ring, the apparent sites of origin were as follows: tonsil, 70; base of tongue, 31; nasopharynx, 24; and multiple areas, 12. In the majority of the cases, the histopathology was diffuse large cell lymphoma (Kong et al. 1984); the breakdown was as follows: diffuse large cell, 116; diffuse mixed, 5; diffuse poorly differentiated lymphocytic, 3; diffuse well differentiated lymphocytic, 3; nodular poorly differentiated lymphocytic, 3; nodular large cell, 5; Burkitt's, 1; and unclassified, 1. Of the 137 patients, disease in 79 was staged by lymphangiography and of these, 11 also had staging laparotomy. In common with their carcinomatous counterparts, extranodal lymphomas generally had associated involvement of neck nodes. The overall incidence of cervical adenopathy was 72%. However, the percentage of patients with disease in neck nodes was related to the extent of the extranodal disease as well as the specific site, as shown by the TNM$_{AJCC}$ staging system, which is correlated with the Ann Arbor in Table 6. Most of the patients were treated with radiotherapy only using the Wal-

Table 6. *Waldeyer's Ring Non-Hodgkin's Lymphomas: Incidence of Small (T_1-T_2-T_X) to Large (T_3-T_4) Disease in 137 Stage IE and IIE Patients*

	T_1-T_2-T_X		T_3-T_4	
Stage IE	IIE	IE	IIE	
16%	28%	12%	44%	

Table 7. *Waldeyer's Ring Radiotherapy Only: Comparisons of Five-Year Disease-Free Survival Figures by Site, TNM$_{AJCC}$ Staging and Ann Arbor Staging*

	T_1-T_2-T_X		T_3-T_4	
Stage	IE	IIE	IE	IIE
Base of tongue	80%	40%	25%	40%
Tonsil	62%	36%	53%	10%
Nasopharynx	0/1	60%	50%	18%
Multiple sites	—	—	35%	0/8

deyer's ring technique, which has been described previously (Wong et al. 1975). The remainder were treated with CHOP-Bleo and radiotherapy or chemotherapy alone in a few instances.

Treatment Results

The survival rate for all patients who were treated with radiotherapy alone was only 34%. However, results for patients with small extranodal lesions (T_X, T_1, or T_2) with no involved neck nodes (stage IE) were significantly better than those for patients with extensive extranodal disease or patients with cervical adenopathy (Table 7). However, the specific site of extranodal disease also influenced results. The best disease-free survival figure of 80% was observed in patients with T_1 and T_2 base of tongue lesions and no cervical adenopathy (Table 7). Age younger than five years was the other important factor that favorably affected results. Patients younger than 50 years who presented with stage IE disease had an 88% disease-free survival rate.

Comparison by treatment modality showed improved results for combination chemotherapy and radiotherapy over that achieved with either one alone (Table 8). The five-year disease-free survival rate of 17 patients treated with CHOP-Bleo and radiotherapy was 69% as compared with 58% for seven patients treated with CHOP-Bleo only ($P = .05$). The difference between results of 69% for treatment with CHOP-Bleo and radiotherapy and 34% for radiotherapy alone was highly significant ($P = .008$).

Table 8. *Waldeyer's Ring: Comparison of Five-Year Disease-Free Survivals by Treatment*

Radiotherapy (XRT) only	34%	
Chemotherapy only*	58%	$P = .05$ — $P = .008$
Chemotherapy and XRT program	69%	

CHOP-Bleo (cyclophosphamide, doxorubicin, vincristine, prednisone, and bleomycin) or COP (cyclophosphamide, vincristine, and prednisone).

Although the numbers of patients treated with either CHOP-Bleo and radiotherapy or chemotherapy alone were small, it would appear that combination treatment with CHOP-Bleo and radiotherapy is optimal for most patients. The exceptions would be patients under age 50 with small T_1 and T_2 lesions and no cervical adenopathy (stage IE). For these patients, the least amount of treatment is important because of their chances for a normal life expectancy and the fact that more intensive treatment tends to be associated with a higher incidence of late complications.

SUMMARY

This retrospective review of the results of treatment of stages IE and IIE lymphomas originating in the three major extranodal sites, namely the stomach, paranasal sinuses, and Waldeyer's ring, has shown that the clinical behavior following local treatment is related not only to the status of adjacent lymph nodes but also to the extent of the primary extranodal disease. The Ann Arbor system of staging has been useful for determining the effect of lymphadenopathy (stage IIE) on results of treatment with localized radiotherapy, chemotherapy, and various combinations. It was not useful for assessing and comparing different treatments for stage IE disease. This is because the size of the extranodal disease or invasion of the adjacent structures has a major impact on results of treatment with any of the treatment modalities used alone. Results for extranodal head and neck disease have been particularly confusing. By using the TNM_{AJCC} system for categorizing the extent of the extranodal head and neck disease, it has been possible to make valid comparisons for different treatment modalities for both stage IE and stage IIE disease. Although we were not able to use specific criteria for staging the extent of extranodal disease in a retrospective study of gastric lymphomas, resectability proved useful for evaluating response to radiotherapy, chemotherapy, surgery, and combinations of the three modalities.

Regardless of the criteria that were used to evaluate the extent of both the extranodal and nodal disease, two important facts emerged from this study. One was that lymphomas arising in extranodal sites are usually extensive regardless of whether the adjacent lymph nodes are involved. The second was that results for neither local radiotherapy nor CHOP-Bleo alone were as satisfactory as those for combined modality treatment of CHOP-Bleo and radiotherapy. However, lesser treatment may be a more appropriate choice for a very small number of patients with prognostically favorable features associated with their disease. To reiterate, local treatment with radiotherapy alone has been very effective (88% disease-free survival) for patients younger than 50 years with stage IE Waldeyer's ring disease. Also, radiotherapy alone was sufficient treatment for patients with small T_1 or T_2 nasal cavity or paranasal sinus disease with no cervical adenopathy. Similarly, CHOP-Bleo alone may be adequate adjunctive treatment after gastrectomy for stage IE disease when the margins are adequate and the disease is not transmural.

ACKNOWLEDGMENT

This investigation was supported by grants CA-06294 and CA-16672 awarded by the National Cancer Institute, United States Department of Health and Human Services.

REFERENCES

American Joint Committee on Cancer. 1983. Manual for Staging of Cancer, 2nd ed. J. B. Lippincott Company, Philadelphia.

Brooks JJ, Enterline HT. 1983. Primary gastric lymphomas: A clinicopathologic study of 58 cases with long-term follow-up and literature review. Cancer 51:701–711.

Connors J, Wise L. 1974. Management of gastric lymphomas. Am J Surg 127:102–108.

Evans HL, Butler JJ, Youness EL. 1978. Malignant lymphoma, small lymphocytic type: A clinicopathologic study of 84 cases with suggested criteria for intermediate lymphocytic lymphoma. Cancer 41:1440–1455.

Fleming ID, Mitchell S, Dilawari RA. 1982. The role of surgery in the management of gastric lymphoma. Cancer 49:1135–1141.

Fuller LM, Banker FL, Butler JJ, Gamble JF. 1975. The natural history of non-Hodgkin's lymphomas stages I and II. Br J Cancer 31(Suppl II):270–285.

Fuller LM, Robbins KT, Vlasak MC, Osborne BM, Velasquez WS, Sullivan JA. 1984. Primary lymphomas of the nasal cavity and paranasal sinuses. Cancer (In press).

Gospodarowicz MK, Bush RS, Brown TC, Chua T. 1983. Curability of gastrointestinal lymphoma with combined surgery and radiation. Int J Radiat Oncol Biol Phys 9:3–9.

Hande KR, Fisher RI, DeVita VT, Chabner BA, Young RC. 1978. Diffuse histiocytic lymphoma involving the gastrointestinal tract. Cancer 41:1984–1989.

Heifetz LJ, Fuller LM, Rodgers RW, Martin RG, Butler JJ, North LB, Gamble JF, Shullenberger CC. 1980. Laparotomy findings in lymphangiogram-staged I and II non-Hodgkin's lymphomas. Cancer 45:2778–2785.

Hertzer NR, Hoerr SO. 1976. An interpretive review of lymphoma of the stomach. Surg Gynecol Obstet 143:113–124.

Kong JS, Fuller LM, Butler JJ, Barton JH, Robbins KT, Velasquez WS, Sullivan JA. 1984. Stages IE and IIE non-Hodgkin's lymphomas of Waldeyer's ring and the neck. Am J Clin Oncol (In press).

Lester JN, Fuller LM, Conrad FG, Sullivan JA, Velasquez WS, Butler JJ, Shullenberger CC. 1982. The roles of staging laparotomy, chemotherapy, and radiotherapy in the management of localized diffuse large cell lymphoma: A study of seventy-five patients. Cancer 49:1746–1753.

Maor MH, Maddux B, Osborne BM, Fuller LM, Sullivan JA, Nelson RS, Martin RG, Libshitz HI, Velasquez WS, Bennett RW. 1984. Stages IE and IIE non-Hodgkin's lymphomas of the stomach: Comparison of treatment modalities. Cancer (in press).

Mill WB, Fransiska AL, Kaarle OF. 1980. Radiation therapy treatment of stage I and II: Extranodal non-Hodgkin's lymphoma of the head and neck. Cancer 45:653–661.

Naqvi MS, Burrows L, Kark AE. 1969. Lymphoma of the gastrointestinal tract: Prognostic guides based on 162 cases. Ann Surg 170:221–231.

Nelson RN, Lanza FL. 1974. The endoscopic diagnosis of gastric lymphoma: Gross characteristics and histology. Gastrointestinal Endoscopy 21:66–68.

Rodriguez V, Cabanillas F, Burgess MA, McKelvey EM, Valdivieso M, Bodey GP, Freireich EJ. 1977. Combination chemotherapy ("CHOP-Bleo") in advanced (non-Hodgkin) malignant lymphoma. Blood 49:325–333.

Rosch W, Hartwich K, Ottenjann R. 1971. Gastric lymphoma. Endoscopy 1:28–33.

Weingrad DN, Decosse JJ, Sherlock P, Straus D, Lieberman PH, Filippa DA. 1982. Primary gastrointestinal lymphoma: A 30-year review. Cancer 49:1258–1265.

Wong DS, Fuller LM, Butler JJ, Shullenberger CC. 1975. Extranodal non-Hodgkin's lymphomas of the head and neck. American Journal of Roentgenology 123:471–481.

UT M.D. Anderson Clinical Conference on Cancer,
Vol. 27, edited by R. J. Ford, L. M. Fuller, and
F. B. Hagemeister. Raven Press, New York © 1984.

Prognostic Factors for Stage III and Stage IV Diffuse Large Cell Lymphoma: Long-Term Follow-Up

William S. Velasquez, Sundar Jagannath, Susan Tucker,*
John Manning,† Peter McLaughlin, K. K. Oh,‡
Fredrick B. Hagemeister, and Lillian M. Fuller**

*Departments of Hematology, *Biomathematics, †Pathology, ‡Internal Medicine, and
**Radiotherapy, The University of Texas M.D. Anderson Hospital and Tumor Institute at
Houston, Houston, Texas 77030*

Advanced diffuse large cell lymphoma is a distinct clinical and pathological entity that may occur in patients of all ages, can present in both nodal and extranodal sites, tends to disseminate rapidly, and has an unfavorable prognosis unless intensive chemotherapy treatment can induce a sustained complete remission (CR). In the new classification proposed by the expert international panel, it falls into the intermediate- and high- (immunoblastic sarcoma) grade category (Non-Hodgkin's Lymphoma Pathologic Classification Project 1982).

More than one-half of the patients with diffuse large cell lymphoma (called diffuse histiocytic lymphoma according to the Rappaport (1966) classification) present with stage III or stage IV disease at the time of initial diagnosis. Several clinical studies have been published on advanced diffuse large cell lymphoma that include these stages. Combination chemotherapy has been the mainstay of treatment, and CR rates of about 16%–75% have been reported (Canellos et al. 1981, McKelvey et al. 1976, Fisher et al. 1977, Ginsberg et al. 1982, Pettingale 1981, Skarin et al. 1977). Patients in these studies who did not achieve CR died within 24 months. A significant proportion of the patients who achieved CR remain in remission longer than five years with a possibility of being cured of the disease (DeVita et al. 1975, Schein et al. 1974, Fisher et al. 1981).

An adequate long-term analysis of this population has not been presented in the literature. Different investigators have included "transformed" large cell lymphoma, patients previously treated, and even other histologic types of lymphoma in their reports (Armitage et al. 1982, Fisher et al. 1981). At UT M.D. Anderson Hospital, patients with advanced large cell lymphoma have been treated with CHOP-Bleo (cyclophosphamide, doxorubicin, vincristine, prednisone, and bleomycin; Rodriguez et al. 1977) combination since 1974, and for patients with stage III disease, radiotherapy has been used for consolidation. We wish to report our experience

357

and determine the biologic characteristics that might be related to prognosis in obtaining complete remission, in maintaining freedom from disease, and ultimately, in achieving survival. This analysis also could identify different prognostic subgroups of patients who could then be selected for different therapies, depending on the risks factors at the time of presentation. Thus, this could lead to a more individualized treatment.

PATIENTS AND METHODS

Patients Characteristics

Stage III

Forty-seven consecutive adult patients with stage III and stage IIIE disease have been entered on the study. The median follow-up was 58 months with a range of 24 to 108 months (Table 1).

The median age for these patients was 55 years (range 20–78 years). Disease was subsequently staged according to the Ann Arbor classification. Lymphangiogram and bone marrow biopsies were included routinely in the initial work up. Seven patients with negative lymphangiogram underwent staging laparotomy that revealed occult abdominal involvement. In 37 of the 47 patients, the involvement

Table 1. *Diffuse Large Cell Lymphoma Patient Characteristics*

Characteristic	Stages III-IIIE No. of patients (%)	Stage IV No. of patients (%)
Total patients	47	61
Sex		
Male	23 (48)	32 (52)
Female	24 (51)	29 (47)
Age		
<56	24 (51)	30 (49)
≥56	23 (48)	31 (50)
Constitutional symptoms		
A	39 (83)	32 (52)
B	8 (17)	29 (47)
Lactic dehydrogenase level*		
Normal	19 (42)	19 (31)
Elevated	26 (57)	41 (68)
Tumor burden		
Minimum nodal involvement	11 (23)	—
Extensive nodal involvement		
1 area	23 (48)	—
≥2 areas	13 (27)	—
Extranodal sites		
1 site	—	28 (45)
≥2 sites	—	33 (54)

*Two patients with stage III or IIIE and one patient with stage IV disease did not have this measured.

was limited to the lymph nodes, and 7 of these patients had constitutional symptoms. The other 10 patients had extranodal extension at a single site in addition to nodal involvement, and only 1 of these patients had constitutional symptoms.

Extensive upper-torso area disease involvement, other than mediastinum, was demonstrated in nine patients, and in three, it was the only area of extensive involvement. Similarly, 15 patients had mediastinum enlargement; in 6 of them, it was the sole area of extensive disease. There were 26 patients with extensive abdominal disease, and 14 showed this as the only area of disease involvement.

Stage IV

Sixty-one consecutive, previously untreated adult patients with stage IV diffuse large cell lymphoma were included in this analysis. Staging procedures were the same as in stage III, with the exception of staging laparotomy. Extranodal biopsies, other than bone marrow, were done when clinically indicated. There were 32 men and 29 women. The median age was 56 years (range 21–78 years). The median duration of patient follow-up was 53 months (range 22–98 months). Several clinical characteristics of the patient population are outlined in Table 1. The most common extranodal sites of involvement were bone marrow, bone, lung, pleura, and skin. Other sites were less commonly involved (Table 2).

Two patients died within one month of initiation of chemotherapy (early deaths); three other patients were lost to follow-up and their remission statuses were not clearly established. Thus, 61 patients were evaluable for survival analysis, but only 56 were evaluable for remission status.

Prognostic Indicators

Stage III

For stage III disease, several factors were analyzed for their influence on survival, on achieving CR, and on probability of relapse. These factors were age, sex, constitutional symptoms, extranodal involvement, lactic dehydrogenase (LDH) level, and extent of tumor burden. Extent of tumor burden was measured by the presence

Table 2. *Frequency of Extranodal Sites of Disease*

Site	No. of patients	Frequency %	Site	No. of patients	Frequency %
Bone	20	33	Skin	11	18
Bone Marrow			Liver	8	13
LCL	10	15	GI	7	11
SCL	11	18	CNS	3	5
Pleura	16	26	Miscellaneous	12	20
Lung	10	16			

LCL–large cell lymphoma; SCL–small cell lymphoma; GI–gastrointestinal tract; CNS–central nervous system.

or absence of extensive disease involvement in a specific nodal area in head, upper torso, or lower torso. In the head, extensive involvement is defined as a mass that qualifies as a T_3 or T_4 lesion according to the TNM classification system. In other nodal areas, such as the neck and axilla, any nodal mass larger than 7 cm in diameter also qualifies as an extensive lesion in upper torso. In addition, the presence of mediastinal adenopathy, seen on chest radiograph, was considered to be extensive disease. Finally, the simultaneous involvement of para-aortic and iliac lymph nodes, the presence of an abdominal mass larger than 7 cm, or both indicated extensive abdominal involvement. The absence of any extensive disease involvement was classified as minimal involvement.

Stage IV

In stage IV disease, in addition to the described risk factors, a further assessment of tumor burden was needed and was made on the basis of the number of extranodal organs or systems (sites) involved with disease at the time of diagnosis. Patients with one site of extranodal lymphoma were compared with patients who had two or more extranodal sites of involvement. Bone marrow involvement and anemia were also included in the assessment of the adverse prognostic indicators.

Treatment

Stage III

The combined modality program was initiated with four cycles of inductive CHOP-Bleo chemotherapy. The drug schedules and dosages were those used in the Southwest Oncology Group studies (Table 3). Thereafter, radiotherapy was administered to the abdomen. Treatment fields were limited to the known areas of disease. The tumor dose was 3,000 rad delivered in 20 fractions over four weeks. The major portion of the liver was not irradiated. The dose to the kidneys was limited to 1,800 rad by appropriate shielding during treatment to the posterior field. The patient was allowed to recover for three to four weeks and then CHOP-Bleo was resumed for another four cycles. Subsequently, radiotherapy was delivered to the next major area of disease involvement. The chemotherapeutic portion of the program was completed with four cycles of COP (cyclophosphamide, vincristine,

Table 3. *CHOP-Bleo Schedule*

	Dose	Day
Cyclophosphamide	750 mg/m² i.v.	1
Hydroxydaunomycin	50 mg/m² i.v.	1
Oncovin*	1.4 mg/m² i.v.	1
Prednisone	100 mg daily p.o.	1–5
Bleomycin	5 mg/m² i.v.	1

*Oncovin = vincristine; dose not to exceed 2 mg total.

and prednisone). Following this, the radiotherapy portion was completed for the remaining sites of initial involvement.

In this program, the treatment schedule was modified in 15 patients. In eight patients, irradiation was administered during the initial assessment, as an emergency measure. This was usually done to prevent respiratory obstruction because of massive or rapidly progressive head and neck or mediastinal disease. In seven other patients, chemotherapy was compromised because doxorubicin had to be either reduced by 50% or eliminated because of severe cardiovascular disease.

Stage IV

CHOP-Bleo chemotherapy was used as in stage III. The limiting dose of doxorubicin that was administered was 450 mg/m² and for bleomycin was 180 units. The courses of chemotherapy were repeated every three or four weeks after recovery from myelosuppression. When total doses of doxorubicin reached the limit, the chemotherapy was continued with COP-Bleo (cyclophosphamide 1 G/m²) to complete one year of therapy.

CR was defined as disappearance of all evidence of disease documented clinically, and normalization of all laboratory and radiological parameters that were abnormal prior to therapy.

A partial remission (PR) was defined as a greater than 50% reduction in measurable disease for at least one month. Periodic restaging was performed, which included performing bone marrow aspiration and biopsies and radiographic and scanning procedures. During treatment, patients were checked closely and reevaluated at regular intervals. Those not achieving PR during the initial three cycles of chemotherapy were withdrawn from the protocol but were included in this analysis.

Pathology

We reviewed all of the pathological material in light of the guidelines of this study. Four patients with stage III and three patients with stage IV disease were classified as having immunologic sarcomas. Further characterization of the histiologic diagnosis of large cell lymphoma was not attempted.

Statistical Methods

Survival was calculated from the day of admission to the last follow-up visit or death. The relapse-free survival was calculated from the time of documented CR until relapse. Survival and relapse-free survival curves were obtained for all the pretreatment characteristics and for remission status using the Kaplan and Meier method (1958). The generalized Wilcoxon test was used to compare results (Gehan 1965). In stage IV disease, the proportional hazards model was used to identify a subset of independent risk factors, other than remission induction, from among those factors that, individually, indicated poor prognosis for survival. When more than one variable with a significant effect on outcome was identified, further analysis was done to examine synergistic effects among the variables. Fisher's exact test was used to compare frequencies in 2×2 tables (Bradley 1968).

RESULTS

Stage III

The calculated eight-year survival for the entire group of the 47 patients was 50% (Figure 1). Thirty-three patients (70%) achieved CR. Ten patients obtained only PR and four progressed. The eight-year survival rate for patients who achieved CR was 71%, median survival not yet reached, compared with a median survival of less than 10 months for patients who did not achieve CR (Figure 2). The difference was statistically significant. Among the factors analyzed, only tumor burden was found to be an independent risk factor in survival.

The 34 patients with minimal disease involvement or having a single area of extensive involvement had an excellent probability of survival of 68% at eight years. In contrast, for the 13 patients with two or more areas of extensive disease involvement, the survival was less than 20% at six years (Figure 3).

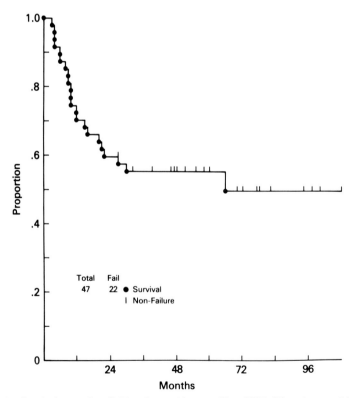

Figure 1. Survival curve for all 47 patients with stage III and IIIE diffuse large cell lymphoma.

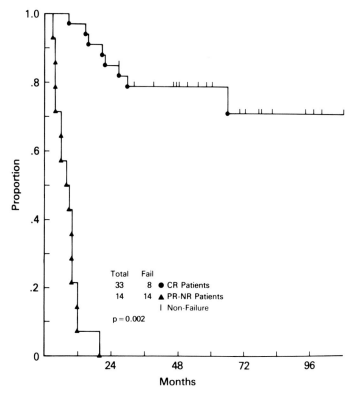

Figure 2. Survival of patients with stage III diffuse large cell lymphoma by response to therapy. CR-complete responders; PR-partial responders; NR-nonresponders.

The probability of achieving CR was then analyzed for patients with different pretreatment characteristics (Table 4). Constitutional symptoms and age did not appear to be significant prognostic indicators. The age of 55 years was selected as the dividing line in our groups, since it was the median age in our population. Patients older than 55 had a CR rate of 62%, while younger patients had a rate of 79%. Among the 39 patients with no constitutional symptoms, 28 obtained CR, as did 5 of the 8 patients with constitutional B symptoms. Serum LDH level, however, was a very important prognostic indicator for achievement of CR, as demonstrated in Table 7.

When tumor burden and LDH level were analyzed together, the interrelationship between these factors became apparent (Table 5). The proportion of patients with elevated LDH levels increases in direct relationship to heavier tumor burden. Whereas, the CR rate was inversely related to tumor burden and elevated LDH levels. Thus, fewer patients with two or more areas of extensive disease involvement and with elevated LDH levels achieved complete remission.

Another important biologic determination for survival is the ability to remain free of disease, since successful treatment of relapsing patients is notoriously poor

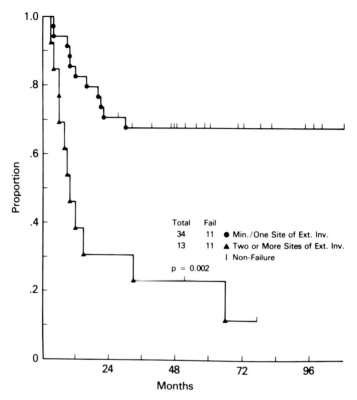

Figure 3. Survival of patients with stage III diffuse large cell lymphoma burden. Ext. Inv.—extensive disease involvement.

(Cabanillas 1983, Hansen 1980). There were four early relapses among the 33 patients who achieved initial CR. Subsequently, nine additional patients suffered relapse, usually in nonradiated areas, after treatment was terminated. In three of the 12, the central nervous system was the only site of relapse. An additional patient who died of a metastatic fibrohistiosarcoma of the thigh was found to have active lymphoma at autopsy. It is pertinent to mention that three patients suffered relapses after three years of continuous CR. Two of them had nodular poorly differentiated lymphocytic lymphoma at the time of relapse at 49 and 80 months (Figure 4), and each of these patients have enjoyed a second remission for longer than one year. This phenomenon has not been recognized in the past and should be further investigated. This could be done by performing lymph node biopsies at the time of relapse.

Among the pretreatment characteristics that are studied as possible prognostic indicators for relapse, the serum LDH level and the tumor burden were again found to be significant predictors for relapse (Table 6). Patients who had minimal disease involvement, or extensive disease in one area only, had low probability of relapse. However, of the five patients with more than one site of extensive involvement who

Table 4. *Stage III Diffuse Large Cell Lymphoma Risk Factors in Relation to Complete Remission*

	No. of patients	CR (%)	P
Age (yr)			
<56	23	18 (79)	NS
≥56	24	15 (62)	
Constitutional symptoms			
A	39	28 (72)	NS
B	8	5 (62)	
Lactic dehydrogenase level*			
Normal	19	19 (100)	.005
Elevated	26	14 (54)	
Tumor burden			
Minimum involvement	11	10 (91)	
Extensive involvement			
1 area	23	18 (78)	.017
2 areas	13	5 (38)	

*Two patients did not have this measured.
NS–Not statistically significant; CR–complete remission.

Table 5. *Stage III Diffuse Large Cell Lymphoma Remission in Relation to Mass Burden and Lactic Dehydrogenase Level*

		LDH level	
Tumor burden	No. of patients (%)	Normal	Elevated
Minimum disease involvement	11*	6	3
Achieving CR	10 (91)		
Extensive disease involvement			
1 area	23	11	12
Achieving CR	18 (78)	11	7
≥2 areas	13	2	11
Achieving CR	5 (38)	2	3

*Serum lactic dehydrogenase (LDH) determination was not performed on two patients, including one who entered complete remission (CR).
The difference between the first two groups and the third was significant $(P = .017)$.

obtained CR, only one has remained in CR longer than 24 months. This difference was found to be significant.

Stage IV

The survival curve for all 61 patients with diffuse large cell lymphoma and treated with CHOP-Bleo is shown in Figure 5. The median survival is 32 months, and 48.5% of all patients were alive at five years.

Fifty-six patients were evaluable for remission status. Forty-one patients (73%) achieved CR, nine patients (16%) achieved PR, and six patients (11%) had pro-

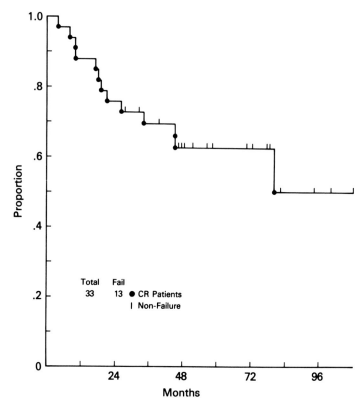

Figure 4. Relapse-free survival for the 33 patients with stage III diffuse large cell lymphoma who were in complete remission (CR). Three patients relapsed after three years; two of them had nodular small cell lymphoma.

Table 6. *Stage III Diffuse Large Cell Lymphoma Risk Factors for Relapse*

Tumor Burden	No. of patients	CR	CCR (%)
Minimum disease involvement	11	10	6 (60)
Extensive disease involvement			
1 area	23	18	13 (73)
≥2 areas	13	5	1 (2)
LDH level			
Normal	19	19	14 (74)
Elevated	26	14	6 (43)

CR–Complete remission; CCR–Number of responders in continuous complete remission longer than 24 months; LDH–Lactic dehydrogenase.

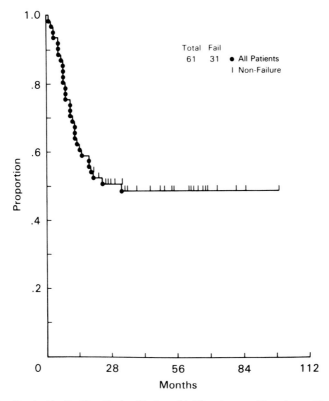

Figure 5. Survival for the 61 patients with stage IV diffuse large cell lymphoma. Median survival was 32 months. All deaths occurred within the first 32 months of observation.

gressive disease. Figure 6 shows that as in stage III disease, achievement of CR is very important for survival. All patients who did not achieve CR died within 24 months. The median survival time among patients who achieved CR (including those who later relapsed) was not reached at eight years. The patients with PR or progressive disease had median survival times of 10 months and 7 months, respectively, which differs significantly from CR patients ($P = .002$).

Nine clinical factors, determined at the time of diagnosis, were analyzed for their possible role as prognostic indicators in stage IV diffuse large cell lymphoma treated with CHOP-Bleo. First, each of the nine factors was examined individually for its relationship to overall survival time. The six factors that have statistical significance are age, constitutional symptoms, mediastinal involvement, LDH level, bone marrow infiltration with large cell lymphoma, and number of extranodal sites (Table 7).

The proportional hazards model was then used to identify an independent subset of the factors that were individually related to differences in survival times. At a

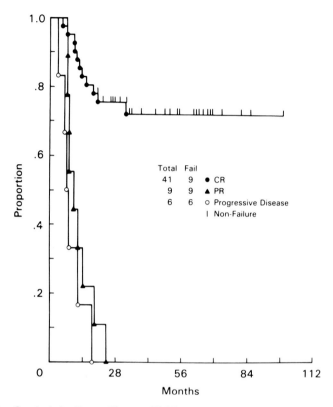

Figure 6. Survival of patients with stage IV diffuse large cell lymphoma according to response to treatment. CR-complete responder; PR-partial responder; a single vertical line may represent one or more patients alive at the given interval.

significance level of $P<.01$, two factors were identified, age and number of extranodal disease sites.

Table 8 illustrates the influence of the combination of these two factors, age and number of sites, on survival rates for this patient population. It also illustrates the tendency toward higher incidence of constitutional symptoms, large cell lymphoma involvement of the bone marrow and elevated LDH level when the four risk groups were listed according to decreasing observed five-year survival times. When interaction terms were included in the model, a significant interaction was found between age and number of sites. The interaction term appeared with a negative coefficient, indicating that the effects of age and number of sites were not additive. That is, older patients with two or more extranodal sites of disease did not fare significantly worse than patients 56 years or older with one extranodal site or than patients younger than 56 with two or more extranodal sites. The proportion of patients alive at five years in the last three groups in Table 8 differ far less from one another than they do from the lowest risk group. The graphic demonstration is shown in

Table 7. *Risk Factors and Their Effect on Survival Time and Complete Response in Patients with Stage IV Diffuse Large Cell Lymphoma*

Risk factor	Group	Number of patients	Median survival (Months)	Proportion surviving at 5 yr	P
Age	<56	30	NR	0.70	.013
	≥56	31	15	0.31	
Sex	Female	29	NR	0.51	.424
	Male	32	19	0.47	
Constitutional symptoms	A	32	NR	0.66	.003
	B	29	12	0.29	
Extranodal sites	1	28	NR	0.67	.026
	≥2	33	13	0.33	
Mediastinal involvement	No	48	NR	0.56	.024
	Yes	13	12	0.23	
Extensive abdominal disease	No	24	NR	0.54	.546
	Yes	37	19	0.46	
Bone marrow involvement	No/SCL	51	NR	0.54	.031
	LCL	10	9.5	0.20	
Lactic dehydrogenase level	Normal	19	NR	0.73	.008
	High	41	15	0.26	
Hemoglobin level	Normal	49	NR	0.53	.590
	Low	12	18.5	0.31	

NR–Median survival time had not been reached; SCL–small cell lymphoma; LCL–large cell lymphoma.

Table 8. *Correlation Among Age, Number of Extranodal Sites, and Other Risk Risk Factors in Patients with Diffuse Large Cell Lymphoma*

	No. of patients	Constitutional B symptoms (%)	BM-LCL (%)	Elevated LDH (%)	Mediastinal involvement (%)	Complete remission (%)	Percentage surviving five yr
Age <56 yr 1 site of involvement	17	18	0	50	6	94	88
Age >56 yr 1 site of involvement	11	46	9	54	36	67	36
Age <56 yr ≥2 sites of involvement	13	69	23	77	31	75	38
Age >56 yr ≥2 sites of involvement	20	60	30	85	20	56	29

BM-LCL–Large cell lymphoma involvement of the bone marrow.

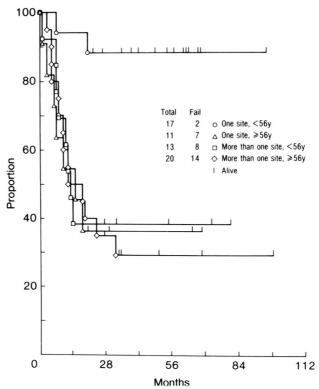

Figure 7. Survival of stage IV diffuse large cell lymphoma patients in different risk groups related to tumor burden and age. There are highly significant differences between survival among the younger patients with only one site of extranodal involvement and the other three subgroups (*P*<.001).

Figure 7. The survival for 17 younger patients with low tumor burdens was 88% at five years. In contrast, the prognosis is much poorer for the other subsets with a calculated five-year survival rate of less than 40%.

Mediastinal involvement with disease was highly correlated with abdominal involvement. Of the 13 patients with mediastinal involvement, 11 (85%) had concomitant extensive abdominal disease, whereas, of the 48 patients without mediastinal disease, only 26 (54.2%) presented with extensive abdominal involvement (*P* = .04). Likewise, patients with mediastinal involvement quite often had constitutional symptoms (69%) and elevated LDH (77%) levels.

Each of the nine clinical factors was also examined for its relationship to remission induction and relapse-free survival. The only factor significantly associated with achievement of CR was age. Table 8 also shows the incidence of CR in each of four subgroups determined by age and number of extranodal sites of disease. Patients younger than 56 years with one extranodal site of disease had a 94% CR rate. As expected, the incidence progressively declines with age and more sites of disease.

There were 11 relapses among the 41 CR patients (Figure 8). Twenty-seven patients (66%) are still alive and in remission. Two patients died of treatment complications and one from an unrelated cause while still in remission. Thus a significant proportion of patients achieving CR are probably cured of the disease.

Age and number of extranodal sites were not significantly related to remission duration, but three other factors were important for relapse-free survival LDH level, constitutional symptoms, and mediastinal involvement with disease. Among 14 patients with normal LDH levels who achieved CR, there have been no relapses. For the 25 patients with A symptoms achieving CR, only three have relapsed, and remission durations ranged from more than 3 to more than 91 months. Fewer patients had mediastinum disease and half of the patients who achieved CR have relapsed.

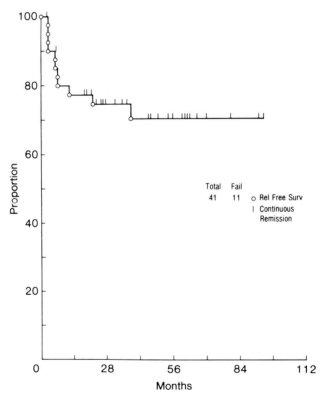

Figure 8. Relapse-free survival for the 41 patients with stage IV diffuse large cell lymphoma who achieved complete remission. A vertical line represents patients in continuous complete remission at the given interval. Rel Free Surv—relapse-free survival.

DISCUSSION

Modern treatment for advanced diffuse large cell lymphoma is associated with high level of CR achievement and long-term survival for a significant proportion of patients with stages III and IV disease. The addition of doxorubicin to the combination known as COP has improved the results observed in previous studies by the Southwest Oncology Group. This combination known as CHOP-Bleo has been the mainstay of therapy at UT M.D. Anderson Hospital since 1973. The rationale for combined modality therapy for stage III disease follows the observation of frequent relapse at the site of extensive nodal involvement.

Stage III

The results for a combined modality program in stage III disease initially demonstrated a calculated five-year survival rate of 64% (Velasquez et al. 1984). With longer follow-up, the overall survival rate has decreased to about 50% at eight years. It is difficult to compare our results with those of other institutions, since data on these patients are frequently analyzed with data on patients with stage IV large cell lymphomas or other histologic aggressive lymphomas. Eighteen patients with stage III grade II histology, as defined by the Manchester group, and who went into CR have also achieved the 60% projected survival at four years with the use of doxorubicin, vincristine, and cyclophosphamide and radiation as consolidation treatment (Blackledge 1980). However, a preliminary National Cancer Institute (NCI) study utilizing a more intensive chemotherapeutic regimen obtained a higher CR rate in 13 patients, and hopefully, better survival will be demonstrated in the future (Fisher 1983).

The benefit of radiotherapy, however, remains unknown. One of the major limiting factors for long-term survival in patients treated with CHOP-Bleo only was disease recurrence at sites of bulky disease (Cabanillas 1978). The administration of radiotherapy to these areas has decreased the probability of disease recurrence in previously irradiated involved areas. However recurrence in nonirradiated areas still remains a serious problem. In addition, 3 of the 13 patients who relapsed suffered recurrence in the central nervous system only.

The prognostic indicators for achievement of CR and relapse-free survival found in this study were LDH level and tumor burden. We also found that these two characteristics are interrelated. The CR rate for patients who have minimal disease involvement or only one site of extensive involvement is excellent, ranging from 78%–91%. Furthermore, 73% of these patients who achieved CR will remain in remission beyond three years if the LDH levels are normal. Likewise, patients who had elevated LDH levels and heavier tumor burdens demonstrated a lower CR rate, 38%, but most important, patients in this category who had elevated LDH levels did not remain in remission. Undoubtedly, the low probability for CR in this subset of patients demands intensification of the chemotherapeutic regimen. A number of chemotherapeutic agents such as VP16 (etoposide) and methotrexate (Fisher et al. 1983, Skarin et al. 1983) can be added to CHOP-Bleo. However, this may increase toxicity and cause unacceptable mortality rates (Fisher et al. 1983). At present, sequential chemotherapy with two different active combinations are given at our institution in an effort to improve overall results and avoid severe toxicity. Similarly, once remission has been obtained, further chemotherapeutic intensification in a bone marrow transplantation program could be considered for patients with high risk of relapse.

Stage IV

Our study comprises a representative sample of patients with stage IV diffuse large cell lymphoma who were treated with the single treatment modality of CHOP-Bleo followed by COP, for a total of one year. The overall survival rate was calculated to be 48.5% at five years, and, as observed previously (DeVita et al. 1975), the survival curve forms a plateau after 30 months. Survival was directly related to CR, which was achieved by 73% of all patients. These parameters compare favorably to data of other investigators in this field. Jones (1979), reporting the experience from the Southwest Oncology Group, demonstrated the superiority of doxorubicin-containing combination in the treatment of diffuse lymphoma. The CR rate of 55% was initially indicated for CHOP. In his most recent analysis, for a larger group of patients, Jones et al. (1983) showed that this CR rate was 49%, and for CHOP-BCG (*Bacillus Calmette-Guerin*) it was 65%. Jones and his colleagues combined data on patients with stages III and IV nodular and diffuse large cell lymphoma, and the survival rates show a 35% level projected at five years. Armitage et al. (1982) have reviewed treatment results of CHOP for stage IV diffuse large cell lymphoma in 48 patients and reported a 44% CR rate and 35% disease-free survival rate at three years. The latter study included previously treated patients with "transformed" large cell lymphoma. However, using the same drugs, Parlier et al. reported a small number of patients with diffuse histiocytic lymphoma 75% of whom had stages III and IV disease and 83% of whom obtained CR (Parlier et al. 1982). Fisher et al. (1977) reported a much lower remission rate in diffuse lymphoma patients treated with similar combination (BACOP–bleomycin, doxorubicin, cyclophosphamide, vincristine, and prednisone). In the initial report, the remission rate was 38% and the overall survival was 25% at five years (Fisher 1977). In a recent update of the experience at NCI, Fisher et al. (1981) reported a 38% CR rate among 76 patients with stage IV diffuse lymphoma. These patients however, were treated with different combinations at different time periods.

Efforts to improve these results have led to intensification of the chemotherapeutic treatment by adding other effective drugs to the combination. ProMACE (cyclophosphamide, doxorubicin, etoposide, and methotrexate) (Fisher et al. 1983) shows a 66% CR rate with 80% of patients who achieve CR remaining free of disease. Skarin et al. (1983) reported that a similar combination but without etoposide (methotrexate, bleomycin, doxorubicin, cyclophosphamide, vincristine, and decadron) produced a 72% CR rate for all stages II to IV diffuse histiocytic and undifferentiated lymphomas, and a recent paper by Cabanillas et al. (1983) showed similar results with sequential chemotherapy. However, Jacobs et al. (1981), found a much lower remission rate using a VP16 and doxorubicin combination. These studies have a short follow-up, but the CR and relapse-free survival rates resulting from these intensive combinations seem to be comparable to the rates reported in our analysis.

Since cost and toxicity have increased in newer regimens (Fisher et al. 1983), it has become imperative to investigate the different variables that may have a prognostic significance and to tailor the chemotherapeutic combination to the individual patient. This approach has been taken by different investigators in the past. Armitage et al. (1982), using a multivariate analysis, reported three independent variables that had significant effects on the chance of achieving CR in 75 patients with diffuse large cell lymphoma treated with CHOP. These variables were the appearance of a histologic conversion (transformed lymphoma), constitutional B symptoms, and large cleaved cell histologic type disease. In addition, they found that the constitutional symptoms were important as prognosticators for relapse. Fisher et al. (1981), using a proportional hazard model of Cox, reported on 151 patients treated for diffuse mixed, histiocytic, and undifferentiated lymphoma and found that sex, constitutional symptoms, bone marrow involvement with disease, and the presence of hugh abdominal masses involving the gastrointestinal tract correlated with poor survival. In this latter study, the histopathologic categories defined by Rappaport (1966) or Strauchen (1978) did not demonstrate any significant difference in survival.

Koziner et al. (1982) have published their experience at the Memorial Sloan-Kettering Cancer Center. Patients treated with a combination different than CHOP had a lower remission rate, and LDH levels were an important factor for achievement of remission, without reaching statistical significance.

In our study, six risk factors, namely age, constitutional symptoms, serum LDH level, mediastinal involvement, and bone marrow infiltrate by large cell lymphoma were shown to affect the overall survival, confirming some of the findings of other investigators (Fisher et al. 1981, Glick et al. 1982). Furthermore, the number of extranodal sites of disease as a measure of tumor burden also has prognostic value. The proportional hazard model, however, identifies only two factors, age and number of extranodal sites, as the independent risk factors.

Thus, this analysis has identified a subset of patients younger than 56 years with low tumor burden who had an excellent probability of survival. The favorable prognosis of primary skin (Fisher et al. 1977) and bone lymphomas (W. S. Velasquez, unpublished data) was recognized in this study, since most of these patients' lymphomatous burdens seem to be limited to one organ or system. Likewise, further analysis shows that this subset of patients have lower frequency of other risk factors such as constitutional B symptoms, elevated LDH levels, or bone marrow involvement with diffuse large cell lymphoma. However, the rest of the population could benefit from additional intensification of the chemotherapy, alternating newer agents with CHOP. Also, there seems to be a need in all patients who achieved CR and have constitutional symptoms and elevated serum LDH levels at diagnosis for consolidation therapy. This therapy might include autologous bone marrow transplantation at the time of complete remission to decrease the chance of relapse.

There is reasonable probability that these factors will have the same significance for patients with stage IV diffuse large cell lymphoma who were treated with other regimens.

REFERENCES

Armitage JO, Dick FR, Corder MP, Garneau SC, Platz CE, Slyman DJ. 1982. Predicting therapeutic outcome in patients with diffuse histiocytic lymphoma treated with cyclophosphamide, adriamycin, vincristine and prednisone (CHOP). Cancer 50:1695–1702.

Blackledge G, Bush H, Chang J, Crowther D, Deakin DP, Dodge OG, Garrett JV, Palmer M, Pearson D, Scarffe JH, Todd IDH, Wilkinson PM. 1980. Intensive combination chemotherapy with vincristine, adriamycin and prednisone (VAP) in the treatment of diffuse histology non-Hodgkin's lymphoma. (A report of 89 cases with extensive disease from the Manchester Lymphoma Group). Eur J Cancer Clin Oncol 16:1459–1468.

Bradley JV. 1968. Distribution-Free Statistical Tests. Prentice-Hall Inc., Englewood, NJ, pp. 195–203.

Cabanillas FC, Burke JS, Smith TL, Moon TE, Butler JJ, Rodriguez V, Freireich EJ. 1978. Factors predicting for response and survival in adults with advanced non-Hodgkin's lymphoma. Arch Intern Med 138:413–418.

Cabanillas FC, Burgess MD, Bodey GP, Freireich EJ. 1983. Sequential chemotherapy and late intensification for malignant lymphomas of aggressive histological type. Am J Med 74:382–388.

Canellos GP, Skarin AT, Rosenthal DS, Moloney WC, Frei E. 1981. Methotrexate as a single agent and in combination chemotherapy for the treatment of non-Hodgkin's lymphoma of unfavorable histology. Cancer Treat Rep 65:125–129.

DeVita VT, Chabner B, Hubbard SP, Canellos GP, Schein P, Young RC. 1975. Advanced diffuse histiocytic lymphoma, a potentially curable disease. Lancet 1:248–250.

Fisher RI, DeVita VT, Hubbard SM, Longo DL, Wesley R, Chabner BA, Young RC. 1983. Diffuse aggressive lymphomas: Increased survival after alternating flexible sequences of ProMACE and MOPP chemotherapy. Ann Intern Med 98:304–309.

Fisher RI, DeVita VT, Johnson BL, Simon R, Young RC. 1977. Prognostic factors for advanced diffuse histiocytic lymphoma following treatment with combination chemotherapy. Am J Med 63:177–182.

Fisher RI, Hubbard SM, DeVita VT, Berard CW, Wesley R, Cossman J, Young RC. 1981. Factors predicting long-term survival in diffuse mixed, histiocytic, or undifferentiated lymphoma. Blood 58:45–51.

Gehan EA. 1965. Generalized Wilcoxon test for comparing arbitrarily singly-censored samples. Biometrika. 52:203–223.

Ginsberg SJ, Crooke ST, Bloomfield CD, Peterson B, Kennedy BJ, Blom J, Ellison RR, Pajak TF, Gottlieb AJ. 1982. Cyclophosphamide, Doxorubicin, vincristine, and low-dose continuous infusion bleomycin in non-Hodgkin's lymphoma: Cancer and leukemia group B study #7804. Cancer 49:1346–1352.

Glick JH, McFadden E, Costello W, Ezdinle E, Berard CW, Bennett JM. 1982. Nodular histiocytic lymphoma: Factors influencing prognosis and implications for aggressive chemotherapy. Cancer 49:840–845.

Hansen MM, Bloomfield CD, Jorgensen J, Ersboll J, Pedersen-Bjergaard J, Blom J, Nissen NI. 1980. VP-16-213 in combination with cyclophosphamide, doxorubicin, vincristine, and prednisone in the treatment of non-Hodgkin's lymphomas. Cancer Treat Rep 64:1135–1137.

Jacobs P, King HS, Cassidy F, Dent DM, Harrison T. 1981. VP-16-213 in the treatment of stage III and IV diffuse lymphocytic lymphoma of the large cell (histiocytic) variety: An interim report. Cancer Treat Rep 65:987–993.

Jones SE, Grozea PN, Metz EN, Haut A, Stephens RL, Morrison FS, Butler JJ, Byrne GE Jr, Moon TE, Fisher R, Haskins CL, Coltman CA Jr. 1979. Superiority of adriamycin containing combination chemotherapy in the treatment of diffuse lymphoma. A Southwest Oncology Group Study. Cancer 43:417–425.

Jones SE, Grozea PN, Metz EN, Haut A, Stephens RL, Morrison FS, Talley R, Butler JJ, Byrne GE, Hartsock R, Dixon D, Salmon SE. 1983. Improved complete remission rates and survival for patients with large cell lymphoma treated with chemoimmunotherapy. A Southwest Oncology Group Study. Cancer 51:1083–1090.

Kaplan EL, Meier P. 1958. Non-parametric estimation from incomplete observations. Journal of the American Statistical Association 53:457–481.

Koziner B, Little C, Passe S, Thaler HT, Sklaroff R, Straus DJ, Lee BJ, Clarkson BD. 1982. Treatment of advanced diffuse histiocytic lymphoma: An analysis of prognostic variables. Cancer 49:1571–1579.

McKelvey EM, Gottlieb JA, Wilson HE, Haut A, Talley RW, Stephens R, Lane M, Gamble JF, Jones SE, Grozea PN, Gutterman J, Coltman C, Moon TE. 1976. Hydroxyldaunomycin (Adriamycin) combination chemotherapy in malignant lymphoma. Cancer 38:1484–1493.

Non-Hodgkin's Lymphoma Pathologic Classification Project. 1982. National Cancer Institute sponsored study of classifications of non-Hodgkin's lymphomas: Summary and description of a Working Formulation for clinical usage. Cancer 49:2112–2135.

Parlier Y, Gorin NC, Najman A, Stachowiak J, Duhamel G. 1982. Combination chemotherapy with cyclophosphamide, vincristine, prednisone and the contribution of adriamycin in the treatment of adult non-Hodgkin's lymphomas. A report of 131 cases. Cancer 50:401–409.

Pettingale KW. 1981. The management of generalized grade 2 non-Hodgkin's lymphomas: Report No. 18. Clin Radiol 32:553–555.

Rappaport H. 1966. Tumors of the hematopoietic system. *In* Atlas of Tumor Pathology. Section III, Fascicle 8. Armed Forces Institute of Pathology, Washington, D.C., pp. 97–161.

Rodriguez V, Cabanillas F, Burgess MA, McKelvey EM, Valdivieso M, Bodey GP, Freireich EJ. 1977. Combination chemotherapy ("CHOP-Bleo") in advanced (non-Hodgkin's) malignant lymphoma. Blood 49:325–333.

Skarin AT, Canellos GP, Rosenthal DS, Case DC, MacIntyre JM, Pinkus GS, Moloney WC, Frei E. 1983. Improved prognosis of diffuse histiocytic and undifferentiated lymphoma by use of high dose methotrexate alternating with standard agents (M-BACOD). J Clin Oncol 1:91–98.

Skarin AT, Rosenthal DS, Moloney WC, Frei E. 1977. Combination chemotherapy of advanced non-Hodgkin lymphoma with bleomycin, adriamycin, cyclophosphamide, vincristine, and prednisone (BACOP). Blood 49:759–770.

Schein PS, Chabner BA, Canellos GP, et al. 1974. Potential for prolonged disease-free survival following combination chemotherapy of non-Hodgkin's lymphoma. Blood 43:181–189.

Strauchen JA, Young RC, DeVita VT, Anderson T, Fantone JC, Berard CW. 1978. Clinical relevance of the histopathologic subclassification of diffuse "histiocytic" lymphoma. N Engl J Med 299:1382–1387.

Velasquez WS, Fuller LM, Oh KK, Hagemeister FB, Sullivan JA, Manning JT, Shullenberger CC. 1984. Combined modality in stage III and stage IIIE diffuse large cell lymphomas. Cancer (In press).

UT M.D. Anderson Clinical Conference on Cancer,
Vol. 27, edited by R.J. Ford, L.M. Fuller, and
F.B. Hagemeister. Raven Press, New York © 1984.

Advances in the Treatment of Diffuse Aggressive Lymphomas

Richard I. Fisher, Vincent T. DeVita, Jr.,* and Robert C. Young

Medicine Branch and *Director, National Cancer Institute, National Institutes of Health,
Bethesda, Maryland 20205

The diffuse aggressive lymphomas have traditionally been considered a rapidly progressive, fatal disease. Included in this category are diffuse mixed lymphoma, diffuse histiocytic or large cell lymphoma, and diffuse undifferentiated non-Burkitt's lymphoma (Berard and Dorfman 1974). Diffuse histiocytic lymphoma has classically been considered the prototype of these diffuse aggressive lymphomas, since it is the most common type. During the 1960s only 10%–20% of patients with diffuse histiocytic lymphoma were alive at five years after diagnosis (Fuks et al. 1973). Radiation therapy led to a 30%–50% five-year survival rate when clinical stage I patients were treated (Peckham 1974). However, in patients with more advanced stages, complete remissions were rarely achieved with either radiation therapy or single-agent chemotherapy. The first report demonstrating that disease-free survival of longer than 5-10 years could be obtained in patients with advanced stages of diffuse histiocytic lymphoma who were treated with combination chemotherapy was published in 1975 (DeVita et al. 1975). Subsequent studies at several other institutions have confirmed that a subset of patients with diffuse histiocytic lymphoma could be cured (Berd et al. 1975, Jones et al. 1979, Skarin et al. 1977, Sweet et al. 1980). Thus, by 1977 it was well established that complete remissions, documented by reevaluation of all initially involved sites, could be achieved in 40%–50% of all patients with advanced stages of diffuse histiocytic lymphoma and that 75%–80% of these complete responders would have long-term disease-free survival. Furthermore, an analysis of prognostic factors in these patients enabled us to predict, with a high degree of accuracy, the ultimate survival rate of certain subsets of patients, based on their initial clinical staging information (Fisher et al. 1977, Fisher et al. 1981).

In 1977, we initiated the third generation of the National Cancer Institute (NCI) studies in the chemotherapy for the advanced stages of the diffuse aggressive lymphomas with a treatment program termed ProMACE-MOPP (cyclophosphamide, doxorubicin, etoposide, methotrexate, and prednisone plus mechlorethamine, vincristine, procarbazine, and prednisone). The results of this clinical trial have recently been published and suggest a significant improvement in the long-term survival rate of these patients (Fisher et al. 1983). Several other studies that were initiated at approximately the same time have also suggested a significant improvement in survival (Cabanillas et al. 1983, Laurence et al. 1982, Skarin et al. 1983). Thus, in the 1980s it may now be possible to achieve long-term disease-free survival in approximately 60% of all patients with advanced stages of the diffuse aggressive lymphomas. Studies are ongoing in an attempt to improve the complete response rate and long-term disease-free survival rate, while at the same time minimizing the toxicity and cost to the patient.

C-MOPP/MOPP CLINICAL TRIALS

As noted previously, DeVita et al. (1975) reported that advanced stage diffuse histiocytic lymphoma was a curable disease in 1975. Twenty-seven patients with stages II-IV disease were treated with either the C-MOPP (cyclophosphamide instead of mechlorethamine in MOPP) regimen consisting of cyclophosphamide at 650 mg/m^2 intravenously on day one and day eight of treatment, vincristine at 1.4 mg/m^2 intravenously on day one and day eight, procarbazine at 100 mg/m^2 orally for 14 days, and prednisone at 40 mg/m^2 orally for 14 days or with the classical MOPP chemotherapy program that had been utilized for the treatment of Hodgkin's disease (DeVita et al. 1980). After the initial two weeks of therapy, the patients received no therapy for the next two weeks, and the monthly cycles were repeated for a minimum of six cycles or at least two cycles after a complete clinical remission had been achieved. One month after chemotherapy had been stopped, the patients were reevaluated to determine whether all disease at previously involved sites had disappeared. Only patients without evidence of disease at that point were considered complete responders. Eleven of the 27 patients (41%) achieved complete remission and 37% of the patients were alive and disease free with no maintenance chemotherapy at five years. The follow-up on these patients now exceeds ten years, and the disease free survival curve remains essentially flat. There was no significant difference in the therapeutic results achieved with C-MOPP (17 patients) or MOPP (10 patients), although the number of patients receiving each regimen was small.

BACOP CLINICAL TRIAL

The second generation of NCI studies of combination chemotherapy for the treatment of advanced diffuse histiocytic lymphoma utilized the BACOP (bleomycin, doxorubicin, cyclophosphamide, vincristine, and prednisone) chemotherapeutic regimen (Schein et al. 1976) and introduced two new agents with significant activity in these diseases, namely doxorubicin and bleomycin. The regimen consisted of cyclophosphamide, 650 mg/m^2, doxorubicin 25 mg/m^2, and vincristine, 1.4 mg/m^2, each given intravenously on days one and eight of treatment. Bleomycin, 5 U/m^2, was then given intravenously on days 15 and 22, while prednisone, 60 mg/m^2, was given orally on days 15 through 28. The cycle was repeated monthly for a minimum of six cycles or until at least two cycles after a clinical remission had been achieved. Restaging procedures were similar to that used in the C-MOPP study. Twelve of 25 patients with stages II–IV diffuse histiocytic lymphoma (48%) achieved pathologically documented complete remission. These complete remissions again proved durable with few relapses after two years.

PROGNOSTIC FACTORS IN DIFFUSE HISTIOCYTIC LYMPHOMAS

In 1981 we analyzed the prognostic factors used to predict long-term survival in 151 patients with diffuse mixed, histiocytic, or undifferentiated non-Burkitt's lymphoma treated at NCI between 1964 and 1977 (Fisher et al. 1981). Twenty percent of these patients had diffuse mixed, 60% had diffuse histiocytic, and 13% had diffuse undifferentiated non-Burkitt's lymphoma. Thirteen percent were classified stage I, 23% stage II, 14% stage III, and 50% stage IV. Twenty-five percent received radiation, 61% received combination chemotherapy, and 11% received combined modality treatment as their initial treatments. The results of this study indicated that a number of factors were associated with poor prognosis. They included male sex, constitutional or B symptoms, advanced stage, bone marrow involvement, abdominal mass greater than ten centimeters with gastrointestinal involvement, hepatic involvement, hemoglobin <12 g/dl or serum lactic dehydrogenase >250 U/L. Furthermore, in contrast to each of these clinical factors, which provide highly significant prognostic information ($P<.001$), the division of patients into diffuse mixed, histiocytic, or undifferentiated lymphoma categories did not provide significant information about their prognoses ($P=0.27$). In addition, it proved difficult for expert hematopathologists, even at the same institution, to consistently separate diffuse mixed, diffuse histiocytic, and diffuse undifferentiated non-Hodgkin's lymphoma. Therefore, the term diffuse aggressive lymphomas was introduced so that this difficult pathologic subdivision was not a critical factor in the assignment of patients to various arms of a clinical trial.

A comparison of the results of the C-MOPP and the BACOP studies demonstrated several important conclusions (Fisher et al. 1977). The complete response rate in each study was 46% and greater than 80% of those complete responders were alive and disease free in excess of five years. Essentially, all of the relapses occurred in the first 24 months after the completion of therapy. Thus, disease-free survival beyond two years was tantamount to cure. In subsequent follow-up, although there has been an occasional late relapse, the disease-free survival curves remain flat with 37% long-term disease-free survival. It was also of interest that, although the partial responders included patients with a 50% reduction in tumor measurement as well as some patients with complete clinical remission who had only microscopic evidence of residual disease at their restaging evaluations, the survival of the partial responders was not significantly different from that of the nonresponders. Therefore, only patients who achieved a complete clinical remission could have long-term disease-free survival. It is also essential to realize that all of the patients in these studies were previously untreated, with the possible exception of local radiation therapy. The chance for a complete remission falls dramatically when the patient has relapsed after previous chemotherapy. In fact, there is no evidence at this time that long-term disease-free survival can be achieved in that circumstance.

Thus, these are diseases in which the initial chemotherapy is of paramount importance. Obviously, the response rates and survival curves for the two regimens (C-MOPP and BACOP) were so similar that it was impossible to determine which of these two chemotherapeutic regimens was more beneficial. Detailed analysis of the prognostic factors of the patients present in each study also revealed great similarity. The only difference between the two studies was that the only patients with exceedingly poor prognostic factors, such as bone marrow involvement and huge gastrointestinal masses, who achieved complete remission were those who were treated with the BACOP regimen. However, it must be noted that the BACOP regimen was more difficult to administer and was associated with more patient complaints of weakness, loss of appetite, and weight loss.

ProMACE-MOPP CLINICAL TRIAL

In 1977, we initiated the third generation of NCI studies for the treatment of diffuse aggressive lymphomas with the ProMACE-MOPP chemotherapeutic regimen. The aim of this study was to develop two potentially non–cross-resistant combination chemotherapeutic regimens that could be used for induction, consolidation, and late intensification therapy (Fisher et al. 1983). In addition, these regimens took advantage of the newly described activity of epipodophyllotoxin VP-16 and high dose methotrexate for use in the lymphomas. Patients were initially treated with induction therapy using the ProMACE regimen and prednisone. They then received MOPP chemotherapy in the second phase and finally were treated with ProMACE chemotherapy again in the late intensification phase. The number of cycles of therapy that a patient received during each phase of his treatment was determined by his rate of tumor response, i.e., the patients were treated with the alternate chemotherapeutic regimen whenever clinically available measurements of tumor area revealed the rate of tumor response had decreased. This was based on the rationale that a decrease in the rate of tumor response indicated either a reduced rate of cell kill or regrowth of cells that were resistant to the chemotherapy being administered. A mathematical model developed by Goldie and Coldman (1979) suggests that tumor resistance to chemotherapy may develop spontaneously based on somatic mutations. This model suggests that the use of multiple non–cross-resistant chemotherapeutic agents would be the best way to treat patients, since this approach would have the highest likelihood of preventing the growth of tumor clones that have spontaneous resistance to a particular drug treatment.

From September 1977 to August 1981, 79 consecutive patients admitted to the Medicine Branch of NCI were entered on this study. Two percent of the patients had diffuse poorly differentiated lymphocytic lymphoma, 18% diffuse mixed, 71% had diffuse histiocytic, and 9% diffuse undifferentiated non-Burkitt's lymphoma. Twenty-three percent of the patients had stage II disease, 16% had stage III, and 61% had stage IV. Among the 18 patients with stage II disease, 7 had gastrointestinal involvement and 4 had large mediastinal masses. None of the patients had prior chemotherapeutic treatment.

In the ProMACE chemotherapeutic regimen (Figure 1) the patients received epipodophyllotoxin VP-16, 120 mg/m^2, cyclophosphamide, 650 mg/m^2, and Adriamycin, 25 mg/m^2, intravenously on days one and eight of treatment. Methotrexate, 1.5 g/m^2, was given intravenously as a 12-hour infusion on day 14, followed by leucovorin, 50 mg/m^2, intravenously q 6 hr for 5 doses beginning 24 hours after the initiation of the methotrexate infusion. All patients received intravenous hydration at a rate of 3,000 ml/m^2/24 hours from 12 hours prior to the methotrexate infusion until the completion of the leucovorin rescue. This methotrexate infusion was, therefore, administered in the hospital. Sodium bicarbonate was added to the intravenous fluid as needed to maintain urinary pH >7.0. The serum methotrexate level was determined 48 hours after the initiation of the methotrexate infusion. If the 48-hour level was $<5\times10^{-7}$ m, the patient was discharged. If the level was $\geqslant5\times10^{-7}$ m, intravenous hydration, alkalinization, and leucovorin rescue were continued until the serum methotrexate was $<5\times10^{-7}$ m. Prednisone, 60 mg/m^2, was given orally every day for the first 14 days of the cycle. No cytotoxic drugs were administered from days 15 to 28, and a complete cycle of ProMACE chemotherapy lasted 28 days. Details of the carefully structured "flexi-therapy" induction schedule are presented elsewhere (Fisher et al. 1983). The doses of chemotherapy administered during each cycle were reduced according to a sliding scale, depending on the patient's white blood cell count and platelet count.

Complete remissions were determined in the same manner as in the C-MOPP or BACOP studies, except that abdominal computed tomographic (CT) scans were routinely employed. The complete remissions were, therefore, more carefully documented in the current study. The complete remission rate for the entire group of patients was 74%. According to the stage of the disease, the complete remission rate was 82% for patients with stage II disease, 92% for stage III, and 66% for

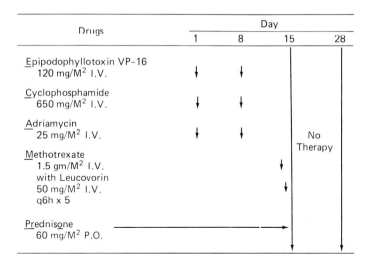

Figure 1. ProMACE chemotherapeutic regimen.

stage IV. In patients with stage III or IV disease, this represents an overall complete remission rate of 72%. Essentially, all patients who achieved complete remission required six or nine cycles of chemotherapy. They appeared to enter complete clinical remission throughout the three phases of their therapy. Forty-five percent of the complete responders entered complete clinical remission during the Pro-MACE induction, 27% during MOPP consolidation, and 15% during late intensification. The durability of these complete remissions was excellent. Actuarial analysis predicts that 66% of the complete responders will remain disease free in excess of three years (Figure 2). Eighteen percent of the complete responders have relapsed. Eight patients relapsed with diffuse lymphoma while two patients who presented with diffuse aggressive lymphoma in one site and nodular lymphoma in another site relapsed with nodular lymphoma. Three of the ten patients have been successfully re-treated and are now disease free from 9 to 30 months.

The survival rate of all patients in the study who were treated with the ProMACE-MOPP chemotherapeutic regimen is shown in Figure 3. Median survival has not been reached at this time. Median follow-up for this study now exceeds two and one-half years. Actuarial analysis predicts that the median survival will be in excess of four years with 65% of all patients alive at that time. As expected, the prolonged survival observed in the entire population is a function of the survival of the complete responders. Eighty-two percent of the complete responders are predicted to be alive at four years while only 10% of the partial responders and none of the nonresponders survived two years.

Myelosuppression was the dose-limiting toxic effect in the ProMACE-MOPP chemotherapeutic regimen. At some time during their therapies, 85% of the patients had white blood cell counts $<1,500/mm^3$ and at some time during therapy 34%

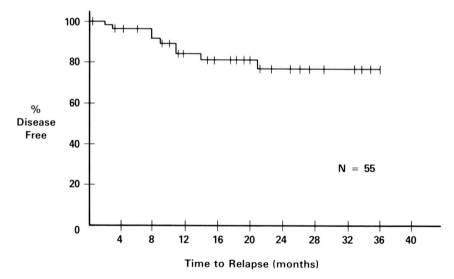

Figure 2. Disease-free survival for all complete responders treated with ProMACE-MOPP.

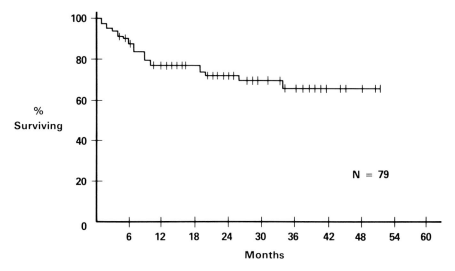

Figure 3. Overall survival rate for all patients treated with ProMACE-MOPP.

had platelet counts of $<50,000/mm^3$. Fever of unknown origin, which required empiric therapy with multiple broad-spectrum antibiotics, occurred in 15% of the cycles. In fact, there was a 10% septic death rate representing eight septic deaths. Four of these patients deserve special comment. In two cases, ProMACE chemotherapy was initiated despite the presence of intraabdominal fistula and abscesses that grew multiple organisms prior to treatment. These patients were treated because of their progressive lymphoma but were unable to survive the leukopenic period. A third patient had an initial pretreatment white blood cell count $<1,000/mm^3$, secondary to extensive bone marrow involvement. This was an extremely unusual severity of bone marrow involvement, and only one other patient in the NCI experience presented with this degree of leukopenia. Finally, a patient with drug-induced pancytopenia and sepsis was treated initially with single-agent antibiotic therapy at his local hospital and died within 12 hours. In spite of the 10% septic death rate, 65% of the patients are predicted to be alive at four years after initiation of treatment.

COMPARISON OF PROMACE-MOPP WITH C-MOPP OR BACOP REGIMENS

Comparison of the therapeutic results achieved with the C-MOPP or BACOP regimens and the ProMACE-MOPP regimen clearly demonstrates a significant improvement in the current study. The complete response rate on the ProMACE-MOPP study of 74% is significantly higher than the complete rate achieved in the C-MOPP or BACOP studies ($P<0.01$). In fact, regardless of the category of patients analyzed, complete remission with the ProMACE-MOPP regimen is always higher than that achieved in the previous studies. For example, complete remission rates for patients with B symptoms in ProMACE-MOPP was 62% versus 43% with C-MOPP or BACOP. For stage II, the complete remission rates were 82% versus 50%, stage III 92% versus 75%, and for stage IV 66% versus 38%. Patients with bone marrow involvement had a 50% complete remission rate on ProMACE-MOPP versus 8% with C-MOPP or BACOP. Patients with gastrointestinal involvement had a 64% complete remission rate with ProMACE-MOPP and 20% with C-MOPP or BACOP. For patients with liver involvement, the respective rates are 55% and 33%. Furthermore, if one plots the survival rate of patients treated with the ProMACE-MOPP program versus all patients on the C-MOPP or BACOP program, a highly significant improvement in survival is shown (Figure 4) ($P = 0.002$). The survival advantage is statistically significant when one considers all patients with diffuse aggressive lymphomas, as in Figure 4, patients with diffuse histiocytic lymphoma only, or patients with stage IV diffuse histiocytic lymphoma only (data not shown). Thus, by any statistical methods, the ProMACE-MOPP therapy appears to provide a significant survival advance over that achieved with our previous studies.

COMPARISON OF CHEMOTHERAPEUTIC REGIMENS FOR DIFFUSE AGGRESSIVE LYMPHOMAS

Table 1 depicts the pathologic complete remission rate and long-term survival figures for chemotherapeutic regimens commonly used in the treatment of the diffuse aggressive lymphomas. The NCI experience with C-MOPP and BACOP have been previously described, and approximately 37% of patients enjoy long-term disease-free survival. These numbers are similar to results achieved at the Dana-Farber Cancer Institute with their BACOP regimen. This regimen includes the same drugs but a different schedule than the one used at the NCI (Skarin et al. 1977).

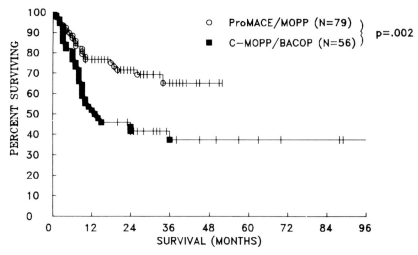

Figure 4. Overall survival rate of all patients with diffuse aggressive lymphomas treated with either the ProMACE-MOPP or C-MOPP/BACOP regimens.

Table 1. *Comparison of Chemotherapeutic Regimens for Aggressive Diffuse Lymphomas*

Regimen (institution)	No. of patients	Pathologic CR	Long-term survivors
MOPP/C-MOPP (NCI)	24	45%	37%
BACOP (NCI)	32	46%	37%
CHOP (SWOG)	112	58%	< 30%
COMLA (Chicago)	42	55%	48%
COP-BLAM (NY)	33	73%	TE
M-BACOD (Boston)	101	72%	59%
ProMACE-MOPP (NCI)	79	74%	65%

NCI–National Cancer Institute; SWOG–Southwest Oncology Group; Chicago–University of Chicago; NY–New York Hospital; Boston–Dana-Farber Cancer Institute; CR–complete remission; TE–Too early to evaluate. (See text for components of chemotherapeutic regimens.)

Probably the most commonly utilized chemotherapy in the United States for the treatment of the diffuse lymphomas is the CHOP (cyclophosphamide, doxorubicin, vincristine, and prednisone) regimen (Jones et al. 1979). Complete remission rates have varied in previous CHOP studies depending on whether restaging of disease in all previously involved sites was performed. In no study has the complete remission rate been greater than 60%. Yet even with pathologic restaging, greater than 50% of the complete responders had relapsed by the end of two years (Jones et al. 1979). This high rate of relapse is in contrast to that seen with any of the other regimens used for the treatment of this disease. Furthermore, there is no evidence of a significant plateau on the disease-free survival curve of patients treated with CHOP chemotherapy. As a result, fewer than 30% of all patients would be expected to have long-term disease-free survival when treated with CHOP.

The COMLA (cyclophosphamide, vincristine, methotrexate, leucovorin, and cytarabine) regimen, which has been utilized at Yale University and the University of Chicago, gives cyclophosphamide and vincristine initially and follows that at weekly intervals with methotrexate and cytarabine (Berd et al. 1975, Sweet et al. 1980). In 42 previously untreated patients from the University of Chicago, a 56% pathologically documented complete remission rate was obtained and 48% of those patients appeared to be long-term disease-free survivors.

The highest complete remission rates that have been achieved have recently been reported with the ProMACE-MOPP, M-BACOD (methotrexate, bleomycin, doxorubicin, cyclophosphamide, vincristine, and decadron), and COP-BLAM (cyclophosphamide, vincristine, prednisone, bleomycin, doxorubicin, and procarbazine) programs (Laurence et al. 1982, Skarin et al. 1983). A 73% complete remission rate has been reported in 33% of patients on the COP-BLAM program at New York University. However, the number of patients is relatively small in this study and the remissions are too short to enable us to predict the long-term disease-free survival. The M-BACOD study appears comparable in many respects to the

ProMACE-MOPP study. The only significant difference between the M-BACOD study and the previously described BACOP study from the Boston group is the addition of the high-dose methotrexate. The M-BACOD study was performed in patients with diffuse histiocytic and diffuse undifferentiated lymphoma. A 72% pathologically documented complete remission rate was achieved with a 59% survival rate at five years. Toxicity was again significant, depending on the method of calculation, and resulted in 4%–6% of the deaths. In fact, the parallels in the results between the M-BACOD study and the ProMACE-MOPP study are quite striking. One of the few significant differences between the two studies is the fact that M-BACOD did not include patients with diffuse mixed lymphoma. Patients with diffuse mixed lymphoma were treated with the M-BACOD regimen and reported in a separate study (Canellos et al. 1982). For unclear reasons, the patients with diffuse mixed lymphoma had a much higher relapse rate in the Boston experience, and the regimen did not produce a high number of long-term disease-free patients. Excellent results have also been obtained at the UT M.D. Anderson Hospital in the treatment of the diffuse aggressive lymphomas using multiple sequential combination chemotherapeutic regimens (Cabanillas et al. 1983).

Thus, it is clear that the long-term survival rates for patients with diffuse aggressive lymphomas may vary from less than 30% to approximately 60%, depending on the chemotherapeutic regimen. The newer regimens, however, are more complicated and not easily applied in nonresearch hospitals or in an office practice setting. As a result of these limitations in the ProMACE-MOPP study, the newest NCI study is a prospective randomized trial comparing ProMACE-MOPP with a regimen termed ProMACE-CytaBOM (cytarabine, bleomycin, vincristine, and methotrexate). The ProMACE-MOPP regimen has been changed in this study to give the ProMACE drugs on day 1, MOPP drugs on day 8 and then methotrexate at a dose of 500 mg/m^2 rather than the original 1.5 g/m^2 on day 15 of treatment. The ProMACE-CytaBOM regimen includes the ProMACE drugs on day one and then the CytaBOM drugs on day eight. Both of these regimens were designed to allow for outpatient administration and to eliminate the need for hospitalization related to methotrexate administration. At the present time, 47 patients have been entered into the trial, 26 on ProMACE-MOPP and 21 on ProMACE-CytaBOM. Preliminary results indicate a complete remission rate of 75% for ProMACE-MOPP and 81% for ProMACE-CytaBOM. Although it is much too early for a definitive conclusion, both regimens appear to be very effective, and the septic death rate and number of hospitalizations for fever and granulocytopenia appear to be significantly reduced. Both regimens can be administered safely to outpatients. If longer follow up proves that they are as effective as the original regimen, these new programs may be extremely useful for the treatment of patients with diffuse aggressive lymphomas.

REFERENCES

Berard CW, Dorfman RF. 1974. Histopathology of malignant lymphoma. Clin Haematol 3:39–76.

Berd D, Cornog J, DeConti R, Levitt M, Bertino JR. 1975. Long term remission in diffuse histiocytic lymphoma treated with combination sequential chemotherapy. Cancer 35:1050–1054.

Cabanillas F, Burgess MA, Bodey GP, Freireich EJ. 1983. Sequential chemotherapy and late intensification for malignant lymphomas of aggressive histiologic type. Am J Med 74:382–388.

Canellos G, Skarin A, Rosenthal D, Anderson R, Leonard G, Pinkus G, McIntyre J. 1982. High dose methotrexate combination chemotherapy (M-BACOD) of advanced favorable and intermediate prognosis histology non-Hodgkin's lymphoma. (Abstract) Proceedings of the American Society of Clinical Oncology 1:159.

DeVita VT, Canellos GP, Chabner BA, Schein P, Hubbard SP, Young RC. 1975. Advanced diffuse histiocytic lymphoma, a potentially curable disease. Lancet 1:248–250.

DeVita VT, Simon RM, Hubbard SM, Young RC, Berard CW, Moxley JH, Frei E, Carbone PE, Canellos GP. 1980. The curability of advanced Hodgkin's disease with chemotherapy: long term followup of MOPP treated patients at the NCI. Ann Intern Med 92:587–594.

Fisher RI, DeVita VT, Johnson BL, Simon R, Young RC. 1977. Prognostic factors for advanced diffuse histiocytic lymphoma following treatment with combination chemotherapy. Am J Med 63:177–182.

Fisher RI, Hubbard SM, DeVita VT, Berard CW, Wesley R, Cossman J, Young RC. 1981. Factors predicting long-term survival in diffuse mixed, histiocytic, or undifferentiated lymphoma. Blood 58:45–51.

Fisher RI, DeVita VT, Hubbard SM, Longo DL, Wesley R, Chabner BA, Young RC. 1983. Diffuse aggressive lymphomas: Increased survival after alternating flexible sequences of ProMACE and MOPP chemotherapy. Ann Intern Med 98:304–309.

Fuks Z, Bull M, Kadin ME, Dorfman HS, Rosenberg SA, Kim H. 1973. Lymphoma IV Clinicopathologic correlations. Cancer 31:806 823.

Goldie JE, Coldman AJ. 1979. A mathematical model for relating the drug sensitivity of tumors to their spontaneous mutation rate. Cancer Treat Rep 63:1727–1733.

Jones SE, Grozea PN, Metz EN, Haut A, Stephens RL, Morrison FS, Butler JJ, Byrne GE, Moon TE, Fisher R, Haskins CL, Clotman CA. 1979. Superiority of adriamycin containing combination chemotherapy in the treatment of diffuse lymphoma. Cancer 43:417–425.

Laurence J, Coleman M, Allen SL, Silver RT, Pasmantier M. 1982. Combination chemotherapy of advanced diffuse histiocytic lymphoma with the six drug COP-BLAM regimen. Ann Intern Med 97:190–195.

Peckham MJ. 1974. Radiation therapy of the non-Hodgkin's lymphomas. Semin Hematol 11:41–58.

Schein PS, DeVita VT Jr, Hubbard S, Chabner BA, Canellos GP, Berard C, Young RC. 1976. Bleomycin, adriamycin, cyclophosphamide, vincristine and prednisone (BACOP) combination chemotherapy in the treatment of advanced diffuse histiocytic lymphomas. Ann Intern Med 85:417–422.

Skarin AT, Rosenthal DS, Maloney WC, Frei E. 1977. Combination chemotherapy of advanced non-Hodgkin's lymphoma with bleomycin, adriamycin, cyclophosphamide, vincristine, and prednisone (BACOP). Blood 49:759–770.

Skarin AT, Canellos GP, Rosenthal DS, Case DC, MacIntyre JM, Pinkus GS, Moloney WC, Frei E. 1983. Improved prognosis of diffuse histiocytic and undifferentiated lymphoma by use of high dose methotrexate alternating with standard agents (M-BACOD). Journal of Clinical Oncology 1:91–97.

Sweet DL, Golomb HM, Ultmann JE, Miller JB, Stein RS, Lester EP, Mintz U, Bitran JD, Streuli RA, Daly K, Roth NO. 1980. Cyclophosphamide, vincristine, methotrexate with leucovorin rescue, and cytarabine (COMLA) combination sequential chemotherapy for advanced diffuse histiocytic lymphoma. Ann Intern Med 92:785–790.

New Drugs and Modalities of Therapy for
Malignant Lymphomas

UT M.D. Anderson Clinical Conference on Cancer,
Vol. 27, edited by R. J. Ford, L. M. Fuller, and
F. B. Hagemeister. Raven Press, New York © 1984.

New Chemotherapeutic Agents and Combinations in the Treatment of Lymphoma

Fernando Cabanillas

Department of Hematology, The University of Texas M.D. Anderson Hospital and Tumor Institute at Houston, Houston, Texas 77030

NEW AGENTS AND COMBINATIONS

Several new chemotherapeutic agents tested during the past 10 years have shown activity against lymphoma. Most of the studies of these new drugs have been conducted on previously treated patients with recurrent or refractory lymphomas. Consequently, investigators might underestimate the true response rate of these drugs if they were to be applied to previously untreated patients. With this in mind, we shall review the activity of new single agents as well as their uses in combination regimens.

VP-16 (Etoposide)

The most extensively studied new agent is VP-16. Four published studies on a total of 116 patients have identified this drug as one of the most active in recurrent or refractory lymphoma (Jacobs 1975, Bender et al. 1978, Dombernowsky et al. 1972, Cecil et al. 1978). These studies, however, differ broadly in the doses used and in the patient population treated. For example, the study by Cecil et al. from the Southwest Oncology Group (SWOG) used a dose that was two thirds of the average maximum tolerated dose. Their population consisted of poor risk, heavily pretreated patients who could not tolerate the usual doses. In 56 patients, 3 (5%) responded representing the lowest recorded response rate for VP-16. On the other hand, Jacobs' study, which showed 6 (60%) responders out of 10 patients with recurrent lymphoma, included patients who received less extensive therapy, most of whom had not been given doxorubicin. The other two studies recorded response rates of 8 (26%) of 31 patients and 8 (42%) of 19 patients responding. The average response to VP-16, if all these studies are considered, is 22%. If the SWOG study that used the low dose of VP-16 is excluded, then the average response rate would be 37%. Only Jacobs' study lists the median response duration, which was 5.5 months.

Methyl GAG (Methylglyoxal Bis-Guanylhydrazone)

This interesting compound has recently received considerable attention. The early studies conducted in the 1960s revealed its activity against leukemia. However, the toxicity was severe and consisted mostly of mucositis and vasculitis. An advantage was its lack of myelosuppression. Administration of methyl GAG once or twice per week has been substantially less toxic than the daily schedule. Two independent studies have shown this drug to be active against lymphoma. Warrell et al. (1981) at Memorial Sloan-Kettering Hospital treated 40 patients with Hodgkin's disease and lymphomas. Sixteen, or 40%, responded, all with partial remissions. The median response duration was three months. The second study was conducted by Kuhn et al. (1982) from the SWOG who treated 23 lymphoma patients. Thirty percent responded. Most of the responses were in patients with the indolent (low grade) lymphomas.

Ifosfamide

Ifosfamide probably deserves more attention than it has received. Its lack of cross-resistance with cyclophosphamide and its mild myelosuppressive effect makes it an attractive compound (Rodriguez 1978). In 1974 we studied this drug and found it to be active in both acute lymphocytic leukemia and lymphomas (Rodriguez 1978). We used a dose of 1.2 gm/m^2 daily for five days every three weeks. Fifteen patients with lymphoma were treated and seven (47%) responded, all with partial remissions. The median response duration was one and one-half months. The dose-limiting toxicity of this compound is hemorrhagic cystitis. Bladder protective agents such as Mesnum have been studied and show promise of being able to inhibit this toxic effect.

Amsacrine

We studied amsacrine (AMSA) in 1979 (Cabanillas et al. 1981). The preliminary results in the first 30 patients were promising. Six patients (20%) responded and three of these responses were complete. Further entries on this protocol revealed that out of 50 patients, 7 (14%) responded (Cabanillas and Bodey 1982). Interestingly, of the three patients who achieved complete remission (CR), two are still free of disease more than 28 and 43 months. Both patients had diffuse large cell lymphoma and are now off treatment. The median response duration in this study was eight months. In view of the steep dose response curve observed in acute myeloblastic leukemia with the use of this drug, it is conceivable that the use of high-dose AMSA and bone marrow transplantation might be beneficial in lymphoma.

Spirogermanium

The most recently introduced agent with activity against lymphomas is a novel heavy metal. It has no myelosuppressive effect, and it is limited only by central nervous system toxicity, mainly dizziness and ataxia. In a study conducted at Georgetown University (Espana 1982), 23 patients were treated and 5 (22%) responded. Two patients achieved CR. In a subset of 13 patients who received a higher dose, 4 (31%) responded. In view of its unusual pattern of toxicity, this drug should be easy to combine with other drugs without overlapping toxicity.

RESCUE COMBINATION CHEMOTHERAPEUTIC REGIMENS

From 1974 to 1977 we used IMV (ifosfamide in combination with methotrexate and vincristine) to treat patients with recurrent lymphoma (Table 1) (Cabanillas et al. 1980). Thirty patients were treated with this combination. We recorded a response rate of 46%, which was not different from our previous experience with ifosfamide as a single agent (Table 2). However, three patients achieved complete remissions with IMV, while none did so with ifosfamide alone. Of these three patients, two have remained free of disease for over 48 months.

Table 1. *Treatment Details of the Rescue Combination Regimens*

Acronym	Drugs and doses*
IMV	Ifosfamide 1 g/m² in 1000cc D/W daily × 5 days
	MTX 30 mg/m² i.v. days 3 and 14
IMVP-16	Ifosfamide 1 g/m² in 1000cc D/W daily × 5 days
	MTX 30 mg/m² days 3 and 10 i.v.
	VP-16 100 mg/m² in 1000cc NS over 2 hr daily × 3 days
AIVP-16	AMSA 80 mg/m² in 100cc D/W over 30 min day 1
	Ifosfamide 1 g/m² in 1000cc D/W daily × 5 days
	VP-16 70 mg/m² in 1000cc NS over 2 hr daily × 3 days
MIME	Methyl GAG 500 mg/m² in 100cc over 45 min, days 1 and 14
	Ifosfamide 1 g/m² in 1000cc D/W daily × 5 days
	MTX 30 mg/m² day 3, i.v.
	VP-16 100 mg/m² in 1000cc NS over 2 hr daily × 3 days

*Courses are all repeated every 21 days if blood counts are recovered (>1000 neutrophils and 100,000 platelets).

D/W–dextrose in water; MTX–methotrexate; VP-16–etoposide; NS–normal saline; AMSA–amsacrine.

Table 2. *Response Rate of Rescue Combination Regimens*

Acronym	Drugs	No. of pts	% CR	% CR + PR
IMV	Ifosfamide, MTX, vincristine	30	10	46
IMVP-16	Ifosfamide, MTX, VP-16	53	38	62
AIVP-16	AMSA, ifosfamide VP-16	46	28	39
MIME	Methyl GAG, ifosfamide, MTX, VP-16	115	24	63

Methyl-GAG–methylglyoxal bis-guanylhydrazone. (See Table 1 for other abbreviations.)

IMVP-16 (Ifosfamide, Methotrexate, and Etoposide)

In view of the mild myelosuppressive qualities of the IMV regimen, we felt it was possible to add a myelosuppressive agent. We became aware, in 1977, of the encouraging results of Jacobs et al. (1975) who used VP-16 to treat patients with recurrent lymphomas, as well as previously untreated patients. The IMV regimen was modified by including VP-16 and deleting vincristine (Table 1) (Cabanillas et al. 1982). Six of the 53 patients in this study were treated with IMVP-16 before they experienced progressive disease. The results are shown in Table 2. Both the overall response rate and CR rate increased with the addition of VP-16. The median relapse-free interval of complete responders was 12 months.

The toxicity of this regimen included gross hemorrhagic cystitis in 8% of patients, documented infections in 19%, and mucositis in 23%.

AIVP-16 (AMSA, Ifosfamide, and Etoposide)

In 1979 we attempted to modify further the IMVP-16 regimen by substituting AMSA for methotrexate. In order to do this, we had to reduce the dose of VP-16 by 30% because of the myelosuppressive properties of AMSA. The dose of AMSA used was also 66% of the single agent dose (Table 2).

Of 46 patients treated, 18 (39%) responded (Cabanillas et al. 1982). The CR rate was 28% (Table 2). Although these results appeared inferior to IMVP-16 results, it was unclear whether the difference was real or was caused by inequities in the distribution of prognostic factors.

Prognostic Factors

No data were available about which factors are associated with response to rescue chemotherapy. We studied 14 pretreatment variables to determine their influence on response rate in the 99 patients treated with IMVP-16 and AIVP-16. With the use of multivariate analysis, the following factors were associated with a higher response rate: previous CR on front-line therapy, intermediate- and high-grade histology, and absence of central nervous system involvement. When the treatment regimen itself was included as a variable in the analysis, the mathematical model selected IMVP-16 as the better regimen.

MIME (Methylglyoxal Bis-Guanylhydrazone, Ifosfamide, Methotrexate, and Etoposide)

In view of the superiority of IMVP-16, we next attempted to improve its activity by adding methyl GAG. Because this drug is not myelosuppressive, we did not have to reduce the dose of VP-16 (Table 1). Table 2 shows the results of the MIME regimen in the first 115 patients treated. The CR and partial remission (PR) rates are very similar to those observed with IMVP-16. The CR rate is lower than the one achieved on IMVP-16, probably because the IMVP-16 regimen included a higher proportion of patients who received treatment while still in PR before they relapsed. Interestingly, the response rate to MIME of patients with indolent histologies was higher than in our previous regimens.

In order to assess more accurately the value of MIME, we applied the mathematical model derived from the multivariate analysis. The overall expected response rate for MIME was 51%, while the observed response rate was 62%, which suggested that it was superior to our previous regimens. A breakdown of the patients receiving MIME according to their level of predicted probability of response was done in order to determine in which prognostic category the improvement took place. A 51% response rate occurred in the group of patients with the lowest (<40%) expected response rate. This group mostly comprised patients with indolent histologies. Methyl GAG, as a single agent, is most active in those histologic groups.

Toxicity

Patients with recurrent lymphoma usually do not tolerate treatment as well as previously untreated patients. Their bone marrow reserve is frequently compromised by prior radiation therapy, extensive chemotherapy, or both. In spite of this, we feel that we should make an effort to deliver the maximum tolerated dose of chemotherapy. There will frequently be complications, especially during the first course. After the first course, the doses can be adjusted according to the side effects observed.

The most frequent toxic effect with MIME has been mucositis, which occurred in 39 (34%) of 115 patients. Usually, it was mild. The second most frequent effect (30%) was fever of unknown origin associated with neutropenia. We documented infections in an additional 28% of the patients. The vast majority of these episodes took place during the first course of therapy.

Another potentially serious complication observed in 18% of patients is hemorrhagic cystitis secondary to ifosfamide administration. We have been able to continue treatment with ifosfamide in most of these patients either by increasing hydration to five liters of fluid i.v. daily or by inserting a Foley catheter. The use of bladder protective agents such as Mesnum could help counteract this problem.

DURATION OF RESPONSE

The relapse-free interval of patients who achieved CR on the IMVP-16, AIVP-16, and MIME studies has been similar (12–16 months) (Table 3). No statistically significant differences were evident among the three treatment groups. From the shape of the curves it appears that approximately 30% of the patients who attain CR on rescue treatment will remain in CR and, most likely, be cured of their recurrent lymphoma.

CONCLUSIONS

In summary, the addition of VP-16 to our rescue treatment program has resulted in an increase in both the CR rate and overall response rates. A modest fraction

Table 3. *Relapse-Free Survival of Patients Who Achieved Complete Remission on Ifosfamide and VP-16 Combinations*

Acronym	No. of pts	75% RFS (months)	50% RFS	25% RFS	P
IMVP-16	20	9	12.5	Not reached	
AIVP-16	15	6	18	Not reached	>.05
MIME	28	12	17	Not reached	

RFS–relapse-free survival. (See text for components of chemotherapeutic regimens.)

of patients, particularly those with intermediate and high-grade histologic types who respond better to our rescue treatments, appear to be curable with ifosfamide and VP-16–based combination regimens.

REFERENCES

Bender RA, Anderson T, Fisher RI, Young RC. 1978. Activity of the epipodophyllotoxin VP-16 in the treatment of combination chemotherapy resistant non-Hodgkin's lymphoma. Am J Hematol 5:203–209.

Cabanillas F, Bodey GP. 1982. Amsacrine current perspectives and clinical results with a new anticancer agent. Proceedings of International Symposium on Amsacrine 55-62.

Cabanillas F, Hagemeister FB, Bodey GP, Freireich EJ. 1982. IMVP-16: An effective regimen for patients with lymphoma who have relapsed after initial combination chemotherapy. Blood 60:693–697.

Cabanillas F, Legha SS, Bodey GP, Freireich EJ. 1981. Initial experience with AMSA as single agent treatment against malignant lymphoproliferative disorders. Blood 57:614–616.

Cabanillas F, Rodriguez V, Bodey GP. 1980. Ifosfamide, methotrexate, and vincristine (IMV) combination chemotherapy as secondary treatment for patients with malignant lymphoma. Cancer Treat Rep 64:933–937.

Cecil JW, Quagliana JM, Coltman CA, Al-Sarraf M, Thigpen T, Groppe CW. 1978. Evaluation of VP-16-213 in malignant lymphoma and melanoma. Cancer Treat Rep 62:801–803.

Dombernowsky P, Nissen NI, Larsen V. 1972. Clinical investigation of a new podophyllum derivative epipodophyllotoxin 4' demethyl-9-(4-6-0-2-thenylidene-B-D-glucopyranoside) (NSC-122819) in patients with malignant lymphomas and solid tumors. Cancer Treat Rep 56:71–82.

Espana P, Kaplan R, Robichaud K, Gustafson P, Wiernik P, Smith F, Woolley P, Schein P. 1982. Phase II study of spirogermanium in lymphoma patients. Proceedings of the American Society of Clinical Oncology (Abstract) 1:166.

Jacobs P, King HS, Sealy GRH. 1975. Epipodophyllotoxin (VP-16-213) in the treatment of diffuse histiocytic lymphoma. South African Medical Journal 49:483–485.

Kuhn JG, Knight WA, McDaniel TM, Coltman CA, Whitecar JP, Fabian C, Costan JJ. 1982. Methylglyoxal bis-guanylhydrazone (methyl-gag) in the management of non-Hodgkin's lymphoma (NHL). Proceedings of the American Society of Clinical Oncology (Abstract No. C-635) 1:163.

Rodriguez V, McCredie K, Keating MJ, Valdivieso M, Bodey GP. 1978. Isophosphamide therapy for hematologic malignancies in patients refractory to prior treatment. Cancer Treat Rep 62:493–497.

Warrell RP, Lee BJ, Kempin SJ, Lacher MJ, Straus DJ, Young CW. 1981. Effectiveness of methyl-gag (methylglyoxal-bis [guanylhydrazone]) in patients with advanced malignant lymphoma. Blood 57:1011–1014.

UT M.D. Anderson Clinical Conference on Cancer, Vol. 27, edited by R. J. Ford, L. M. Fuller, and F. B. Hagemeister. Raven Press, New York © 1984.

Immunotoxins and Allogeneic Bone Marrow Transplantation for Treatment of Human Leukemia and Lymphoma

Daniel A. Vallera,*† Richard J. Youle,§ Alexandra H. Filopovich,‡
David M. Neville, Jr.,§ Esmail D. Zanjani,**
Christine C. B. Soderling,* Susan M. Azemove,*
and John H. Kersey*†

*Departments of Therapeutic Radiology, †Laboratory Medicine/Pathology, ‡Pediatrics
and **Medicine, University of Minnesota, Minneapolis, Minnesota 55455; and §Section
on Biophysical Chemistry, Laboratory of Neurochemistry, National Institutes of
Mental Health, Bethesda, Maryland 20205

Immunotoxins (IT) are the product of hybridoma technology and, more recently, biochemical cross-linking procedures employing heterobifunctional cross-linking reagents. Because of their availability, homogeneity, and exquisite specificity, monoclonal antibodies have proved to be excellent targeting agents for catalytic toxins (Youle and Neville 1980, Thorpe et al. 1982, Jansen et al. 1982, Raso et al. 1982, Vallera et al. 1982a,b). Use of these reagents in vivo has been limited by their nonspecific reactivity with tissue. In contrast, in vitro studies have shown that IT can eliminate select antigen-positive target cells at concentrations of 700-fold less than antigen-negative control cells (Youle and Neville 1980). The high degree of selective potency of these reagents in vitro has prompted us to define their role as potential reagents for use in bone marrow treatment for allogeneic transplantation.

A variety of severe and life-threatening hematological disorders such as immunodeficiency diseases and, more recently, leukemia can be aggressively treated by bone marrow transplantation. Even when donors and recipients are HLA matched, graft-versus-host disease (GVHD) may develop due to immunocompetent T cells in the donor graft that recognize and react against the recipient's minor histocompatibility antigens. The role of T cells in GVHD has been well established in mice and can be prevented by eliminating T cells (Vallera et al. 1981, Tyan 1973, Cantor 1972, von Boehmer and Sprent 1976, Rodt et al. 1974). In man, the consensus is that T cells play a major role in the development of GVHD. Anti-T-cell monoclonal antibodies have been used to treat donor cells prior to infusion. The results of such studies have been disappointing (Prentice et al. 1982, Filopovich et al. 1982). Other approaches, such as antibody plus complement treatment (Hayward et al. 1982,

Reinherz et al. 1982), have been used to deplete bone marrow of T cells. However, complement treatment has posed severe limitations in man.

A new approach, which is simple, rapid, and highly reproducible, is to use IT that are capable of selectively killing T cells. We have shown that such reagents can be successfully used in mice (Vallera et al. 1982a,b). We have now extended our studies to the human system (Vallera et al. 1983, Vallera et al. 1984, Quinones et al. 1984). IT have been used to pretreat cell suspensions in vitro and inhibit T cells at doses that minimally affect the stem cells. More important, these reagents have been used to pretreat histocompatible donor bone marrow in patients undergoing bone marrow transplantation for acute lymphocytic leukemia.

MATERIALS AND METHODS

Synthesis and Purification of Immunotoxins

A complete description of the procedure for covalent linkage of a monoclonal antibody to intact ricin employing the cross-linking agent M-maleimidobenzoyl-N-hydroxysuccinimide (MBS) ester has been previously reported (Youle and Neville 1980). Briefly, ricin was reacted with MBS ester to link maleimide residues to ricin. The monoclonal antibody was then prepared for cross linking by partial reduction of disulfide bonds. The maleimide-linked ricin was mixed with the sulfydryl-containing antibodies, which formed a nonreducible thioether linkage between the two species.

Antibody and Ricin

We selected three monoclonal antibodies reactive against different molecules on the surface of T lymphocytes. T101 is an IgG2a monoclonal antibody recognizing a 65 kilodalton glycoprotein (Royston et al. 1979). UCHT1, an IgG1, precipitates a 19 kilodalton glycoprotein (Beverley and Callard 1981). TA-1, an IgG2a, recognizes a dimeric non-covalently linked glycoprotein complex of 170 and 95 kilodaltons (LeBien and Kersey 1980). Ricin was purified from the seeds of *Ricinus communis* (kindly supplied by Anthony Huang), according to the methods of Nicholson and colleagues (1974).

Treatment of Cells with Immunotoxins

Human peripheral blood mononuclear cells (PBMC) or bone marrow mononuclear cells (BMMC) were obtained by separating normal blood and bone marrow on Ficoll-Hypaque density gradients, as described (Vallera et al. 1983). Washed cells were adjusted to 10^7/ml and pretreated with IT (300 ng/ml) for 2 hr at 37°C, 5% CO_2/95% air in RPMI 1640 + 2% human serum albumin (HSA) plus antibiotics. Medium was made 100 mM lactose (isoosmotic) since lactose will block the native galactosyl-binding site of ricin B chain and render IT antibody specific. Following IT treatment, suspensions were washed twice and then resuspended for in vitro assays.

Bone Marrow Transplants

Two girls ages 6.5 and 12.9 years with non-T, non-B acute lymphoblastic leukemia (ALL) underwent transplantation during third remission. Both recipients received conditioning before transplantation with cyclophosphamide (60 mg/kg/d × 2) and fractionated total body irradiation (bid 165 rad × 8). Donor bone marrow was obtained from HLA-matched siblings and treated with IT, as described above. Immediately following treatment, donor marrow was tested in various T-cell assays, phytohemagglutinin (PHA), mixed lymphocyte reaction (MLR), and cell-mediated lympholysis (CML). Neither patient received conditioning following transplantation. Therefore, IT pretreatment was the sole method of GVHD prophylaxis.

PHA Assay

To measure polyclonal T-cell proliferation, PBMC were stimulated with the T-cell mitogen (PHA). PBMC, 10^5/well, were added to 96-well flat-bottomed microtiter plates (Linbro Chem. Co, Hamden, CT) in 0.2 ml culture medium (RPMI 1640 + antibiotics + 15% pooled human serum). Two μg PHA (Difco Chem. Co, Detroit, MI) were added to each well. Cultures were incubated in 5% CO_2/95% air for three days and then pulsed with 1 μCi tritiated thymidine (^{3}H-TdR) 18 hr prior to harvest. The ^{3}H-TdR incorporation was quantitated by standard scintillation counting techniques. The addition of PHA resulted in average stimulation of 120-fold compared to non–PHA-stimulated cultures. In IT experiments, mean data from triplicate samples were calculated as "percent control responses" as follows:

$$\text{percent control} = \frac{\begin{array}{c}(\text{cpm stimulated PBMC} + \text{IT} \\ -\text{ cpm unstimulated PBMC} + \text{IT})\end{array}}{\begin{array}{c}(\text{cpm stimulated PBMC untreated} \\ -\text{ cpm unstimulated PBMC untreated})\end{array}} \times 100$$

The CML and MLR assays were previously reported (Quinones et al. 1984, Vallera et al. 1984).

CFU-GEMM Assay

We used an in vitro colony-forming unit (CFU) assay for detecting mixed colonies containing cells committed to granulocytic and monocytic, erythroid and megokaryocytic differentiation (CFU-GEMM). We used the assay developed by Fauser and Messner (1979) modified by Ash and Zanjani (1981). Briefly, 2.5×10^5 BMMC were suspended in Iscove's modified Dulbecco's minimum essential medium containing 30% fetal calf serum (FCS), 5% PHA-conditioned media, 5×10^{-5} 2-mercaptoethanol, and 1 IU erythropoietin in a 0.9% methyl-cellulose support matrix. Triplicate suspensions in Petri dishes were cultured for 15 days in 5% CO_2/95% air atmosphere and were then examined under a microscope for the presence of CFU-GEMM colonies. In IT experiments, data were expressed as percent of control response.

Assay for Leukemia Cell Growth

HPB/MLT, a human T-cell ALL cell line, KOPN-1, a pre-B ALL cell line, and REH, non-T, non-B ALL cell line were cultured and passaged by standard tissue culture techniques. Cells in log phase were washed once with RPMI 1640 + 10% FCS + antibiotics and then added (1 to 2×10^5/well) to 96-well flat-bottom culture plates in 0.15 ml medium. All wells were fed with 50 μl medium on day 2. Cells were assayed daily by adding 0.04% trypan blue dye to triplicate wells and counting viable cells (those excluding dye) microscopically with a hemacytometer. Data were plotted linearly as cells/well $\times 10^{-5}$ versus days of culture. The HPB/MLT cell line was selected for these assays because it bound T101 antibody by indirect immunofluorescence assay. KOPN-1 and REH were not reactive with T101.

RESULTS AND DISCUSSION

In previous studies using a murine model, we have shown that anti–T-cell IT display marked potency and selectivity against T lymphocytes in functional assays (Vallera et al. 1982, Vallera et al. 1981). When used to pretreat murine lympho-hematopoietic grafts, IT protected lethally irradiated mice from the development of lethal GVHD, despite bone marrow transplantation across major histocompatibility barriers. Data derived from serotyping showed that these animals were fully chimeric several months after transplantation. Skin grafting experiments demonstrated that they were specifically unresponsive, since third party, but not donor-type grafts, were rejected. Pretreatment of bone marrow in this manner offers several major advantages: (1) the majority of IT can be washed from the cells prior to infusion into the patient, which decreases the risk of ricin toxicity; (2) this approach is technically simple as compared to other mechanical manipulations of bone marrow used to eliminate T cells; thus, the marrow spends a shorter time period outside the patient and there is less risk of complication; and (3) use of IT circumvents the need for complement activation. Many problems are associated with the in vitro use of complement.

Our studies in mice have led to the synthesis and testing of three anti–T-cell IT with potential for use in human allogeneic bone marrow transplantation (Vallera et al. 1983). A representative experiment illustrating the potency and selectivity of one of these IT, T101 ricin is shown in Figure 1. When human PBMC were pretreated with T101 ricin in the presence of a lactose blockade and then stimulated with a mitogen PHA, the proliferative response to mitogen was inhibited greater than 95% at 300 ng IT/ml. In contrast, an identical pretreatment of human BMMC with the same concentration of IT plus lactose did not inhibit clonal formation of multipotent stem cells that were measured in the CFU-GEMM assay.

It should be noted that 60 kilodalton ricin is composed of two 30 kilodalton subunits, the A and B chains. The A chain is the toxic enzyme, inhibiting protein synthesis. The A chain cannot penetrate the cell membrane and thus by itself is not toxic (Olsnes and Pihl 1973). The B chain has a galactose binding site, which binds galactosyl receptors on the cell and facilitates A-chain entry into the cytosol (Youle and Neville 1980). In its native configuration, ricin is an extremely potent,

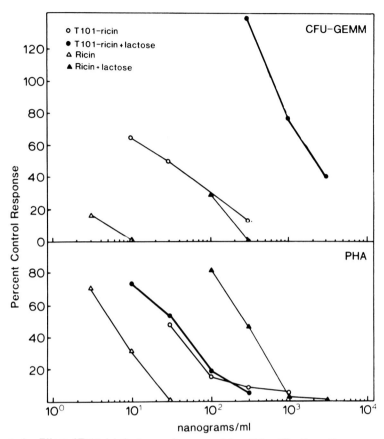

Figure 1. Effect of T101 ricin/lactose on human peripheral blood T cells and bone marrow stem cells. PBMC (10⁷/ml) from normal donors were pretreated with T101 ricin/lactose, T101 ricin, ricin/ lactose, or ricin alone. Cells were cultured and tested on day 3 in a PHA assay. Unstimulated control cultures averaged 848 ± 538 counts per minute while addition of PHA resulted in stimulation of 108-fold. Data are expressed as "percent control lactose response." BMMC from the same donor were pretreated identically and simultaneously tested in a CFU-GEMM assay. Lactose control cultures averaged 9.3 ± 3.0 CFU-GEMM/10⁵ plated cells.

catalytic phytotoxin. When linked to an antibody we must block the B-chain site with lactose to render IT antibody specific. As shown in Figure 1, T101 ricin plus lactose was about 70-fold more toxic to T cells than to stem cells. T101 ricin without lactose was similarly toxic to both T cells and stem cells. The degree of IT selectivity can vary from individual to individual.

Because of their selectivity against T lymphocytes, it would also be possible to use IT as purgative reagents for human autologous bone marrow transplantation for T-cell leukemia and lymphoma. Thus, we tested IT against various leukemic cell lines with known cell surface phenotypes. HPB/MLT is a human T-cell leukemic line that binds T101. Neither KOPN-1, a pre–B-cell leukemia, nor REH, a non-T, non-B leukemia, binds T101, according to immunofluorescence studies. These leukemic cell lines were preincubated with T101 ricin and lactose. The number of surviving cells was determined by a trypan blue dye exclusion over a five-day culture interval (Figure 2). In two independent experiments, our data show that as little as 30 ng of T101 ricin inhibited HPB/MLT growth in bulk culture assays. Even 100-1000 ng/ml T101 ricin did not inhibit KOPN-1 or REH cells. More recent studies in our laboratory employing a more sensitive clonogeneic assay (Stong R, unpublished data) have demonstrated nonspecific toxicity for all leukemic cell lines

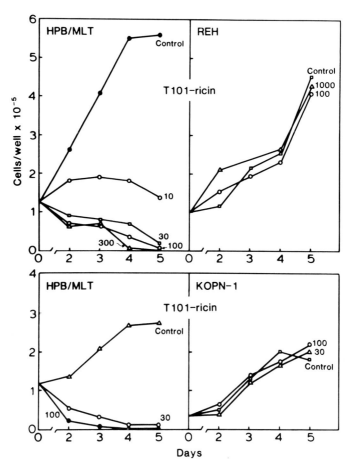

Figure 2. The selective reactivity of T101 ricin/lactose with human ALL cell lines. Prior to assay, lines were screened for the presence of the cell surface structure binding T101 by indirect immunofluorescence. HPB/MLT bound T101, but REH and KOPN-1 did not. The cell lines were preincubated as previously described. Cells in RPMI + 10% FCS + antibiotics were suspended in flat-bottomed culture plates (1-2 × 10⁵/well). Aliquots of triplicate samples were removed daily and diluted in trypan blue dye. Only living cells that excluded dye were counted and data were expressed as living cells/well × 10⁻⁵. Control cultures contained culture media plus 100 mm lactose. Lactose had no inhibitory effect on the cell lines.

at higher concentrations of IT. Such findings may be attributed to the fact that we have reached the limitations of our lactose blockade at 100 mm. Increasing the lactose concentration may provide additional protection from the nonspecific toxic effects of ricin.

Taken together, these data show that T101 ricin in the presence of lactose is a highly selective reagent, which, when used at certain concentrations, disrupts T-cell function and inhibits the growth of cells expressing at T101 antigen but is not toxic to stem cells. We have extended our studies (Vallera et al. 1983) and have synthesized other IT that are selectively toxic to T lymphocytes. We have found that a cocktail of TA-1 ricin, UCHT1 ricin, and T101 ricin is more potent in the elimination of T-cell function than any of the individual IT alone. The added effect of these IT prompted us to select a dose that was effective against T cells, but not against stem cells and to enter into phase I clinical trial, employing IT as reagents for GVHD prophylaxis in allogeneic bone marrow transplantation.

In vitro experiments with ^{125}I-labeled IT and toxicity studies in mice showed that the risk of ricin toxicity would be extremely low (Vallera et al. 1983). We chose two patients with third remission ALL. The patients were selected because bone marrow was available from a histocompatible sibling donor and thus were not high risk for GVHD. Evaluation before transplantation confirmed normal renal, hepatic, cardiac, and neurologic functions. As shown in Table 1, patient 1 received 1.81×10^8 bone marrow cells/kg containing approximately 20% T lymphocytes, as determined by immunofluorescence. Patient 2 was given 0.94×10^8 bone marrow cells/kg containing 34% T lymphocytes. Engraftment occurred on day 17 in patient 1 and day 16 in patient 2. Studies on the patients' T-cell depleted bone marrow showed that MLR and CML responses were inhibited greater than 99%, while there was much less toxicity directed at CFU-GEMM. No GVHD had occurred in either patient several months following transplantation. There were no renal, hepatic, cardiac, or neurologic complications.

Our initial experience with T-cell depletion of bone marrow using IT showed that these reagents were extremely efficient in the elimination of T-cell function. At the same time, the procedure involved less technical manipulation than other methods of T-cell depletion tried to date. Little cell loss occurred so that it was possible to return a maximum number of donor bone marrow cells to the immuno-suppressed recipient. The IT were safe and had little or no effect on pluripotent stem cells, since engraftment in these two patients occurred without delay. Since our reagents can be prepared in large batches and they remain stable at $-20°C$, reagents can be prepared with a high degree of quality control.

In our opinion, preclinical and clinical studies using antibody ricin conjugates show that IT are both safe and effective in their activity against T lymphocytes and that these reagents show great promise as purgative reagents for GVHD prophylaxis in human allogeneic bone marrow transplantation. They have great potential in transplanting bone marrow in future leukemia and lymphoma patients for whom histocompatible sibling donors are not available.

Table 1. *Pretreatment of Human Bone Marrow with an Equimolar Mixture of Three Immunotoxins: Two ALL Patients Undergoing Transplantation at the University of Minnesota*

	Patient 1	Patient 2
Date of transplantation	3/25/83	5/6/83
Patient information		
Age (yr)	6	12.9
Weight (kg)	21.3	44.8
Sex	F	F
Leukemia	ALL 3rd remission	ALL 3rd remission
Donor information		
Age (yr)	3.9	2.1
Sex	M	F
HLA disparity	Matched sibling	Matched sibling
BM cells given/kg	1.81×10^8	0.94×10^8
Contaminating T cells		
OKT 3 positive (%)	20	34
OKT11 positive (%)	21	ND
Studies on patient's T-cell depleted bone marrow		
MLR assay	+	+
CTL assay	+	+
CFU-C assay	−	−
GVHD	None	None
Engraftment	Day 17	Day 16

BM–Bone marrow; MLR–Mixed lymphocyte reaction; CML–Cell mediated lympholysis; CFU-C–A clonogenic assay measuring granulocytic and monocytic precursors from bone marrow; + inhibited >99%; − inhibited <35%; ND–Not done.

ACKNOWLEDGMENT

This investigation was supported by grant ROICA-31618, CA-36725, and CA-25097 awarded by the National Cancer Institute, United States Department of Health and Human Services. We wish to thank Dr. Tucker W. LeBien, Dr. Peter C. L. Beverley, and Hybritech, Inc. for generously supplying anti-human T-cell antibodies. Dr. Vallera is a Scholar of the Leukemia Society of America.

REFERENCES

Ash RC, Detrick RA, Zanjani ED. 1981. Studies of human pluripotential hematopoietic stem cells (CFU-GEMM) in vitro. Blood 58:309–316.

Beverley PCL, Callard RE. 1981. Distinctive functional characteristics of human T lymphocytes defined by E rosetting or a monoclonal anti-T cell antibody. Eur J Immunol 11:329–333.

Cantor H. 1972. The effects of anti-theta antiserum upon graft-versus-host activity or spleen and lymph node cells. Cell Immunol 3:461–469.

Fauser AA, Messner HA. 1979. Identification of megakaryocytes, macrophages, and eosinophils in colonies of human bone marrow containing granulocytes and erythroblasts. Blood 53:1023–1027.

Filopovich AH, McGlave PB, Ramsay NKC, Goldstein G, Warkentin P, Kersey JH. 1982. Pretreatment of donor bone marrow with monoclonal antibody OKT3 for prevention of acute GVHD in allogeneic histocompatible bone marrow transplantation. Lancet 1:1266–1268.

Hayward AR, Murphy S, Githens J, Troup G, Ambruso D. 1982. Failure of panreactive anti-T cell antibody, OKT3 to prevent GVHD in severe combined immunodeficiency. J Pediatr 100:665–668.

Jansen FK, Blythman H, Carriere D, Casellas P, Gros O, Gros P, Laurent J-C, Paolucci E, Pau B, Poncelet P, Richer G, Vidal R, Viosin G. 1982. Immunotoxins: Hybrid molecules combining high specificity and potent cytotoxicity. Immunol Rev 62:185–216.

Krolick A, Uhr J, Vitetta E. 1982. Selective killing of leukemia cells by antibody-toxin conjugate: Implications for autologous bone marrow transplantation. Nature 295:604–605.

LeBien TW, Kersey JH. 1980. Monoclonal antibody (TA-1) reactive with human T lymphocytes and monocytes. J Immunol 125:2208–2214.

Nicolson GL, Blaustein J, Etzler M. 1974. Characterization of two plant lectins from Ricinus communis and their quantitative interaction with murine lymphoma. Biochemistry 13:196–203.

Olsnes S, Pihl A. 1973. Different biological properties of the 2 constituent peptide chains of ricin. Biochemistry 12:3121–3126.

Prentice HG, Blacklock HA, Janossy G, Bradstock KF, Skeggs D, Goldstein G, Hoffbrand AV. 1982. Use of anti-T-cell monoclonal antibody OKT3 to prevent acute graft-versus-host disease in allogeneic bone-marrow transplantation for acute leukemia. Lancet 1:700–703.

Quinones RR, Youle RJ, Kersey JH, Zanjani ED, Azemove SM, Soderling CCB, LeBien TW, Beverley PCL, Neville Jr DM, Vallera DA. 1984. Anti-T-cell monoclonal antibodies conjugated to ricin as potential reagents for human GVHD prophylaxis: Effect on the generation of cytotoxic T cells in both peripheral blood and bone marrow. J Immunol 132:678–683.

Raso V, Ritz J, Busala M, Schlossman S. 1982. Monoclonal antibody-ricin A chain conjugate is selectively cytotoxic for cells bearing the common acute lymphoblastic leukemia antigen. Cancer Res 42:457–464.

Reinherz EL, Geha R, Rappeport JM, Wilson M, Penta AC, Hussey RE, Fitzgerald KA, Daley JF, Levine H, Rosen FS, Schlossman SF. 1982. Reconstitution after transplantation with T-lymphocyte-depleted HLA haplotype-mismatched bone marrow for severe combined immunodeficiency. Proc Natl Acad Sci USA 79:6047–6051.

Rodt HV, Theirfelder S, Eulitz M. 1974. Antilymphocytic antibodies and marrow transplantation. III. Effect of heterologous anti-brain antibodies on acute secondary disease in mice. Eur J Immunol 4:25–29.

Royston I, Majda A, Baird SM, Meserve BL, Griffiths JC. 1979. Monoclonal antibody specific for human T lymphocyte-identification of normal and malignant T-cells. Blood 54 (Suppl. 1):1069.

Thorpe PE, Mason D, Brown A, Simmonds F, Ross W, Cumber A, Forrester J. 1982. Selective killing of malignant cells in a leukemic rat bone marrow using an antibody/ricin-conjugate. Nature 297:594–596.

Tyan ML. 1973. Modification of severe graft-versus-host disease with antisera to the theta antigen or to whole serum. Transplantation 15:601–604.

Vallera DA, Ash RC, Zanjani ED, Kersey JH, LeBien TW, Beverley PCL, Neville Jr DM, Youle RJ. 1983. Anti-T cell reagents for human bone marrow transplantation ricin linked to three monoclonal antibodies. Science 222:512–515.

Vallera DA, Quinones RR, Azemove SM, Soderling CCB. 1984. Monoclonal antibody toxin conjugates reactive against human T lymphocytes: A comparison of antibody linked to intact ricin toxin to antibody linked to ricin A chain. Transplantation 37:387–392.

Vallera DA, Soderling CCB, Carlson GJ, Kersey JH. 1981. Bone marrow transplantation across major histocompatibility barriers in mice: The effect of elimination of T cells from donor grafts by treatment with monoclonal Thy 1.2 plus complement or antibody alone. Transplantation 31:218–222.

Vallera DA, Youle RJ, Neville Jr DM, Kersey JH. 1982a. Bone marrow transplantation across major histocompatibility barriers. V. Protection of mice from lethal graft-versus-host disease by pretreatment of donor cells with monoclonal anti-Thy-1.2 coupled to the toxin ricin. J Exp Med 155:949–954.

Vallera DA, Youle RJ, Neville Jr DM, Soderling CCB, Kersey JH. 1982b. Anti-T cell monoclonal antibody-toxin conjugates as reagents for experimental GVHD prophylaxis are not selectively reactive with murine stem cells. Transplantation 36:73–79.

von Boehmer H, Sprent J. 1976. T cell function in bone marrow chimeras: Absence of host reactive T cells and cooperation of helper T cells across allogeneic barriers. Transplant Rev 29:3–21.

Youle RJ, Neville Jr DM. 1980. Anti-Thy-1.2 monoclonal antibody linked to ricin is potent cell type specific toxin. Proc Natl Acad Sci USA 77:5483–5486.

UT M.D. Anderson Clinical Conference on Cancer,
Vol. 27, edited by R. J. Ford, L. M. Fuller, and
F. B. Hagemeister. Raven Press, New York © 1984.

Bone Marrow Transplantation in Lymphoma

Gary Spitzer, Sundar Jagannath, Karel Dicke, Axel Zander,
Nizar Tannir, Lijda Vellekoop, Fernando Cabanillas,
Fredrick B. Hagemeister, William Velasquez, Peter McLaughlin,
and Dharmvir Verma

*Department of Hematology, Bone Marrow Transplantation and Lymphoma Sections,
The University of Texas M.D. Anderson Hospital and Tumor Institute at Houston,
Houston, Texas 77030*

The results of allogeneic bone marrow transplantation for patients with acute myeloid leukemia (AML) and acute lymphocytic leukemia (ALL) in remission and relapse, benign- and accelerated-phase chronic myeloid leukemia (CML), and other hematopoietic diseases are most promising (Thomas 1983, Thomas et al. 1977, 1979, Johnson et al. 1981, Doney et al. 1978, McClave et al. 1981). Elimination of leukemic disease is possible due to these aggressive chemotherapy–radiotherapy programs. However, without infusion of allogeneic bone marrow cells, death would occur secondary to treatment-induced bone marrow toxicity. Allogeneic transplantation requires an HLA-identical, mixed lymphocyte culture, nonreactive bone marrow donor in order to minimize the risk of acute and chronic graft-versus-host disease (GVHD), a major life-threatening complication. Allogeneic bone marrow transplantation is also associated with other serious complications, such as interstitial pneumonitis and other infections secondary to immunodeficiencies (Thomas et al. 1975, Sullivan et al. 1980, Neiman et al. 1980, Meyers and Thomas 1982). Because of these complications, the most successful results have been in patients younger than 20 years and have been achieved at an early stage in the disease before the cumulative effects of chemotherapy make administration of aggressive cytoreductive therapy practically impossible. Thus, allogeneic bone marrow transplantation is, so far, limited to young patients with good performance status, and it should be used in subsets of patients who have undergone transplantation early in the natural history of their disease because there is a propensity to early relapse.

There is an important difference in the natural history of lymphoma, compared to that of AML. A high cure rate with conventional therapies is seen, and in some lymphomas, combination chemotherapy can still rescue approximately 10% of patients who have relapsed. Allogeneic bone marrow transplantation in patients in relapse or second (or subsequent) remissions has played a major role only in ALL, where patients usually have been younger than 20 years.

The majority of patients with either Hodgkin's disease or lymphoma who are eligible for transplantation studies are either in relapse, possibly failing to respond even to alternative therapies for that relapse, or are in second complete remission with a poor outlook for a maintained remission. Therefore, allogeneic bone marrow transplantation will have a small role to play because of the amount of prior chemotherapy and the age of the patient.

Bone marrow transplantations between identical twins has led to long-term survival in patients with recurrent acute leukemia (Fefer et al. 1981), benign-phase CML (Fefer et al. 1982a), lymphoma (Appelbaum et al. 1981), or multiple myeloma (Fefer et al. 1982b). Although the number of donors is small, it does provide an ideal model for evaluating what the most ideal outcome could be with autologous bone marrow transplantation. Transplantation between identical twins is not associated with the problems of GVHD because the donor and the recipient are immunologically identical. There is also a decreased incidence of interstitial pneumonitis. Bone marrow transplantation between identical twins has a number of theoretical advantages over autologous bone marrow transplantations (ABMT). The donor-twin's bone marrow is not contaminated with either leukemia or lymphoma cells. The donor has also not had chemotherapy, which would affect the quality of the aspirated bone marrow.

The absence of suitable allogeneic donors for most patients with leukemia and lymphoma, the many life-threatening complications of allogeneic bone marrow transplantation in the lymphoma patients who would undergo transplantation and the rare availability of bone marrow from an identical twin has precipitated the recent investigation of ABMT as a more generally applicable transplantation approach for patients with lymphoma.

This review will focus on clinical studies of allogeneic and identical twin transplantations and particularly ABMT in lymphoma patients. We will attempt to be somewhat critical of transplantation in these disorders so the potential of this approach relative to alternative rescue therapies can be determined (Cabanillas 1984).

Lymphomas are sensitive tumors. With aggressive combination chemotherapy, Hodgkin's disease, diffuse large cell and undifferentiated lymphomas such as Burkitt's lymphoma, and lymphoblastic lymphoma have significant chance of being cured. The exact role of very high-dose chemotherapy either for rescuing relapsed patients with resistant lymphoma or as an intensification therapy for patients at high risk of relapse is difficult to define. The treatment of lymphoma is changing dramatically. Recently, several new drugs have been identified that are active in lymphoma. These include VP-16 (etoposide), high-dose methotrexate, methyl GAG, (methylglyoxal bis-guanylhydrazone), isophosphamide, cisplatin, (cis-diamminedichloroplatinum), and cytosine arabinoside. Such a large number of active drugs offers the potential for successful combination chemotherapy at fully tolerated doses that may rescue relapsed or initially resistant patients.

AUTOLOGOUS BONE MARROW TRANSPLANTATION IN HODGKIN'S DISEASE

Table 1 summarizes the results of high-dose cytoreductive therapy with ABMT in Hodgkin's disease. Hodgkin's disease represents the most attractive model of all of the lymphoma subgroups. In nodular sclerosing lymphoma, the most common subtype, there is only a small chance of bone marrow or blood contamination. To date, a total of 31 patients have undergone transplantation, after varying conditioning regimens, with an impressive complete response rate of 65% and an equally impressive anticipated rescue rate of approximately 16% (12 months or longer disease-free unmaintained survival). It is impossible to delineate the prior chemotherapy in all these patients, but the majority, particularly in the first three studies listed in Table 1, had received both MOPP (mechlorethamine, vincristine, procarbazine, and prednisone) and ABVD (doxorubicin, bleomycin, vinblastine, and dacarbazine) therapy at the very least. The most promising outcome certainly was in these three studies; the chemotherapy was well known and included a large dose (300 mg/m^2 or greater) of BCNU (1,3-bis-(2 chloroethyl)1-nitrosourea).

There is very little published about the response rate with alternative therapies in MOPP- and ABVD-resistant Hodgkin's disease patients. Amiel et al. (1981) achieved only one CR (complete remission) in 10 MOPP- and ABVD-resistant Hodgkin's disease patients using a combination of vindesine followed by a bleomycin infusion. Bonadonna and co-workers (1982) reported using CEP (CCNU[chloroethyl cyclohexyl nitrosourea], etoposide, and prednimustine) in

Table 1. *High-dose Cytoreductive Therapy with ABMT in Relapsed Hodgkin's Disease*

Author	Cytoreductive therapy	No. of patients	CR	Long-term disease-free survival	Months
M. D. Anderson Hospital	CBV	7	5	1:	25+
Carella et al. 1983	BCNU ±†CTX ± Vinblastine	5	4	2:	11+, 27+
Philip et al. 1983	BACT ± TBI	6	5	2:	9+, 18+
Phillips 1983	CTX + TBI	3	1	0	
Phillips 1983	BCNU	2	1	0	
Bensinger et al. 1983	CTX + TBI	4	0	0	
Barbasch et al. 1983	CTX ± BCNU	2	0	0	
Gorin 1981	TACC	1	1	0	
Gale 1980	Vinblastine, CTX, TBI	1	—	0	
Total		31	17* (65%)	5 (16%)	

CR—Complete remission. CBV—Cyclophosphamide, BCNU, VP-16. BCNU—1,3-bis-(2 chloroethyl)1-nitrosourea. BACT—Carmustine, cytosine arabinoside (ARA-C), cyclophosphamide (CTX), and thioguanine. TBI—Total body irradiation.
*Evaluable patients only.
† With or without.

MOPP- and ABVD-resistant patients. This induced CR in 26% of patients who had relapsed after MOPP, ABVD, or MOPP-ABVD therapy (Bonadonna 1982, Santoro et al. 1982). Similar complete response results have also been reported in patients given MIME (methyl GAG, ifosfamide, methotrexate, and etoposide) who had failed to respond to MOPP-ABVD (Cabanillas et al. 1984).

These high complete response rates (65%) achieved using high-dose chemotherapy and ABMT in such heavily pretreated Hodgkin's disease patients in whom alternative rescue therapy had not achieved equal complete response rates (approximately 20%–30%) suggest that the use of high doses of drugs, particularly incorporating BCNU with marrow support, could have a definite role in treating this disease.

BURKITT'S LYMPHOMA AND DIFFUSE SMALL-CELL NONCLEAVED LYMPHOMA

One of the most quoted studies that forms the background for the use of ABMT in lymphoma was the original tumor report of BACT (carmustine, cytosine arabinoside, cyclophosphamide, and thioguanine) therapy in Burkitt's lymphoma by Appelbaum (Appelbaum et al. 1978, Appelbaum and Thomas 1983). This was a study involving 18 Burkitt's lymphoma patients, most of whom had not received Adriamycin-containing programs and several of whom received only high-dose chemotherapy without bone marrow transplantation. In this group of patients, there were four long-term disease-free survivors, all of whom are alive more than five years after therapy. Of interest also is the fact that one of these patients had prior bone marrow involvement; his bone marrow was collected during complete remission. This experience in Burkitt's or diffuse undifferentiated lymphomas of childhood has been reproduced by a number of groups. Detailed in Table 2 is a summary of the long-term survivors after the use of high-dose chemotherapy or chemotherapy plus total body irradiation (usually with the support of ABMT) in 42 Burkitt's or diffuse undifferentiated lymphoma patients who relapsed. In these patients, there was a 70% complete response rate and the potential of nine long-term disease-free survivors, for a 23% rescue rate. This is a very impressive outcome, and there are no data in the literature on rescue therapy in relapsed Burkitt's lymphoma patients to refute that this approach is the preferred therapy.

Neither is there reason not to consider high-dose chemotherapy and ABMT as intensification therapy for those patients with Burkitt's lymphoma who have achieved only partial remission or who have particularly bulky disease and are therefore most likely to relapse. Table 3 gives the number of Burkitt's lymphoma patients who were treated during partial remission after incomplete responses to induction therapy. Early outcome seems promising, and all the patients achieved complete responses with high-dose therapy.

However, today, initial chemotherapy for Burkitt's lymphoma patients is much more aggressive and consists of alternating drugs, including Adriamycin (Brecher et al. 1981, Weinstein and Link 1979, Wollner et al. 1979, Link et al. 1983). A recent report on a study incorporating doxorubicin and CHOMP (cyclophospha-

Table 2. *High-Dose Cytoreductive Therapy with ABMT in Relapsed Burkitt's or Diffuse Undifferentiated Lymphoma Patients*

Author	Cytoreductive therapy	No. of patients	CR	Long-term disease-free survival	Months
Appelbaum et al. 1978-1983	BACT	18	12	4	ALL 60 +
Phillips 1983	CTX-TBI	9	7	1	32 +
M. D. Anderson Hospital	CTX-TBI	2	1	0	
Eckert et al. 1982	CTX, DOX, VCR, ARA-C, MTX	3	2	1	16 +
Barbasch et al. 1983	CTX + BCNU	1	1	1	24 +
Kaizer et al. 1979	DOX, CTX, TBI	1	1	1	25 +
Gale 1980	Vinblastine, CTX, TBI	2	2	1	27 +
Philip et al. 1983	BACT ± TBI	2	2	0	
Total		38	28* (74%)	9 (24%)	

DOX–Doxorubicin. VCR–Vincristine sulfate. MTX–Methotrexate. (See Table 1 for other abbreviations.)
*Evaluable patients only.

Table 3. *High-Dose Cytoreductive Therapy for Lymphoma: Partial Response Only to Induction Therapy*

Author	Cytoreductive therapy	No. of patients	Diagnosis	Long-term disease-free survival (months)
Philip et al. 1983	BACT ± TBI	2	DHL 1 BL 1	30 +, 20 +
Gulati et al. 1983	CTX + TBI	3	DHL 3	3 +, 4 +, 11 +
Gorin et al. 1983	TACC	1	BL 1	6 +

DHL–Diffuse histocytic lymphoma. BL–Burkitt's lymphoma. (See Table 1 for other abbreviations.)

mide, vincristine, high-dose methotrexate, and prednisone) revealed an 88% complete response rate with only a 23% relapse rate. The central nervous system (CNS) was the site of recurrence for the five patients who relapsed; no relapses occurred after one year (Magrath et al. 1981). It should be noted that none of the original patients reported by Appelbaum, nor did the majority of the patients reported by the other investigators listed in Table 2, had received Adriamycin. All long-term responders in Appelbaum's study received only cyclophosphamide, vincristine, and normal-dose methotrexate. Results of allogeneic bone marrow transplantation in lymphoma patients are given in Table 4. There are long-term disease-free survivors with Burkitt's lymphoma from the group of patients reported by O'Leary et al. (1983). Two of these patients underwent transplantation in their first remissions; however, one patient underwent transplantation in his third remission and, depending on the chemotherapeutic history, this may have been a favorable outcome.

Table 4. Allogeneic Bone Marrow Transplantation for Lymphoma

Author/Diagnosis	No. of patients	Treatment	Long-term disease-free survival	Months	Relapse status at transplantation of long-term disease-free survivors
Appelbaum et al. 1978, 1983					
Lymphoblastic (LL)	7				
Diffuse small cleaved	7				
Burkitt's (BL)	2	Cyclophosphamide, TBI	2-Diffuse small cleaved	6+, 8+, 27+	2 in 2nd CR and 1 in 3rd CR
Diffuse large cell	2				
Other intermediate and high grade	4		1-LL		
O'Leary et al. 1983					
Burkitt's stage IV	2				
Burkitt's stage III	4	CRAB	3-BL	18+, 28+, 29+, 49+, 73+	2 in 1st CR, 2 in 3rd CR, 1 LL in 1st relapse
Lymphoblastic stage III	3		2-LL		
Lymphoblastic stage IV	1				
M. D. Anderson Hospital 1983					
Lymphoblastic	2	CTX, BCNU, VP-16	1-LL	8+, 27+	1 DUL in 2nd CR, 1 LL in 3rd relapse
Diffuse undifferentiated (DUL)	1	Melphalan, BCNU, VP-16, CTX + TBI	1-DUL		

CRAB–BCNU, cyclophosphamide, ARA-C, and TBI. (See Table 1 for other abbreviations.)

LYMPHOBLASTIC LYMPHOMA

Allogeneic bone marrow transplantation (Table 4) has rescued two lymphoblastic lymphoma patients in relapse and intensified response in two patients, one in second and the other in third remission. However, ABMT for relapse of this condition (using bone marrow usually collected in the first remission) has achieved a complete response in 7 out of 10 patients or a 70% complete response rate (Table 5), but these responses have been short, one to two months, except in one patient who has had complete remission for more than 13 months. Such an outcome, that is, a high rate of complete but short responses suggests that bone marrow contamination may be a significant problem.

Shown in Table 6 are the results of high-dose cytoreductive therapy followed by ABMT for lymphoma patients in second complete remission. These are a miscellaneous group of lymphomas and not many conclusions can be drawn. However, the most interesting results are those of Kaizer et al. (1982) who employed a cyclophosphamide and a total body irradiation cytoreductive program but used bone marrow that had been treated in vitro with an anti–T-cell antibody (Leu-1). Two patients had longer second complete remissions than their first complete remissions. This disease may, therefore, warrant in vitro manipulation of the bone marrow with either antibody or chemotherapy.

There was a time when bone marrow transplantation may have been recommended therapy during first complete remission for lymphoblastic lymphoma because it was felt that most patients would relapse. However, recently Coleman treated 13 patients with a modified CHOP (cyclophosphamide, doxorubicin, vincristine, and prednisone) induction, L-asparaginase, intrathecal and high-dose systemic metho-

Table 5. *High-Dose Cytoreductive Therapy with ABMT for Relapse of Lymphoblastic Lymphoma*

Author	Cytoreductive therapy	No. of patients	CR	Long-term disease-free survival (months)
M. D. Anderson Hospital	CTX + TBI	2	2	0
Philip et al. 1983	BACT ± TBI	2	1	0
Gorin et al. 1981	TACC	2	1	0
Kaizer et al. 1979	DOX, CTX, TBI	1	0	0
Gulati et al. 1983	CTX, TBI BCNU 400- 1000 mg/m^2	1	1	0
Carella et al. 1983	± CTX ± Vincristine	1	1	1 (13 +)
Phillips 1983	CTX, TBI	1	1	0
Total		10	7* (70%)	1 (10%)

DOX–Doxorubicin. (See Table 1 for other abbreviations.)
*Evaluable patients only.

Table 6. *High-Dose Cytoreductive Therapy for Lymphoma: Bone Marrow Transplantation in Second Complete Remission*

Author	Cytoreductive therapy	No. of patients	Diagnosis	Long-term disease-free survival (months)
Philip et al. 1983	BACT ± TBI	7	BL 4 IS 2 LL 1	2-BL (4+, 16+)
Baumgartner et al.* 1984	VCR, DOX, CTX and TBI	2	DUL 2	—
Gorin et al. 1981	TACC	1	Mixed diffuse T-cell	1 (17+)
Kaizer et al. 1982	CTX + TBI	4	Leukemia or LL	3 (5+, 10+, 22+)

*Monoclonal antibody–treated bone marrow and posttransplantation chemotherapy.
BL–Burkitt's lymphoma; IS–immunoblastic sarcoma; LL–lymphoblastic lymphoma; VCR–vincristine sulfate; DOX–doxorubicin; DUL–diffuse undifferentiated lymphoma. (See Table 1 for other abbreviations.)

trexate consolidation, and CNS prophylatic irradiation (Coleman et al. 1982). This was followed by 6-mercaptopurine and methotrexate maintenance treatment for one year. He achieved complete remissions in all 13 patients. Only four have relapsed, three with CNS disease and one with an intraabdominal mass. There were two drug-related deaths. At three years after treatment, 56% of the survivors had been in continuous complete remission, and the actuarial survival rate is 61%. Promising results have also been achieved by other investigators (Levine et al. 1983, Weinstein et al. 1979). Thus, combination chemotherapeutic regimens administered with the intensity of antileukemic treatment appeared to be capable of improving the outlook of these patients too. Unpublished data from the Childrens' Leukemia Group suggest that even patients with bone marrow disease at presentation may have an approximately 50% chance of cure. Because of their good initial prognosis, patients with this disease are no longer a suitable group for intensification therapy with allogeneic bone marrow transplantation in first complete remission. Instead, relapsed patients should be the group investigated. Because of the better results with initial induction therapy, these patients will be more resistant to chemotherapy than the first patients reported. It also appears that some form of in vitro bone marrow manipulation will have to be performed in an attempt to eradicate any contaminating tumor cells.

DIFFUSE LARGE CELL LYMPHOMA

Relapsed diffuse large-cell lymphoma patients probably represent the most common subgroup of patients with aggressive lymphomas who are potentially eligible for bone marrow transplantation. Most relapsed patients being considered are resistant to such programs as CHOP or BACOP (bleomycin, doxorubicin, cyclophosphamide, vincristine, and prednisone). Although approximately 60% of CHOP-treated patients achieve CR, about one half relapse within the first three years (McKelvey and Moon 1977, Jones et al. 1979, Schein et al. 1976).

Recent data suggest that higher complete response rates, on the order of 60% to 75%, can be achieved with programs such as ProMace-MOPP (cyclophosphamide, doxorubicin, etoposide, high-dose methotrexate, and MOPP) or COP-BLAM, a variant of the MOPP and C-MOPP regimens consisting of cyclophosphamide, vincristine, prednisone, procarbazine, bleomycin, and doxorubicin (Fisher et al. 1982, Laurence et al. 1982). Complete remission rates are higher and more durable in stage III than in stage IV disease, and therefore, a significant percentage of the patients relapsing would be unsuitable to undergo transplantation because of either poor performance status, age, or bone marrow involvement. Cabanillas et al. (1983a) have published data on patients failing to achieve initial complete responses with CHOP. They can be induced into durable CR with alternating non–cross-resistant regimens including cytosine arabinoside or, alternatively, IMVP-16 (isophosphamide, methotrexate, and etoposide). This suggests that even partially responding patients can be rescued with alternative programs but without recourse to high-dose chemotherapy and ABMT. Finally, Cabanillas (Cabanillas et al. 1982b) reported high complete response rates (38%) in 34 relapsed large-cell lymphoma patients when he used the combination of isophosphamide, methotrexate, and VP-16. Four of the 13 responders have the potential of being cured. Ng et al. (1982) reported two complete responses in five CHOP-resistant patients after using a combination of prednisone, cytosine arabinoside, and BCNU. More recently, Cabanillas reported a similar complete response rate in patients with diffuse large-cell lymphoma relapsing after CHOP therapy with MIME. At one to two years after treatment, 10% to 20% of these patients are considered long-term disease-free survivors (Cabanillas et al. 1983b). A review of rescue studies in diffuse large-cell lymphoma patients suggests that the highest CR rates achievable are approximately 30% and the best rescue rate approximates 10%.

Most of these studies, however, did not produce a significant percentage of complete responses, particularly those using only single agents (Berkman et al. 1983, Cabanillas et al. 1981, Cavalli et al. 1981, Espana et al. 1982, Keller et al. 1982, Kaplan et al. 1981, Kroner et al. 1983, Lachant et al. 1981, Pavlosky et al. 1981, Rodriquez et al. 1978, Segal et al. 1982, Takvorian and Canellos 1983, Wallach et al. 1983, Warrell et al. 1981a, 1981b, Weick and Jones 1983). All of these studies are difficult to evaluate because of lack of detailed prognostic information such as the initial chemotherapy, initial response, number of prior chemotherapies, bulk of disease, B symptoms, and lactic dehydrogenase (LDH) levels. In diffuse large-cell lymphoma, we are faced with a problem of the ever-changing effective rescue chemotherapy that will probably induce more initial complete responses and maintain more of those complete responses, and, because of less toxicity, may be the first priority for relapsing diffuse large-cell lymphoma patients.

With this background of chemotherapeutic results in diffuse large-cell lymphoma, how then do the few studies of patients treated with high-dose chemotherapy and ABMT compare? Listed in Table 7 are the results of high-dose cytoreductive

Table 7. *High-Dose Cytoreductive Therapy in Relapsed Diffuse Large-Cell Lymphoma Patients*

Author	Cytoreductive therapy	No. of patients	CR	Long-term disease-free survival (months)
M. D. Anderson Hospital	CBV CTX + TBI AMSA, BCNU, VP-16	8	0	0
Phillips 1983	CTX, TBI	13	6	3 (12+, 13+, 32+)
Bensinger et al. 1983	CTX, TBI	5	1	0
Gulati et al. 1983	CTX ± TBI	2	1	0
Appelbaum et al. 1978	BACT	3	?	0
Armitage J. (unpublished data)	CTX, ARA-C, TBI	11	6	1 (1+, 1+, 7+)
Total		42	14* (36%)	4 (10%)

AMSA–Amsacrine. (See Table 1 for other abbreviations.)
*Evaluable patients.

Table 8. *High-Dose Cytoreductive Therapy for Lymphoma: Bone Marrow Transplantation in First Complete Remission*

Author	Cytoreductive Therapy	No. of Patients	Diagnosis	Long-term disease-free survival (months)
Philip et al. 1983	BACT ± TBI	4	BL 1 DHL 2 IS 1	BL (13+) IS (14+)
Baumgartner et al.* 1984	VCR, DOX, CTX + TBI	8	DUL	(5+, 5+, 20+, 23+, 35+)
Gorin et al. 1978	TACC	4	DUL 2 LL 1 IS 1	IS (30+) DHL (6+) LL (2)
Carella et al. 1983	BCNU	1	NOD	(19+)

*Monoclonal antibody–treated bone marrow and posttransplantation chemotherapy.
BL–Burkitt's lymphoma; DHL–diffuse histiocytic lymphoma; IS–immunoblastic sarcoma; DUL–diffuse undifferentiated lymphoma. VCR–vincristine sulfate; DOX–doxorubicin; NOD–nodular lymphoma. (See Table 1 for other abbreviations.)

therapy with the use of ABMT in 42 relapsed patients with diffuse large-cell lymphoma. Our eight patients are given first on this list because all of these patients received VP-16 combinations prior to being considered for transplantation. This, we feel, is the chemotherapeutic history of patients that will be referred in the future for ABMT, when VP-16 is commercially available. Using a number of cytoreductive regimens in this group of patients, we were unable to induce a single complete response. A few groups have reported complete responses with long-term disease-free survival (Table 7). Unfortunately, the nature of the prior chemotherapy and the patients' exact resistance to chemotherapy cannot be determined. If we

Table 9. *High-Dose Cytoreductive Therapy for Lymphoma: Bone Marrow Transplantation at Diagnosis*

Author	Cytoreductive therapy	No. of patients	Diagnosis	Long-term disease-free survival (months)
Gorin et al. 1981	TACC	4	BL 1 DML 1 NOD 1 HD 1	1 NOD (36 +)

BL–Burkitt's lymphoma; HD–Hodgkin's disease; DML–diffuse malignant lymphoma; NOD–nodular lymphoma.

look at the complete response rate to high-dose chemotherapy in this group of patients, it is lower than the rate in other subgroups of aggressive lymphoma patients. The overall complete response rate of 38% is disappointing and suggests a low projected percentage of long-term disease-free survivors. Excluding our cases in which patients received VP-16 combinations prior to transplantation, the complete response rate was 45% to 50%, probably marginally higher than that of the best alternative rescue therapy of IMVP-16 or MIME.

It may be difficult to identify drugs that will be active in this group of patients. We feel that the most ideal patients for whom to consider high-dose chemotherapy would be those achieving second CR or good partial remissions with MIME therapy and who have poor prognoses for continuing such a remission. Such poor prognostic features would be initial bulky disease, high LDH level at relapse, and relapse during or shortly after initial chemotherapy. Patients who are initially treated with combination chemotherapies that incorporate VP-16 therapy or, at least, whose regular treatment is alternated with it could be considered for bone marrow transplantation if they relapse. It is uncertain if adequate rescue therapy exists for such a patient group.

MARROW CONTAMINATION

Patients who are most likely to relapse and who have the worst prognosis are those with diffuse large-cell lymphoma and initial bone marrow involvement, lymphoblastic and undifferentiated lymphoma with initial bone marrow and CNS involvement, and Hodgkin's disease with bone marrow involvement. It is clear, therefore, that bone marrow involvement is a serious hazard in ABMT. Studies done by a number of investigators have documented the usual B-cell origin, a less frequent T-cell origin, and a proportion of unmarked cases in diffuse large-cell lymphoma (Bloomfield et al. 1977, 1979, Foon et al. 1982, Greaves et al. 1981, Janossy 1982, Nadler et al. 1982, 1981a, Nadler 1981b, Warnke 1980). Other studies have shown that lymphoblastic lymphoma, as distinct from acute T-cell leukemia, is usually a disease of the common thymocyte or late thymocyte cells (Bernard et al. 1981, Bradstock et al. 1980, Foon et al. 1982, Greaves et al. 1981, Janossy et al. 1982, Nadler et al. 1982, Roper et al. 1981). Nodular and Burkitt's lymphoma and non-Burkitt's undifferentiated lymphoma are also of B-cell origin (Foon et al. 1982, Greaves et al. 1981, Janossy et al. 1982, Nadler et al. 1982).

A number of monoclonal antibodies that could be used singly, but preferably in combinations, to treat the autologous bone marrow from lymphoblastic lymphoma patients have been described. These include the Leu-1 antibody, which may also have potential for purging bone marrow in T-cell leukemia (Kaizer et al. 1982). This antibody is reactive against T-cell leukemia and lymphoblastic lymphoma, as well as a number of B-cell leukemias (Foon et al. 1982). It appears that it is reactive in more T-cell diseases than any other monoclonal antibody. Another group recently described monoclonal antibody termed 4H9, which reacted with all 36 cases of T-cell ALL and T-cell non-Hodgkin's lymphoma (Link et al. 1983). In 30 of 36 cases, more than 50% of the blast cells were reactive with 4H9 and 20 of those cases showed reactivity with greater than 75% of the cells. All T-cell lines tested have been reactive. Furthermore, the fluorescent intensity was much greater than that obtained with Leu-1. The 4H9 antibody did not react with any other cell lineage tested. It identified a 40,000 molecular weight surface antigen similar to that recognized by another T-cell monoclonal antibody, 3A1 (Haynes 1981). Naito and co-workers (1983) have also described monoclonal antibodies, termed 3-3, specific for T-cell ALL that react against a 35,000-40,000 dalton surface receptor, have a similar distribution to 3A1, and are not reactive against cutaneous T-cell lymphoma, adult T-cell leukemia, and T-cell chronic lymphocytic leukemia. Other antibodies that could react with a large number of lymphoblastic lymphomas include the antibody against the E-rosette receptor T-11, the one against the common thymocyte antigen T-6, and possibly other T-series monoclonal antibodies (such as T-4, T-8, and T-3) against more mature T cells, (Nadler et al. 1982, Reinherz et al. 1980). Monoclonal antibodies reactive against hematopoietic cells, such as T-9 and T-10, would not be suitable because of their reactivity with the bone marrow progenitor cells. Many of these antibodies have not been tested against the cells involved in the marrow microenvironment. There has been poor hematopoietic recovery after in vitro treatment of bone marrow with the J-5 monoclonal antibody. A reason for this could be its reactivity against the marrow microenvironment. This antibody reacts against the adherent cells in long-term human bone marrow cultures (Izaguirre et al. 1982, Keating et al. 1982, Ritz et al. 1982). Before these antibodies are used routinely to purge bone marrow, we suggest that their reactivity with adherent cells in marrow cultures should first be determined.

It is not sufficient to use monoclonal antibodies that are reactive against malignant cells at the time of diagnosis because of the changing antigenic patterns of the relapsed patient (Bernard et al. 1982). This could be of particular concern if patients most likely to relapse are those without T- or B-cell markers. Antibodies would not be available to purge the bone marrow. Alternatively, the relapse could be associated with a low percentage of blast cells reactive with monoclonal antibodies or weakly reactive to monoclonal antibodies. In lymphoma, monoclonal antibodies reactive with specific lymphoid antigens should be used to detect bone marrow contamination (Ault 1979). Terminal transferase-positive cells with thymocyte T-cell markers can be detected when these cells are present at 0.5% or less in the bone marrow, by the use of fluorescent-labeled monoclonal antibodies and fluorescent activated cell sorter analysis (Bradstock et al. 1980).

There are also some recently developed B-cell monoclonal antibodies reactive against virtually all nodular lymphomas, the majority of diffuse large-cell lymphomas, and chronic lymphatic leukemia. This includes the B-1 antibody (Nadler et al. 1982, 1981a, 1981b) and the BA-1 antibody (Abramson et al. 1981, Ash et al. 1982, Jansen et al. 1982, Kersey et al. 1982). The BA-1 antibodies have been tested against granulocyte, erythroid, and mixed colony-forming cells and were nonreactive (Ash et al. 1982, Jansen et al. 1982, Kersey et al. 1982). However, lessons learned from the J-5 antibody experience suggest that these antibodies should be tested for possible reactivity against bone marrow microenvironment cells. Antibody against surface immunoglobulin could also be used in the panel to separate lymphoma stem cells. Again, as in leukemia, these antibodies should be reactive against lymphoma stem cells, which may be more primitive than suspected. For instance, in multiple myeloma, idiotypic surface markers have been documented on pre-B cells; yet, multiple myeloma is much more differentiated than the B-cell neoplasms under consideration for treatment with ABMT (Kubagowa et al. 1981, Vogler 1982). We have documented unsuspected possible T-cell involvement in B-cell lymphoma, which suggests that even the stem cell in this disease may be common to both B and T cells (Costa et al. 1981). It is conceivable that antibodies reactive against B cells may not be reactive against the antigenic determinants of the true stem cells of these diseases; if they are, then these may be cross-reactive with multipotential normal stem cells. As in leukemia, in vitro drug treatment of bone marrow cells may be an alternative method of eliminating bone marrow contamination.

SHOULD WE START CLINICAL TRIALS IN LYMPHOMA WITH IN VITRO-TREATED AUTOLOGOUS BONE MARROW?

As in acute leukemia, it will be difficult to prove the biological effectiveness of monoclonal antibody or other in vitro manipulation of autologous bone marrow. One way to evaluate monoclonal antibody treatment will be first to establish the natural history of ABMT without monoclonal manipulation either in remission or relapse. Next, in a similar patient group, we would need to determine whether monoclonal antibody-treated bone marrow is associated with a more favorable outcome. For instance, in relapsing AML it is accepted that long-term disease-free unmaintained remissions are very rare with the use of unmanipulated ABMT. However, some preliminary results suggest that, even though the likelihood of bone marrow contamination exists, leukemic cells may not necessarily engraft when transplanted during first remission or may not engraft successfully if mild posttransplantation maintenance chemotherapy is administered. It is theoretically possible that if we transplant autologous bone marrow during remission, the bone marrow microenvironment (particularly if mild cycle-specific chemotherapy is administered simultaneously) would favor the establishment of normal hematopoiesis. Transplantation during relapse may allow the establishment of leukemic clones that will eventually lead to clinical relapse.

These questions must be answered in a stepwise approach; what is the true reactivity of antibodies against cells other than clonogenic normal cells and the natural history of ABMT for lymphoma in different stages of that disease and in different lymphoma subtypes, and can such a natural history be changed by using monoclonal antibody-treated marrow? What seems obvious and simple may turn out to be quite the contrary.

CONCLUSION

The results of high-dose chemotherapy with ABMT in lymphoma patients is encouraging, considering the extensive prior therapy of those patients we have treated so far. The use of monoclonal antibodies to purge the marrow is of interest and is being investigated. The effect of monoclonal antibodies on marrow engraftment and the role of ABMT in modifying hematopoietic toxicity is discussed in other reviews (Spitzer et al. 1983a, 1983b). However, the marrow infusion appears to be important in modifying the granulocytopenia of high-dose chemotherapy and is responsible for marrow recovery after lethal doses of irradiation. The next few years should add to our knowledge of the correct role of bone marrow transplantation for lymphoma patients.

ACKNOWLEDGMENT

This investigation was supported by grants CA 28153 and CA 14528, awarded by the National Cancer Institute, United States Department of Health and Human Services. Gary Spitzer is a recipient of a scholarship from the Leukemia Society of America.

REFERENCES

Abramson CS, Kersey JH, LeBien TW. 1981. A monoclonal antibody (BA-1) reactive with cells of human B lymphocyte lineage. J Immunol 126:83–88.

Amiel JR, Tursz T, Droz JP. 1981. Chemotherapies for resistant lymphomas. Nouv Presse Med 10:1939.

Appelbaum FR, Diesseroth AB, Graw RG Jr, Herzig GP, Levine AS, Magrath IT, Pizzo PA, Poplack DG, Ziegler JL. 1978. Prolonged complete remission following high-dose chemotherapy of Burkitt's lymphoma in relapse. Cancer 41:1059–1063.

Appelbaum FR, Fefer A, Cheever MA. 1981. Treatment of chronic granulocytic leukemia with chemoradiotherapy and transplantation of marrow from identical-twins. Blood 306:63–68.

Appelbaum FR, Sullivan K, Thomas ED. 1983. Treatment of non-Hodgkin's lymphoma (NHL) with chemoradiotherapy and allogeneic bone marrow transplantation (BMT). (Abstract) Proceedings of the American Society of Clinical Oncology C859:220.

Appelbaum FR, Thomas ED. 1983. Review of the use of marrow transplantation in the treatment of non-Hodgkin's lymphoma. J Clin Oncol 1:440–447.

Ash RC, Jansen J, Kersey JA, LeBien TW, Zanjani ED. 1982. Normal human pluripotential and committed hematopoietic progenitors do not express the P24 antigen detected by monoclonal antibody BA 2: Implications for immunotherapy of lymphocyte leukemia. Blood 60:1310–1316.

Ault KA. 1979. Detection of small numbers of monclonal B lymphocytes in the blood of lymphoma. N Engl J Med 300:1401–1405.

Barbasch A, Higby DJ, Brass C. 1983. High-dose cytoreductive therapy with autologous bone marrow transplantation in advanced malignancies. Cancer Treat Rep 67:143–148.

Baumgartner C, Bleher E, Bundel RG, Burcher U, Deubelbeiss KA, Greiner R, Hirt A, Imbach P, Luthy H, Rankg O, Wagner HP. 1984. Autologous bone marrow transplantation in the treatment of children and adolescents with advanced malignant tumors. Med Pediatr Oncol (In press).

Bensinger W, Buckner CD, Stewart P, Appelbaum FA, Thomas ED. 1983. Autologous bone marrow transplantation for end-stage lymphomas. (Abstract) J Cell Biochem 0141:58.

Berkman A, Lenhard R, Trump D. 1983. Intensive chemotherapy with cyclophosphamide (C), M-AMSA (AM) and VP-16 (CAMP) as treatment for refractory and relapsing non-Hodgkin's lymphoma (NHL). (Abstract) Proceedings of the American Society of Clinical Oncology C826:211.

Bernard A, Boumsell L, Reinherz EL. 1981. Cell surface characterization of malignant T cells from lymphoblastic lymphoma using monoclonal antibodies. Evidence of phenotypic differences between malignant T cells from patients with acute lymphoblastic leukemia and lymphoblastic lymphoma. Blood 57:1100–1105.

Bernard A, Raynal, B, Lemerle J, Boumsell L. 1982. Changes in surface antigens on malignant T cells from lymphoblastic lymphomas at relapse: An appraisal with monoclonal antibodies and microfluorometry. Blood 59:809–815.

Bloomfield CD, Gajl-Peczalska KJ, Frizzera G, Kersey JH, Goldman AI. 1979. Clinical utility of lymphocyte surface markers combined with the Lukes-Collins histologic classification in adult lymphoma. N Engl J Med 301:512–518.

Bloomfield CD, Kersey JH, Brunning RD, Gajl-Peczalska KJ. 1977. Prognostic significance of lymphocytic surface markers and histology in adult non-Hodgkin's lymphoma. Cancer Treat Rep 61:963–970.

Bonadonna G. 1982. Chemotherapy strategies to improve the control of Hodgkin's disease. Cancer Res 42:4309–4320.

Bradstock KF, Janossy G, Pizzolo G. 1980. Subpopulations of normal and leukemic human thymocytes: An analysis with the use of monoclonal antibodies. JNCI 65:33–42.

Brecher ML, Gardner R, Ettinger LJ, Green D, Freeman AI. 1981. Intensive chemotherapy for treatment of advanced Burkitt's lymphoma. (Abstract) Proceedings of the American Society of Clinical Oncology 22:406.

Cabanillas F. 1984. New chemotherapeutic agents and combinations in the treatment of lymphoma. *In* Ford RJ, Fuller LM, Hagemeister FB, eds., UT M. D. Anderson Clinical Conference on Cancer, Vol. 27. Raven Press, New York, pp 391–396.

Cabanillas F, Burgess MA, Bodey GP, Freireich EJ. 1983a. Sequential chemotherapy and late intensification for malignant lymphomas of aggressive histologic type. Am J Med 74:382–388.

Cabanillas F, Hagemeister FB, Bodey GP, Freireich EJ. 1982. Ifosfamide, Methetrexate, VP-16 (IMVP-16) an effective salvage regimen for lymphoma. Blood 60:693–697.

Cabanillas F, Hagemeister FB, McLaughlin P, Riggs S, Salvador P, Smith TL, Bodey GP, Freireich EJ. 1983b. Long-term outcome of complete responders (CR) to salvage chemotherapy for recurrent or refractory lymphoma. (Abstract) Proceedings of the American Society of Clinical Oncology C833:213.

Cabanillas F, Hagemeister FB, Salvador P. 1982b. Factors predicting for complete remission (CR) in patients (PTS) with recurrent lymphoma treated with salvage combination chemotherapy. (Abstract) Proceedings of the American Society for Clinical Oncology C653:167.

Cabanillas F, Legha SS, Bodey GP 1981. Initial experience with AMSA as a single agent treatment against malignant lymphomproliferative disorders. Blood 57:614–616.

Carella AM, Santini G, Frassoni F. 1983. Autologous bone marrow transplantation (ABMT) without cryopreservation in haematological malignancies and solid tumors. Pilot study in 22 patients. 13th International Congress of Chemotherapy SS76 232:25–33.

Cavalli F, Jung WF, Nissen NJ 1981. Phase II trial of cis-dichlorodiammine-platinum (II) in advanced malignant lymphoma. Cancer 48:1927–1930.

Coleman CN, Rosenberg SA, Cohen JR, Burke JS. 1982. Lymphoblastic lymphoma (LL) in adults: Comparison of two protocols. (Abstract) Proceedings of the American Society of Clinical Oncology C640:164.

Costa RN, Davis F, Kusky C, Verma DS, Spitzer G. 1981. E-rosette forming cell colonies (ERFC-C) with malignant markers in B-cell neoplasms myeloid leukemia. (Abstract) Proceedings of the American Society of Clinical Oncology 103:27.

Doney K, Buckner CD, Sole GE, Ramber R, Boyd C, Thomas ED. 1978. Treatment of chronic granulocyte leukemia by chemotherapy, total body irradiation and allogeneic bone marrow transplantation. Exp Hematol 6:738–747.

Ekert H, Ellis WM, Waters KD. 1982. Autologous bone marrow rescue in the treatment of advanced tumors of childhood. Cancer 49:603–609.

Espana P, Kaplan R, Robichaud K, Gustafson P, Wiernik P, Smith F, Woolley P, Schein P. 1982. Phase II study of spirogermanium (SpiroG) in lymphoma patients. (Abstract) Proceedings of the American Society of Clinical Oncology C647:166.

Fefer A, Cheever MA, Greenberg PD. 1982a. Treatment of chronic granulocytic leukemia with chemoradiotherapy and transplantation of marrow from identical-twins. Blood 306:63–68.

Fefer A, Cheever MA, Thomas ED, Appelbaum FR, Buckner CD, Clift RA, Glucksberg H, Greenberg PD, Johnson FL, Kaplan HG, Sanders JE, Storb R, Weiden PL. 1981. Bone marrow transplantation for refractory acute leukemia in 34 patients with identical twins. Blood 57:421–430.

Fefer A, Greenberg PD, Cheever MA, Appelbaum FR, Bluming AZ, Storb R, Thomas ED. 1982b. Identical-twin bone marrow transplantation (BMT) for multiple myeloma (MM). Blood 60:168.

Fisher RJ, DeVita VT, Hubbard SM, Jaffe ES, Cossman J, Wesley R, Chabner BA, Young RC. 1982. Improved survival of diffuse aggressive lymphomas following treatment with pro-MACE chemotherapy. (Abstract) Proceedings of the American Society of Clinical Oncology C627:161.

Foon KA, Schroff RW, Gale PW. 1982. Surface markers on leukemia and lymphoma cells: Recent advances. Blood 60:1–19.

Gale RP. 1980. Autologous bone marrow transplantation in patients with cancer. JAMA 243:540–542.

Gorin NC, David R, Strachowiak J. 1981. High-dose chemotherapy and autologous bone marrow transplantation in acute leukemias malignant lymphomas and solid tumors. Eur J Cancer 17:557–568.

Greaves MF, Delca D, Robinson J, Sutherland R, Newman R. 1981. Exploitation of monoclonal antibodies: A "Who's Who" of hemapoietic malignancy. Blood 7:257–280.

Gulati S, Langleben A, Jain K, Yopp J, Straus D, Koziner B, Gee T, Lee B, Shank B, Mertelsmann R, Dinsmore R, O'Reilly R, Clarkson B. 1983. Autologous stem cell transplantation (ASCT) after total body irradiation (TBI) and high-dose cytoxan for poor prognosis lymphoma. (Abstract) Proceedings of the American Society of Clinical Oncology C854:218.

Haynes B. 1981. Human T lymphocyte antigens as defined by monoclonal antibodies. Immunol Rev 57:127.

Izaguirre CA, Katz FE, Greaves MF. 1982. Origin of marrow microenvironmental stromal cells in hemopoietic pluripotent stem cells (CFU-stroma). Blood 60:99.

Janossy G, Bollum FJ, Bradstock KF, Ashley J. 1982. Cellular phenotypes of normal and leukemia hemapoietic cells determined by analysis with select antibody combination. Blood 56:430–440.

Jansen J, Ash RC, Zanjani ED, LeBien TW, Kersey JH. 1982. Monoclonal antibody BA 1 does not bind to hematopoietic precursor cells. Blood 59:1029–1035.

Johnson FL, Thomas ED, Clark BS, Chard RL, Hartman JR, Storb R. 1981. A comparison of marrow transplantation with chemotherapy for children with acute lymphoblastic leukemia in second or subsequent remission. N Engl J Med 305:845–851.

Jones SE, Grozea PN, Metz EN, Hout A, Stephens RL, Morrison FS, Butler J, Byrne GE, Moon TE, Fisher R, Haskins CL, Coltman CA. 1979. Superiority of adriamycin-containing combination chemotherapy in the treatment of diffuse lymphoma: A Southwest Oncology Group study. Cancer 43:417–425.

Kaizer H, Levy R, Cote JP, Johnson RJ, Fuller D, Santos GW. 1982. Autologous bone marrow transplantation in lymphoblastic lymphoma and T-cell leukemia. (Abstract) Blood 60:169A.

Kaizer H, Wharam MD, Munoz RJ. 1979. Autologous bone marrow transplantation in the treatment of selected human malignancies: The Johns Hopkins Oncology Center Program. Exp Hematol 7:(Suppl 5)309–320.

Kaplan RS, Bishop JF, Diggs CH, Wiernik PH. 1981. VM-26 and bleomycin plus adriamycin or cis-dichlorodiammineplatinum-II (DDP) in previously treated patients with non-Hodgkin's lymphoma (NHL). (Abstract) Proceedings of the American Society of Clinical Oncology C704:512.

Keating A, Singer JW, Killen PD, Striker GE, Solo AC, Sanders J. 1982. Donor origin of the in vitro haematopoietic microenvironment after marrow transplantation in man. Nature 298:280–282.

Keller AM, Schnetzer GW III, Sexauer JM, Segler SS. 1982. Phase III study with CCNU/VP-16/MTX/prednisone for refractory CLL and malignant lymphoma. (Abstract) Proceedings of the American Society of Clinical Oncology C651:167.

Kersey J, Goldman A, Abramson C. 1982. Clinical usefulness of monoclonal antibody phenotyping in childhood acute lymphoblastic leukemia. Lancet 2:1419–1423.

Kroner TH, Jungi WF, Obrecht JP. 1983. Refractory malignant lymphoma: Effective combination chemotherapy with vindesine, iphosphamide and prednisone (VIP). (Abstract) Proceedings of the American Society of Clinical Oncology C822:210.

Kubagowa H, Vogler L, Conrad M. 1981. Studies on the clonal origin of multiple myeloma: Use of individually specific idiotypes antibodies to trace the oncogenic expression of B cell differentiation. J Exp Med 150:792–807.

Lachant NA, Cooper MR, Bloomfield CD, Ginsberg SJ, Gottlieb AJ, Pajak TF. 1981. Methotrexate VM-26, procarbazine and dexamethasone (MV PD) in the treatment of refractory lymphoma. (Abstract) Proceedings of the American Society of Clinical Oncology C728:518.

Laurence J, Coleman M, Allen SL, Silver RT, Pasmantier M. 1982. Combination chemotherapy of advanced diffuse histiocytic lymphoma with the six-drug COP-BLAM regimen. Ann Intern Med 97:190–195.

Levine AM, Forman SJ, Meyer PR, Koehler SC, Liebman H, Paganini-Hill A, Pockros A, Lukes RJ, Feinstein DJ. 1983. Successful therapy of convoluted T-lymphoblastic lymphoma in the adult. Blood 61:92–98.

Link M, Berberich R, Donaldson S, Mott M, Wilbur J, Burke J, Glader B. 1982. Improved prognosis for children with advanced non-Hodgkin's lymphoma. (Abstract) Proceedings of the American Society of Clinical Oncology C630:162.

Link M, Warnke R, Finlay J, Amylon M, Miller R, Dilley J, Levy R. 1983. A single monoclonal antibody identifies T-cell lineage of childhood lymphoid malignancies. Blood 62:772–728.

Magrath IT, Spiegel RJ, Edwards BK, Janus C. 1981. Improved results of chemotherapy in young patients with Burkitt (BL), undifferentiated (UL), and lymphoblastic lymphomas (LL). (Abstract) Proceedings of the American Society of Clinical Oncology C736:520.

McClave PB, Miller J, Hurd DP, Arthur DC, Kim T. 1981. Cytogenetic conversion following allogeneic bone marrow transplantation for advanced chronic myelogenous leukemia. Blood 58:1050–1052.

McKelvey EM, Moon TE. 1977. Curability of non-Hodgkin's lymphomas. Cancer Treat Rep 61:1185–1190.

Meyers JE, Thomas ED. 1982. Infection complicating bone marrow transplantations. *In* Young LS, Rubin RH, eds., Clinical Approach to Infection in the Immunocompromised Host. Plenum Press, New York, pp. 507–551.

Nadler LM, Ritz J, Griffin JD, Todd RF III, Reinherz EL, Schlossman SF. 1981a. Diagnosis and treatment of human leukemias and lymphoma utilizing monoclonal antibodies. *In* Brown E, ed., Progress in Hematology. Grune and Stratton, Inc., New York, pp. 187–225.

Nadler LM, Ritz J, Reinherz EL, Schlossman SF. 1982. Cellular origins of human leukemias and lymphomas. *In* Brown E, Knapp W, eds., Leukemia Markers. Academic Press, New York, pp. 1–17.

Nadler LM, Stashenko P, Ritz J, Hardy R, Pesando JM, Schlossman SF. 1981b. A unique cell surface antigen identifing lymphoid malignancies of B-cell origin. J Clin Invest 67:134–140.

Naito K, Knowles RW, Red FX, Morishima Y, Kowashima K, DuPont B. 1983. Analysis of two new leukemia-associated antigens detected on T-cell acute lymphoblastic leukemia using monoclonal antibodies. Blood 62:852–865.

Neiman PE, Meyers JD, Medeiros E, McDougall JK, Thomas ED. 1980. Interstitial pneumonia following marrow transplantation for leukemia and aplastic anemia. *In* Gale RP, Fox CF, eds., Biology of Bone Marrow Transplantation. Academic Press, New York, p. 75.

Ng BP, Todd D, Khoo RKK. 1982. Salvage chemotherapy for non-Hodgkin's lymphoma. Cancer Treat Rep 66:1977–1979.

O'Leary M, Ramsay NKC, Nesbit ME, Hurd D, Woods WG, Krivit W, Kim TH, McGlave P, Kersey J. 1983. Bone marrow transplantation for non-Hodgkin's lymphoma in children and young adults. Am J Med 74:497–501.

Pavlosky S, Wooley PV, Garay A. 1981. Phase II study of chlorozotocin in leukemia and other hematologic malignancies. Cancer Treat Rep 65:1109–1111.

Philip T, Biron P, Herve P, Maraninchi D, Le Mevel A. 1983. Massive BACT chemotherapy with autologous bone marrow transplantation in 17 cases of non-Hodgkin's malignant lymphoma with a very bad prognosis. Eur J Cancer Clin Oncol 19:1371–1379.

Phillips GL. 1983. Current clinical trials with intensive therapy and autologous bone marrow transplantation (ABMT) for lymphomas and solid tumors. *In* Gale RP, ed., Recent Advances in Bone Marrow Transplantation. Alan R. Liss, Inc., New York, pp. 567–597.

Reinherz EL, Kung PC, Goldstein G, Levey RH, Schlossman SF. 1980. Discrete stages of human intrathymic differentiation: Analysis of normal thymocytes and leukemic lymphoblasts of T-cell lineage. Proc Natl Acad Sci USA 77:1588–1592.

Ritz J, Sallan SE, Bast RC. 1982. Autologous bone marrow transplantation in cALLa positive acute lymphoblastic leukemia after in vitro treatment with J5 monoclonal antibody and complement. Lancet 1:60–63.

Rodriquez V, McCredie KB, Keating MJ, Valdivieso M, Bodey GP, Freireich EJ. 1978. Isophosphamide therapy for hematologic malignancies in patients refractory to prior treatment. Cancer Treat Rep 62:493–497.

Roper M, Crist W, Metzgar R. 1981. Immune phenotypes in childhood T cell lymphoid malignancies. (Abstract) Proceedings of the American Society of Clinical Oncology 374:167.

Santoro A, Bonfante V, Bonadonna G. 1982. Third-line chemotherapy with CCNU, etoposide and prednimustine (CEP) in Hodgkin's disease (HD) resistant to MOPP and ABVD. (Abstract) Proceedings of the American Society of Clinical Oncology C642:165.

Schein PS, DeVita VT, Hubbard S, Chabner BA, Canellos GP, Berard C, Young RC. 1976. Bleomycin, adriamycin, cyclophosphamide, vincristine, and prednisone (BACOP) combination chemotherapy in the treatment of advanced diffuse histiocytic lymphoma. Ann Intern Med 85:417–422.

Segal ML, Grever MR, Ungerleider J, Balcerzak SP. 1982. Treatment of refractory non-Hodgkin's lymphoma (NHL) with ifosfamide (IF) and VP-16 (VP). (Abstract) Proceedings of the American Society of Clinical Oncology C621:159.

Spitzer G, Vellekoop L, Zander A, Tannir NM, Verma D, Kanojia M, Jagannath S, Dicke K. 1983a. Autologous bone marrow transplantation in leukemia and lymphoma. Journal of Experimental Clinical Cancer Research 3:317–332.

Spitzer G, Zander A, Tannir N, Farha P, Vellekoop L, Verma D, Kanojia M, Jagannath S, Dicke K. 1983b. Autologous bone marrow transplantation in human solid tumors. *In* Gale RP, ed., Recent Advances in Bone Marrow Transplantation. Alan R. Liss, Inc., New York, pp. 567–597.

Sullivan KM, Shulman HM, Weiden PL, Storb R, Tsoi M-S, Thomas ED. 1980. The spectrum of chronic graft-vs-host disease in man. *In* Gale RP, Fox CF, eds., Biology of Bone Marrow Transplantation. Academic Press, New York, pp. 69–74.

Takvorian T, Canellos GP. 1983. High-dose cytosine arabinoside (ARA-C) in advanced non-Hodgkin's lymphoma and chronic myelogenous leukemia (ML). (Abstract) Proceedings of the American Society of Clinical Oncology, C848:217.

Thomas ED. 1978. Treatment of chronic granulocyte leukemia by chemotherapy, total body irradiation and allogeneic bone marrow transplantation. Exp. Hematol. 6:738–747.

Thomas ED. 1983. Marrow transplantation for malignant diseases. Journal of Clinical Oncology 1:516–531.

Thomas ED, Buckner CD, Banaji M, Clift RA, Fefer A, Flournoy N, Goodell BW, Hickman RO, Lerner KG, Neiman PE, Sale GE, Sanders JE, Singer J, Stevens M, Storb R, Weiden PL. 1977. One hundred patients with acute leukemia treated by chemotherapy, total body irradiation, and allogeneic marrow transplantation. Blood 49:511–533.

Thomas ED, Sanders JE, Flournoy N, Johnson FL, Buckner CD, Clift RA, Fefer A, Goodell BW, Storb R, Weiden PL. 1979. Marrow transplantation for patients with acute lymphoblastic leukemia in remission. Blood 54:468–478.

Thomas ED, Storb R, Clift RA, Fefer A, Johnson FL, Neiman PE, Lerner KG, Glucksberg H, Buckner CD. 1975. Bone-marrow transplantation. N Engl J Med 292:832–895.

Vogler LB. 1982. Bone marrow B-cell development. Clin Hematol 11:509–529.

Wallach SR, Huberman MS, Lokich JJ, Bern MM. 1983. Treatment of resistant lymphoma with ARA-C and continuous infusion VP-16-213. (Abstract) Proceedings of the American Society of Clinical Oncology C851:218.

Warnke R, Miller R, Grogan T, Rederson M, Dilley J, Levy R. 1980. Immunologic phenotype in 30 patients with diffuse large cell lymphoma. N Engl J Med 303:294–300.

Warrell RP Jr, Lee BJ, Kempin SJ. 1981a. Effectiveness of methyl-GAG (Methylglyoxal-bis[guanylhydrazone]) in patients with advanced malignant lymphomas. Blood 57:1011–1014.

Warrell RP Jr, Lee BJ, Kempin SJ, Straus DJ, Lacher MJ, Young CW. 1981b. Clinical evaluation of methyl-GAG (methylglyoxal-bis[guanylhydrazone]) alone and in combination with VM-26 (teniposide) in advanced malignant lymphoma. (Abstract) Proceedings of the American Society of Clinical Oncology C738:521.

Weick JK, Jones SE. 1983. Vindesine, BCNU, adriamycin and prednisone (EBAP) in malignant lymphoma. (Abstract) Proceedings of the American Society of Clinical Oncology C818:209.

Weinstein HJ, Link MP. 1979. Non-Hodgkin's lymphoma in childhood. Clin Haematol 8:699–716.

Weinstein HJ, Vance Z, Jaffe N, Buell D, Cassady J, Nathan D. 1979. Improved prognosis for patients with mediastinal lymphoblastic lymphoma. Blood 53:687–694.

Wollner H, Exelby PR, Lieberman PH. 1979. Non-Hodgkin's lymphoma in children: A progress report on the original patients treated with the LSA$_2$-L$_2$ protocol. Cancer 44:1990–1999.

UT M.D. Anderson Clinical Conference on Cancer,
Vol. 27, edited by R. J. Ford, L. M. Fuller, and
F. B. Hagemeister. Raven Press, New York © 1984.

Summary and Perspectives

Emil Frei III

Dana-Farber Cancer Institute, Boston, Massachusetts 02115

In 1965 I joined a National Cancer Institute program-project-grant study section. An outstanding basic scientist member of the study section emphasized, with considerable regularity, that no progress was possible in clinical cancer research, particularly in treatment, without an understanding of the disease at a fundamental (molecular) level. Fortunately, he did not prevail because he was only partially right. Perhaps in no other form of cancer have both basic and clinical science moved so rapidly as in the lymphomas, as witnessed by this monograph. Almost all categories of Hodgkin's disease, and many categories of non-Hodgkin's lymphoma, can now be treated with curative intent. Such progress at a clinical level has had a profound influence on basic science studies. Equally important has been the impact of cell biology, molecular biology, immunology, and other aspects of fundamental and tumor biological studies on our understanding of the disease. It is particularly the integration of such clinical and basic science in the study of lymphoma that makes these extraordinarily exciting times for the investigator. Further, an accelerating progress in our knowledge concerning the prevention and treatment of these diseases seems assured.

THE HODGKIN'S DISEASE CELL

Although the nature of the neoplastic cell in almost all of the lymphomas has been identified in terms of lineage and differentiation level, the neoplastic cell in Hodgkin's disease remains elusive. Dr. Olsson presented data concerning a Hodgkin's cell line that had monocyte-macrophage characteristics, including Fc receptor, nonspecific esterase, and the capacity to present antigen. Dr. Ford came to the same general conclusion by similar studies, including ones involving lymphokine production and phagocytosis. Dr. Stein, using the L428 Hodgkin's cell lines of Diehl and a panel of monoclonal antibodies, found that the Hodgkin's cell did not share characteristics of any known cell lineage or level of differentiation and so concluded that that cell represents either a new cell or a new differentiation state. Using Ki monoclonal antibodies to the Hodgkin's cell, he found varying degrees of cross-reactivity with large cells in the normal tonsil, around normal follicles in the lymph nodes, and in some patients with non-Hodgkin's lymphoma. These studies and seeming discrepancies must be qualified in their interpretation by the fact that the tissues and cell lines isolated and studied may not, in fact, represent the neoplastic cell of Hodgkin's disease.

TREATMENT OF HODGKIN'S DISEASE

Chemotherapy, often in a multimodality setting, has achieved greater progress against Hodgkin's disease than any form of neoplasia save testicular cancer. Using multistep regression analysis techniques, it has been possible, through the pioneering work of Dr. Gehan, to sort out the quantitative power and independence of prognostic factors, including the effects of treatment. For patients with clinical stages I and II Hodgkin's disease, Dr. Bergsagel has found that independent prognostic factors include the pathology, age, bulk disease, and B symptoms. For low-risk patients, radiotherapy alone provides a cure rate in excess of 90%; for high-risk patients, chemotherapy combined with radiotherapy also produces cure rates approaching 90%. Radiotherapy alone in such patients may provide only 25%–50% disease-free survival. Even in this circumstance, the effectiveness of rescue chemotherapy with MOPP (mechlorethamine, vincristine, procarbazine, and prednisone) or other programs is such that the ultimate cure rate approaches 90%.

Strategies for advanced Hodgkin's disease were exemplified by the presentations of Dr. Straus, representing Memorial Sloan-Kettering, and Dr. Prosnitz. Dr. Bonadonna, from the Instituto Nazionale Tumori in Milan, has found that ABVD (doxorubicin, bleomycin, vinblastine, and dacarbazine) is as effective as MOPP, in terms of cure rate for patients with advanced Hodgkin's disease. It has the significant advantage in that reasonable, albeit not definitive, follow-up showed that ABVD is better tolerated in terms of producing a lower incidence of secondary acute myelogenous leukemia (AML) and has less effect on the gonadal system in both males and females. Using a hypothesis based on theoretical and preclinical biologic studies of the development of resistance, the two comparably active but qualitatively different programs (ABVD and MOPP) in an alternating program produced a superior complete remission rate and duration in a controlled study reported from the Milan group. Dr. Straus has studied the same combination and added a third non–cross-resistant drug program consisting of a combination of CCNU (chloroethyl cyclohexyl nitrosourea), melphalan, and vindesine. These drug combinations with follow-up radiotherapy have resulted in high complete remission rates and very low relapse rates.

The other therapeutic hypothesis employed by these groups in designing treatment programs relates to the fact that recurrence of Hodgkin's disease after complete remission occurs predictably at pretreatment sites of bulky disease. Therefore, both the Straus and Prosnitz studies employed radiotherapy to these areas after patients entered complete remission on chemotherapy. Since other variables were involved and control groups were not included, it is difficult to determine the contribution of adjuvant radiotherapy to the results and the perturbations in the effect of chemotherapy. Nevertheless, in both studies of relatively large numbers of patients, complete remission rates in excess of 80% were achieved. Relapse rates were in the range of 10%. This compares to a cure rate of 40%–50% by MOPP only for stages III B and IV disease.

An ominous aspect of the treatment of Hodgkin's disease has been the production of second primaries in the form of AML. Chemotherapy, particularly MOPP, appears to be the major offender, producing by actuarial analysis incidences of secondary AML ranging from 3%–10%, and in patients treated after the age of 40, as high as 20%. Moreover, a plateau in the incidence over time has not yet been reached, and it is possible that the risk will increase in time after 10 years.

Strong indirect evidence indicates that the offender is procarbazine. Experimentally, it is a potent carcinogen. In patients with breast cancer receiving CMF (cyclophosphamide, methotrexate, and 5-fluorouracil), which includes an alkylating agent (cyclophosphamide), an excess of AML has not been seen, nor does it occur after treatment for acute lymphocytic leukemia, which includes programs that do not contain alkyating agents. An increased incidence of AML (but lower than that following MOPP) is seen, for example, in ovarian cancer, where alkylating agents such as melphalan may be administered over a long period of time. Finally, ABVD has not been associated with an excess of AML. Since there are now at least 11 agents that are active against Hodgkin's disease, and since it has been demonstrated that very substantial variation in components of the MOPP program can be tolerated without loss of therapeutic effect, high priority should be given to the development and use of curative regimens that exclude procarbazine.

The first section under non-Hodgkin's lymphoma was devoted to studies of the etiology and immunology of that disease. Major basic scientific contributions of clinical relevance were made in areas involving virology, molecular biology, immunology, and cytogenetics. Some of the highlights include the following. A transforming gene has been isolated from chicken B-cell lymphoma DNA. This gene (ChBlym-1) encodes for a small protein with sequence homology to the growth factor transferrin. That oncogenes should produce growth factors is of considerable interest and is consistent with the discovery by computer matching that certain oncogenes produce platelet-derived growth factor. DNA was isolated from human Burkitt's lymphoma cells, and a calcium precipitate of the DNA was applied to mouse 3T3 cells. Transformation of these fibroblasts occurred as a result of this transfection with oncogene-containing DNA. In fact, the DNA of almost 50% of patients with human tumors will transform this mouse cell. By restriction enzyme mapping, gene isolation, and cloning, a cDNA probe was developed that annealed in in situ hybridization studies to chromosome 1 in Burkitt's lymphoma cells. ChBlym-1 does not exhibit sequence homology with other known oncogenes, nor is chromosome 1 abnormal in Burkitt's lymphoma cells. In view of the multistep nature of transformation, it seems possible that the t(8;14) translocation of the *myc* gene and the ChBlym-1 oncogene are separate and distinct, and yet may represent steps in the progression to neoplasia.

Dr. Nowell reviewed the increasing evidence for specific cytogenetic abnormalities in human neoplastic diseases, emphasizing particularly reciprocal translocations and other evidence for relatively gross genetic changes such as transposons and sister chromatid exchanges. The t(8;14) translocation juxtaposes the *mu* gene for IgM production and the *myc* gene. This was inferred from cytogenetic studies and conclusively demonstrated by DNA sequencing. While the exact mechanism of gene activation, phenotypic expression, and frank neoplasia that derives from such juxtapositions remains to be determined, the evidence that they are important in the etiology of the disease is most compelling.

Dr. Wong-Staal reviewed the current status of the human T-cell leukemia virus (HTLV) story with emphasis on the molecular mechanism of induction by HTLV and T-cell proliferation and neoplasias; the observation that there are several types of HTLV; and the possibility that subtypes may produce somewhat different forms of neoplasia.

Dr. Korsmeyer applied the techniques of molecular biology to the B-cell system. The genetic basis for antibody heterogeneity results from rearrangements in the B-cell lineage of the various genes for the variable, joining, and constant regions (V, J, and C genes and their subunits). For certain lymphocytic neoplasms, a large proportion are non-T, but they are not conclusively B on the basis of immunologic phenotyping. This is true, for example, for acute lymphocytic leukemia. By DNA sequencing studies, it was found that the rearrangements of the above genes consistent with immunoglobulin synthesis were ongoing, compared with that of stem lines, and that the rearrangements in B-cell neoplasias were relatively fixed, consistent with a monoclonal origin for acute lymphocytic leukemia (ALL). Similar studies of lymphoid CML and hairy cell leukemia indicated conclusively the B-cell nature of these diseases. Such studies are moving at an extraordinary pace, and some of the techniques of molecular biology are becoming readily and increasingly adaptable to clinical studies. It seems certain that their application to the study of rearrangements of immunoglobulin genes to the various oncogenes and differentiation genes in clinical material will continue to increase.

Dr. Butcher addressed the issue of the determinants of the distribution of lymphoid cells. He studied the interactions involving specific recognition by normal recirculating lymphocytes of endothelial determinants expressed at high levels by the specialized high endothelial venules and Peyer's patches in lymph nodes. Through monoclonal antibody technology, he demonstrated lymphocyte surface "homing" receptors. Thus, the distribution of normal and neoplastic lymphocytes may well be determined by homing receptors between the cells and the endothelium of an organ in question, reminiscent of the interactions in the pathogenesis of metastases.

Dr. Nadler analyzed normal B-cell differentiation using primarily monoclonal antibody technology and is in the process of applying such technology to neoplasms of the B-cell system. His results are consistent with clonal expansion of a given differentiation step, but he emphasized that the differentiation block is not absolute. For example, differentiation can be nudged substantially for neoplastic B-cells by phorbol. Such studies provide avenues to the genetics and the molecular biology of differentiation. Thus, working back through the differentiation antigens, the genes could be identified and their sequence of activation, possible juxtaposition, and rearrangement, could be determined. Finally, such antibodies allow for the isolation of cells at various differentiation steps and therefore definitive studies of their function, mediator production, response to various treatment, and other perturbations.

Dr. Ford discussed the potential of a truly tumor-specific antigen in relation to the nucleolar-associated antigen, identified by heteroantisera, as well as studies relating to the immunobiology of non-Hodgkin's lymphoma. Drs. Kadin and Bloomfield discussed relatively early studies relating to immunologic phenotyping of lymphoid neoplasms and their pathology, and particularly their clinical correlations. As these studies mature and are conducted prospectively, it can be anticipated with reasonable certainty that fundamental pathogenetic data, such as the level of differentiation and monoclonal expansion, will have important clinical and therapeutic correlates.

THERAPY OF NON-HODGKIN'S LYMPHOMA

The proportion of patients with stages I and II non-Hodgkin's lymphoma, after vigorous staging, is small, probably less than 10%. Some patients with carefully determined stage I disease may be cured by radiographic therapy only, but the proportion is probably not even 50%. While the issue is controversial, evidence strongly favors systemic treatment (often in addition to localized radiotherapy) for patients with stage II disease and probably for those with stage I disease. The chemotherapy to be employed has not been well worked out in the context of clinical trials. In view of experimental data, and data derived from other systems, the approach that is most attractive would be to use optimal chemotherapy, BACOP (bleomycin, doxorubicin, cyclophosphamide, vincristine, and prednisone) and CHOP (cyclophosphamide, doxorubicin, vincristine, and prednisone), or its derivatives with the expectation that a long duration of treatment will probably not be necessary. Thus, for such patients with minimal disease, no compromise in the quality of the chemotherapy is indicated, but probably some shortening of the duration of chemotherapy, as compared to that required for stages III and IV disease, would be a reasonable subject for clinical trial.

The recurrence and survival dynamics differ markedly for diffuse and nodular disease, and this point was emphasized. The hazard function for nodular disease does not appear to change with time, partly because of the rate of transition to diffuse disease. Experience with diffuse histiocytic lymphoma derived from nodular disease indicates that it is less responsive to chemotherapy. Dr. Levine emphasized the distinction between small, noncleaved Burkitt's and non-Burkitt's lymphoma. Both show immunoglobulin monoclonality in the majority of patients. Burkitt's patients tend to be younger and have a somewhat improved survival. The cure rate for T-cell lymphoblastic lymphoma in both pediatric and young adult patients treated with advanced chemotherapy protocols is relatively high.

Dr. Thomas Miller from the Arizona group described the advantage of initial treatment with chemotherapy only for localized non-Hodgkin's lymphoma of unfavorable histology (86% disease-free at a median follow-up time of 41 months).

The status of the chemotherapy of patients with stages III and IV unfavorable histologies were reviewed. Using CHOP-Bleo, Dr. Velasquez at UT M. D. Anderson Hospital reported an overall 50% disease-free survival. Dr. Fisher, for the NCI group, reported on the ProMace-MOPP (cyclophosphamide, doxorubicin, etoposide, methotrexate, and MOPP) program, which addresses the Goldie-Skipper hypothesis concerning mutation to resistance, as well as the adjustments of treatment to the kinetics of tumor regression. They reported a 60%–65% disease-free survival plateau. Another program that has been comparably effective is high-dose methotrexate with rescue, interposed between courses of BACOP. Such issues as the dose of methotrexate, the need for procarbazine (in view of its carcinogenic potential), and the relative merits of CHOP-Bleo (CHOP plus bleomycin) versus the newer programs are important. Approaches to improving the complete remission rate and disease-free survival plateau were discussed (see below).

Dr. Ziegler, in his Heath Award Lecture, reviewed the extraordinary progress, clinical and basic, that derived from the discovery of the Burkitt's tumor in Africa. We are close to a fundamental understanding of the etiology of this disease. A multistep process occurs. The initiating event may be Epstein-Barr virus (EBV) infection, which results in polyclonal expansion of the B-cell system. This expansion is stimulated (or promoted) by holoendemic malaria. Perhaps the very large number of rapidly turning over cells that are EBV infected leads to an increased risk of changes in fragile chromosomes, which results in the t(8;14) reciprocal translocation, a process that juxtaposes the *mu* gene with the *myc* gene. Such a translocation is found in almost all Burkitt's lymphoma cells but does not occur in human cord blood lymphocytes transformed and immortalized by EBV. An additional integrated event that is presumably an essential step to neoplasia in man is the newly discovered activation of the ChBlym oncogene on chromosome 1.

New Drugs and Combinations for Recurrent Lymphoma

Dr. Cabanillas, for the UT M. D. Anderson Hospital group, reported particularly on the activity of etoposide (VP16), ifosfamide, methyl-GAG (methylglyoxal bisguanylhydrazone), amsacrine (AMSA), and spirogermanium. In patients with refractory disease, VP16 produces a response rate of 21%, methyl-GAG 37%, and ifosfamide, 40%–50%. AMSA and spirogermanium produce response rates in the range of 10%–20%. A combination based on the above was developed for refractory patients that included MIME (methyl-GAG, ifosfamide, methotrexate, and etoposide). Overall response rates in excess of 60% and complete response rates of 30%–40% were achieved. This program is being incorporated into current programs for unfavorable histology non-Hodgkin's lymphomas in an effort to further increase the complete response and the cure rates.

The use of varying techniques in bone marrow transplantation for patients with non-Hodgkin's lymphoma were reviewed by the Minnesota and UT M. D. Anderson Hospital groups. Approaches to "cleaning up" autologous marrow with immunotoxins in the form of ricin and with various monoclonal antibodies, plus rabbit complement, were reviewed. Some degree of in vitro effectiveness was clearly demonstrated, but quantitative in vitro techniques sufficient to predict eradication of such cells are lacking. Interpretation of data to date is difficult because of patient selection problems, particularly in terms of extensive prior treatment, the heterogeneity of non-Hodgkin's lymphoma, the transplantation of overt as compared to microscopic disease, and the need to develop models and approaches to the study of optimal cytoreductive chemotherapy with or without total body radiotherapy.

ADDITIONAL COMMENTS

It is clear from this monograph that the investigation of non-Hodgkin's lymphoma has produced major progress in our understanding of this disease at a fundamental and clinical level, as well as in the treatment of the disease. In addition to some of the aforementioned, I would add the following areas that are under early investigation, and might be expected to have an impact on the non-Hodgkin's lymphomas in the near future.

Oncogene products, including various membrane and cytoskeletal proteins, tyrosine protein kinases, and growth factors are being increasingly identified and may be expected to serve as targets for chemotherapeutic approaches. Analogs of substrates for tyrosine protein kinase have been developed, and antibodies to receptors of growth hormones produced by oncogenes have been prepared. Current hypotheses indicate that a sequence of oncogenes must be activated for the multistep neoplastic process to develop. For at least some forms of cancer, a continuum of increasing neoplastic behavior occurs not only in the preneoplastic period, but also following the development of cancer in the form of clonal evolution. For example, the conversion of chronic myelogenous leukemia to blastic crisis was the first form of clonal evolution identified; similar evolution occurs in the nodular lymphomas as they transit to diffuse lymphoma. The genetic events involved include cytogenetic abnormalities, and could relate to post-neoplastic oncogene activation.

It was emphasized at this meeting that the non-Hodgkin's lymphomas are not fixed in terms of differentiation, and indeed can be induced to some degree of maturation by differentiating agents such as phorbol. The process of differentiation is under intensive study at a molecular level, as well as at an applied level. Methylation of DNA after replication inhibits transcription, and drugs that inhibit DNA methylation, such as azacytidine, at least in some experimental systems, will promote differentiation. Other candidate agents for induction of differentiation are or will be undergoing clinical investigation.

Extraordinary progress has been achieved in the area of molecular biology of drug action and drug resistance. The good news in almost all forms of lymphoma is that we can attain a high rate of initial response. The bad news is that a substantial fraction of patients relapse. A major contribution to this bad news is drug resistance. The prevention or circumvention of drug resistance by molecular and classical pharmacologic techniques in the antimicrobial area has been highly successful, and such approaches are being readied at the laboratory level for the clinic.

Extraordinary advances in our understanding of signaling between mammalian cells in the microenvironment by polypeptide hormones, including the various interleukins, growth factors, and interferons, are under way. The therapeutic implications of these are obvious, and their production by recombinant DNA technology is advancing rapidly.

At a more clinical level, we must become increasingly aware of the implications of the "false-negative" syndrome. For diffuse histiocytic lymphoma, for example, 50%–60% of patients can be cured. However, a substantial proportion of patients who fail, have a short and poor prognosis, and the evaluation of new treatment programs in this setting is difficult. This is becoming an increasing problem, generally, in chemoresponsive tumors. Reliable preclinical modeling systems are needed. At a clinical level, multivariant prognostic factor analysis should be increasingly applied to aid in the interpretation of clinical trials in patients with advanced disease. Novel designs for the evaluation of agents deserve major priority.

Heath Memorial Award Lecture

The Heath Memorial Award

The Heath Memorial Award is presented at the UT M. D. Anderson Hospital Annual Clinical Conference to a clinician for outstanding contributions to the care of patients with cancer. It was established in 1965 by William W. Heath, a former chairman of The University of Texas System Board of Regents, to honor his brothers Guy H., Dan C., and Gilford G. Heath.

This year's recipient of the Heath Memorial Award is Dr. John L. Ziegler, an outstanding clinician who has made numerous outstanding contributions to the understanding and treatment of Burkitt's lymphoma.

John Ziegler graduated from Amherst College in 1960 and received his medical degree from Cornell University Medical College in 1964. After serving his internship and residency at Bellevue Hospital in New York, he joined the National Cancer Institute as a clinical associate.

In 1967, Dr. Ziegler traveled to Uganda under the auspices of NCI and Makerere University in Kampala to help establish the Uganda Cancer Institute. During his five years there, he was involved in the study and implementation of chemotherapeutic treatment of Burkitt's lymphoma. As a result of the regimens established by Dr. Ziegler and his colleagues, the cure rate for Burkitt's lymphoma increased from 20% to more than 50%.

John Ziegler and his team at the Uganda Cancer Institute, in collaboration with researchers from the United States and Sweden, helped establish the etiologic association of the Epstein-Barr virus and African Burkitt's lymphoma. In addition, with Dr. Ian T. Magrath, Dr. Ziegler developed the staging classification for Burkitt's lymphoma that is now used in the United States.

Dr. Ziegler returned to the United States in 1972 to develop a pediatric oncology branch at NCI. During this time, he and his colleagues were among the first to study the use of intensive chemotherapy and autologous bone marrow infusion as treatment for lymphoma. It was effective for patients who suffered relapse and no longer responded to conventional doses of chemotherapeutic agents.

In 1975, Dr. Ziegler was named deputy clinical director of the NCI and later was appointed director of the Clinical Oncology Program in the Division of Cancer Treatment. From 1980 to 1981, he served as editor-in-chief of the prestigious *Journal of the National Cancer Institute*. John Ziegler left NCI in 1981 to assume the responsibilities of associate chief of staff for education at the Veterans Administration Medical Center in San Francisco. In addition to his duties as educator, he continues his study of lymphoma in a National Institutes of Health-sponsored investigation of the acquired immune deficiency syndrome.

UT M.D. Anderson Clinical Conference on Cancer,
Vol. 27, edited by R. J. Ford, L. M. Fuller, and
F. B. Hagemeister. Raven Press, New York © 1984.

Burkitt's Lymphoma: Lessons for the Oncologist

John L. Ziegler

*Veterans Administration Medical Center; and University of California,
San Francisco, California 94143*

The history of Burkitt's lymphoma provides a glimpse at the phenomenal development in our knowledge of malignant lymphomas. Viewed through this small window, I wish to explore the landscape of Burkitt's lymphology over the past 25 years.

I must begin with reflections on the remarkable accomplishments of Sir Denis Burkitt, a British surgeon who started his career in a district hospital in Uganda in the 1940s. His account of "a sarcoma involving the jaws in African children" published in the *British Journal of Surgery* in 1958 alerted the world to the existence of an unusual tumor, later determined by Davies, O'Conor, and Wright (Burkitt 1958) to be an undifferentiated lymphoma. The propensity of the tumor for the jaws and abdomen, but sparing the lymph nodes and bone marrow, were unexpected features. Searching the records of Sir Albert Cook, founder of the Mengo Mission Hospital, Burkitt found similar clinical descriptions as far back as 1910.

His curiosity piqued, Burkitt then sent printed leaflets and a questionnaire to his colleagues in other parts of Africa, only to discover that the tumor was geographically confined. He confirmed this by taking a "tumor safari" with two companions in an old Ford station wagon and a research budget of £25 ($75). This project disclosed a remarkable "tumor belt" with rainfall and altitude limitations. Examining Burkitt's map, Professor Alexander Haddow of the Entebbe Virus Research Institute noted the similarity to yellow fever, and a mosquito-vectored virus was suggested as a possible cause. In the meantime, workers in Kenya, Papua-New Guinea, and West Africa began to report their experiences with Burkitt's lymphoma.

In 1961, a biopsy from a Ugandan patient was sent to Professor M. A. Epstein in Great Britain. Electron microscopic examination of the derived cell line revealed a virus particle, and the discovery of the Epstein-Barr virus (EBV) was announced. The remarkable worldwide collaboration that helped characterize the EBV is another story unto itself, but early discoveries did not fit Burkitt's original hypothesis: the virus was not vectored and was equally prevalent in areas where the tumor was uncommon or rare. Undaunted, Burkitt offered an alternate hypothesis stimulated by suggestions from Dalldorf and O'Conor. He showed that the "lymphoma belt" also coincided with malaria endemism, not only on a world scale, but also in individual countries. The coincidence of EBV and malaria affected millions of African children, however, and yet another factor must account for the ultimate development of the tumor in the population at risk.

Burkitt is also credited with the early discovery of the sensitivity of this lymphoma to chemotherapy. Curative surgery was hopeless in this multicentric, rapidly growing tumor, and Burkitt turned to Dr. Joseph Burchenal for advice. Cyclophosphamide was provided, but because of the rapid patient turnover in the pediatric ward, Burkitt was forced to consolidate the recommended 40 mg/kg into a single dose. The clinical response was incredibly dramatic, and some durable responses were achieved (Figure 1). The dramatic remissions and potential for cure prompted yet another important observation by Burkitt: the immune system has a potential role in the control of tumors.

Sir Denis Burkitt has been recognized with a number of awards for these remarkable accomplishments. With characteristic humility, he credits his many colleagues for "turning a small footpath into a major highway" (Sir Denis Burkitt, personal communication). There are important lessons to be cited from these early discoveries (Table 1), but Burkitt (1983, p. 1785.) states:

> ...unquestionably the most important lesson of all is the enormous importance of good personal relationships and communications between workers.

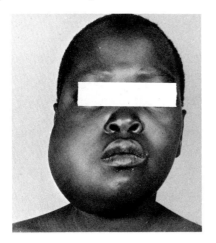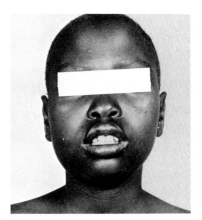

Figure 1.   Dramatic regression of Burkitt's lymphoma of the right mandible in a 10-year-old Ugandan girl before **(left)** and after **(right)** treatment with cyclophosphamide.

Table 1. *Some Lessons Learned—Sir Denis Burkitt*

1. The importance of clinical observation
2. The defects of specialization
3. The role of simple observation followed by deductive reasoning
4. The fallacy that fact finding is directly related to funding

This rather distant vista of Burkitt's lymphoma in the early 1960s fortunately favored the prepared minds of Joseph Burchenal, David Karnofsky, Paul Carbone, Gordon Zubrod, Tom Frei, Emil Freireich, and others who were searching for ways to control cancer with chemotherapy. Some "cures" of acute leukemia and other childhood solid tumors were reported, and the dramatic response of choriocarcinoma began a growing list of tumors that could be cured with drugs. Since Burkitt's lymphoma could be added to this list, the National Cancer Institute sought a collaborative effort with Makerere University in Kampala, Uganda, and in 1967, the Uganda Cancer Institute was born.

The next phase of research in Burkitt's lymphoma moved rapidly and on many fronts—natural history and treatment, immunology and etiology. The hazy outlines in the distant landscape came into sharper focus, and the provocative questions raised by this unusual lymphoma reverberated from East Africa to Stockholm, Philadelphia, Nigeria, New York, London, New Guinea, Bristol, Washington, and Ghana. The skills and discoveries of many specialists—the virologist, chemotherapist, radiotherapist, biologist, immunologist, pathologist, epidemiologist, and statistician—became interwoven into a fascinating and ever-changing tapestry. In the remainder of this paper I shall point out some specific milestones on this terrain and highlight lessons for the modern oncologist.

TREATMENT ADVANCES

Early studies from Africa by Burkitt (1967), Clifford et al. (1967), and Ngu (1968) showed that, in addition to cyclophosphamide, methotrexate, cytarabine, vincristine, and orthomelphelan could produce complete responses. Many patients relapsed, however, and limited follow-up studies disclosed a survival rate of 20%. A strategy was needed to increase the remission rate and prevent relapse. Experience at the Uganda Cancer Institute showed that multiple high doses of cyclophosphamide could induce complete remission in over 90% of the patients, but relapse supervened in over half (Ziegler et al. 1972). Some patients developed cyclophosphamide-resistant tumors during therapy but responded to other agents. Others, with longer remissions, developed tumors at new sites and responded well to the original therapy. Still others relapsed with involvement of the central nervous system, and intrathecal chemotherapy was required (Figure 2). Thus, treatment was adjusted to prevent recurrences by: (1) introduction of cyclic, non–cross-resistant chemotherapy (Ziegler 1972); (2) use of prophylactic intrathecal chemotherapy and neuraxis radiotherapy (Ziegler and Bluming 1971); and (3) development of combination chemotherapy (Olweny et al. 1976). These strategies, combined with improved surveillance, better peritreatment medical management, especially recognition of the acute tumor lysis syndrome (Cohen et al. 1980), and prompt therapy of relapse, raised the overall survival rate to over 50%. These approaches were also applied successfully to American patients with Burkitt's lymphoma and similar cure rates were achieved (Ziegler 1977). Prognosis was directly related to tumor burden and a workable staging system was devised (Magrath et al. 1980).

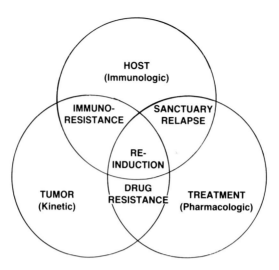

Figure 2. Venn diagram of the mechanisms of relapse in Burkitt's lymphoma based on immunologic, pharmacologic, and kinetic considerations (See text).

In this regard, a dramatic improvement in survival is evident when at least 90% of tumor bulk can be resected surgically.

Cell kinetic studies showed Burkitt's lymphoma to be the fastest growing human tumor; it has a doubling time of 24 hours (Iversen et al. 1974). This growth rate undoubtedly explained the exquisite sensitivity to cytotoxic drugs, the rapid tumor regression, and early emergence of drug-resistant clones. It also explained why conventional radiotherapy was less effective than superfractionated dose schedules (Norin et al. 1971).

The steep dose-response curve for Burkitt's lymphoma led to a successful trial of very high dose cyclophosphamide (the BACT regimen: carmustine, cytosine arabinoside, cyclophosphamide, and thioguanine) (Appelbaum et al. 1978) that required a bone marrow autograft to foreshorten the period of marrow aplasia. Several patients with cyclophosphamide-resistant tumors were cured using this regimen.

Maintenance chemotherapy following complete remission was a therapeutic concept introduced in the management of childhood acute lymphoblastic leukemia and was carried over to the treatment of other tumors. The concept of maintenance is challenged by experience in Burkitt's lymphoma, Hodgkin's disease, and a number of other drug-responsive tumors (Young et al. 1973, Drasga et al. 1982), and it is also shaky on theoretical grounds because of the potential for selection of drug-resistant clones (Skipper et al. 1978). There is little current evidence for prolonged therapy (>6 months) in patients with responsive tumors. The weight of the data persuades therapists to continue treatment for several courses after complete remission is achieved and then to stop therapy.

In summary, Burkitt's lymphoma is a prototypic high growth-fraction tumor that provides a number of treatment lessons (Table 2). These principles have been applied successfully to the treatment of other tumors and confirm many of the predictions made by the experimental chemotherapists who use murine tumor models. We may be approaching the limits of effective chemotherapeutic permutations and combinations in this tumor and must seek additional biologic approaches to successful treatment (Berard et al. 1981).

IMMUNOLOGIC STUDIES

The scope of progress in immunobiology over the past two decades would fill several volumes. For purposes of this discussion, a journey on the research trail of Burkitt's lymphoma reveals some instructive insights and mistakes.

The fortuitous ease with which Burkitt's lymphoma cells could be grown in tissue culture provided a rich opportunity for laboratory observation and experimentation. It soon became apparent that fresh tumor cells were coated with immunoglobulin, some of which eluted with time (IgG) (Klein et al. 1968) and some of which appeared to be synthesized by the cell (IgM) (Fahey et al. 1966). This latter discovery, plus the advent of additional cell markers, allowed full characterization of B-cell lineage and identified Burkitt's lymphoma as a monoclonal outgrowth at an early stage of differentiation (Hansen et al. 1981). Traces of the secreted monoclonal IgM from such tumors have been found in the serum and cerebrospinal fluid (Magrath et al. 1983). Because Burkitt's lymphoma cells retain many of the phenotypic characteristics of their progenitor, it is possible that tumor cells will respond to normal biological control signals, such as suppressor T cells, anti-idiotypic antibody, or various lymphokines. Already there is clinical evidence that such biotherapeutic approaches are feasible and occasionally effective (Miller et al. 1982).

Over the past two decades there was much speculation that tumor-directed immune reactions contribute to origin, regression, and cure of cancer. In the 1970s, Burnet's immunosurveillance hypothesis persuaded many investigators to embark on immunotherapy trials (Burnet 1971). Early work in Burkitt's lymphoma strengthened this notion. Spontaneous regressions, long remissions following min-

Table 2. *Treatment Lessons from Burkitt's Lymphoma*

---

1. Effectiveness of high-dose intermittent therapy
2. Characterization of tumor lysis syndrome
3. Combination therapy better than single agent
4. No need for maintenance therapy
5. Need of sanctuary therapy and prophylaxis
6. Pathogenesis of relapse
7. Prognosis is dependent on tumor burden
8. Effectiveness of surgical debulking
9. Successful rescue therapy for relapse
10. Effectiveness of increased radiation dose fractions

---

imal chemotherapy, improvement following serotherapy, correlation of prognosis with cutaneous anergy to tumor-associated and recall antigens, and serologic evidence of tumor-directed antibody were among the more compelling observations. Burkitt's lymphoma seemed an ideal candidate for immunotherapy.

Since anergy was associated with a poor prognosis and *Bacillus Calmete-Guérin* vaccination (BCG) could significantly improve tumor-associated anergy, we elected to try BCG immunotherapy in patients with Burkitt's lymphoma who were in complete remission after two doses of cyclophosphamide. We reasoned that stimulated, tumor-directed immunocytes might stand a good chance of eliminating residual tumor cells. The results of this study were instructive. First, BCG, as predicted, stimulated an early recovery of the anergic state. Regrettably, remission duration, relapse frequency, and survival were unaffected (Magrath and Ziegler 1976). Of considerable interest was the observation that anergy was a consequence of a large tumor burden and not related causally to the development of relapse (Magrath 1974). In view of a more sophisticated understanding of immunoregulation and the protean effects of BCG, it is hardly surprising that this naive experiment had failed. But new knowledge and new tools now point to other directions in immunotherapy. Some of these involve the removal of immune complexes or suppressor substances that inhibit or block the access of sensitized immunocytes to the tumor. The use of biological immunoregulators, tumor-targeted antibodies armed with cytotoxic agents, or sensitized T lymphocytes grown up in vitro are other possible approaches.

In summary, the laboratory immunology of Burkitt's lymphoma has permitted a closer look at the B cell. The cell literally bristles with receptors that mediate function and immunoregulatory control. Receptor expression has provided a useful tool to demonstrate B-cell lineage and differentiation and discloses the point at which B cells may transform into malignant lymphomas. Clinical immunology of Burkitt's lymphoma showed that cutaneous anergy was related to a large tumor burden, that tumor-associated hypersensitivity could be demonstrated, and that immune reactions may participate in tumor regression.

ETIOLOGY

The discovery of EBV was hailed initially as a long-sought human cancer virus, since, for 30 years, animal viruses were known to cause cancer. Surprisingly, the research trail has led elsewhere. While Burkitt's lymphoma patients (and subsequently, patients with carcinoma of the nasopharynx) had elevated EBV antibody titers, the virus was ubiquitous. In Henle's laboratory, credited with much of the serologic characterization of EBV, a seronegative technician became ill with a classic case of infectious mononucleosis. Her EBV antibody then converted to positive, and the discovery of EBV as a cause for infectious mononucleosis was established. The mononucleosis turned out to be activated suppressor T cells that limit the proliferative B-cell infection. The link to Burkitt's lymphoma still remained circumstantial, however, and even the identification of EBV-DNA in the tumor cell genomes of 90% of the cases, the production by EBV of lymphoproliferative malignancy in primates, and the observation that EBV could immortalize lymphocytes in tissue culture, did not establish a cause-and-effect relationship (Ziegler et al. 1977). A remarkable seroepidemiology survey in the West Nile District of Uganda, wherein children at risk were bled and followed for tumor development, showed elevated EBV antibody titers as long as two years prior to the onset of tumor (de Thé et al. 1978). Even the discovery of strain differences in EBV isolates from West Africans with Burkitt's lymphoma did not shed light on the etiology. Some patients with an x-linked immunodeficiency disorder developed an EBV-related, polyclonal, lymphoproliferative malignancy, presumably as a result of an inherited inability to suppress the virus (Purtilo 1980). Finally, while endemic cases of Burkitt's lymphoma were highly EBV associated, EBV genomes were detected in only 20%–25% of American cases of Burkitt's lymphoma (Ziegler et al. 1976).

While the oncogenic properties of EBV were being pursued, the recent discovery of cellular transforming genes (proto-oncogenes) that are homologous to acute retrovirus *onc* genes directed attention to genomic origins of cancer. Some oncogenes apparently code for a protein kinase with a predilection for phosphorylation of tyrosine or threonine residues (Duesberg 1983). Could this "enemy within" become activated in some way and result in neoplastic transformation? This molecular discovery came on the heels of observations of chromosomal translocations in lymphomas that appeared to be tumor specific but unrelated to EBV (Dalla-Favera et al. 1982). Most recently, the t(8;14), t(8;2), and t(8;22) reciprocal translocations associated with Burkitt's and other lymphomas involve the shift of the *myc* oncogene from chromosome 8 to a new location. Moreover, the translocation is in proximity to the genes coding for IgM (14q), κ light chain (2p), or λ light chain (22q). Thus, a specific oncogene translocation became an additional etiologic factor in Burkitt's lymphoma.

The most recent piece of the puzzle was put in place by the discovery of yet another transforming gene, Blym, unrelated to the *onc* gene, by DNA transfection experiments. Blym may code for a transferrinlike growth factor (Diamond et al. 1983).

These advances in the molecular virology of B-cell transformation now permit an etiologic model that parallels the multistep process in experimental carcinogenesis. Susceptible B cells must be "primed" to a preneoplastic state. In Africa, the high frequency of EBV infection in childhood perhaps aggravated in some way by hyperendemic malaria, initiates the process. Two, probably random, additional steps are then necessary: activation of an *onc* gene (presumably by chromosomal transformation of *myc* to a new site) and activation of a transforming gene Blym. The sequence of the latter genetic changes and the phenotypic consequences of gene rearrangement, mutation, or activation are subjects of ongoing research in many laboratories.

SUMMARY

Burkitt's lymphoma has been a model for understanding the principles of chemotherapy, immunobiology, and viral oncology. In exploring this model, we have travelled from the vistas of East Africa through laboratories around the world, examining this unusual tumor through binoculars at the bedside, under the microscope, and ultimately by molecular dissection. It is worth a final look at the lessons Burkitt outlined (Table 1). It will always be in the province of the clinician to pose problems to the laboratory investigator. Most major medical advances in this century began with simple clinical observations, and, despite our impressive technology, this fundamental lesson will prevail for centuries to come. By defects of specialization, Burkitt implies that tunnel vision will not allow investigators to make connections between events or phenomena. He is actually referring to one of the major breakthroughs in cancer research over the past two decades—the interdependence of multiple disciplines. The specialist tends to be myopic and will miss the unexpected and provocative connections that are more apparent to the generalist, who uses simple observation and deductive reasoning as his main tools. Finally, Burkitt warns that research funding and good ideas are not necessarily related. Many a Nobel prize has been awarded to investigators whose only laboratories were their surroundings and whose only tools were their brains.

REFERENCES

Appelbaum FR, Deisseroth AB, Graw RG Jr, Herzig GP, Levine AS, Magrath IT, Pizzo PA, Poplack DG, Ziegler JL. 1978. Prolonged complete remission following high dose chemotherapy of Burkitt's lymphoma in relapse. Cancer 41:1059–1063.

Berard CW, Greene MK, Jaffe ES, Magrath I, Ziegler J. 1981. A multidisciplinary approach to understanding non-Hodgkin's lymphomas. Ann Intern Med 94:218–235.

Burkitt DP. 1958. A sarcoma involving the jaws of African children. Br J Surg 46:218–223.

Burkitt DP. 1967. Long-term remissions following one and two-dose chemotherapy for African lymphoma. Cancer 20:756–759.

Burkitt DP. 1983. The discovery of Burkitt's lymphoma. Cancer 51:1777–1786.

Burnet FM. 1971. Immunological surveillance in neoplasia. Transplant Rev 7:3–25.

Clifford P, Singh S, Stjernsward J, Klein G. 1967. Long-term survival of patients with Burkitt's lymphoma: an assessment of treatment and other factors which may relate to survival. Cancer Res 27:2578–2615.

Cohen LF, Balow JE, Magrath IT, Poplack DG, Ziegler JL. 1980. Acute tumor lysis syndrome: a review of 37 patients with Burkitt's lymphoma. Am J Med 68:486–491.

Dalla-Favera R, Bregni M, Erikson J, Patterson D, Gallo RC, Croce CM. 1982. Human C-myc onc gene is located on the region of chromosome 8 that is translocated in Burkitt lymphoma cells. Proc Natl Acad Sci USA 79:7824–7827.

de Thé G, Geser A, Day NE, Tukei PM, Williams EH, Peri DP, Smith PG, Dean AG, Bornkamm GW, Feorina P, Henle W. 1978. Epidemiological evidence for causal relationship between Epstein-Barr virus and Burkitt's lymphoma from Ugandan prospective study. Nature 274:756–761.

Diamond A, Cooper GM, Ritz J, Lane M. 1983. Identification and molecular cloning of the human Blym transforming gene activated in Burkitt's lymphoma. Nature 305:112–116.

Drasga RE, Einhorn LH, Williams SO. 1982. The chemotherapy of testicular cancer. CA 32:66–91.

Duesberg PH. 1983. Retroviral transforming genes in normal cells. Nature 304:219–226.

Fahey JL, Rinegold J, Rabson AS, Manaker RA. 1966. Immunoglobulin synthesis in vitro by established human cell lines. Science 452:1259–1261.

Hansen H, Koziner B, Clarkson B. 1981. Marker and kinetic studies in the non-Hodgkin's lymphomas. Am J Med 71:107–123.

Iversen OH, Iversen U, Ziegler JL, Bluming AZ. 1974. Cell kinetics in Burkitt's lymphoma. Eur J Cancer 10:155–163.

Klein E, Klein G, Nadkarni JJ, Nadkarni JS, Wigzell H, Clifford P. 1968. Surface IgM-Kappa specificity on a Burkitt lymphoma cell in vivo and in derived cultured lines. Cancer Res 28:1300–1310.

Magrath I, Lee YJ, Anderson T, Henle W, Ziegler JL, Simon R, Schein P. 1980. Prognostic factors in Burkitt's lymphoma: importance of total tumor burden. Cancer 45:1507–1515.

Magrath IT. 1974. Immunosuppression in Burkitt's lymphoma. I. Cutaneous reactivity to recall antigens: alterations induced by a tumour burden and by BCG administration. Int J Cancer 13:839–849.

Magrath IT, Benjamin D, Papadopoulos N. 1983. Serum monoclonal immunoglobulin bands in undifferentiated lymphomas of Burkitt and non-Burkitt types. Blood 61:726–731.

Magrath IT, Ziegler JL. 1976. Failure of BCG immunostimulation to affect the clinical course of Burkitt's lymphoma. Br Med J 1:615–618.

Miller RA, Maloney DG, Warnke R, Levy R. 1982. Treatment of B cell lymphoma with monoclonal anti-idiotype antibody. N Engl J Med 306:517–522.

Ngu VA. 1968. The treatment of Burkitt tumour. West African Medical Journal 17:273–277.

Norin T, Clifford P, Einhorn J, Einhorn N, Hohansson B, Klein G, Onyango J, DeSchryver A, Walstam R. 1971. Conventional and superfractionated radiation therapy in Burkitt's lymphoma. Acta Radiol [Oncol] 10:545–557.

Olweny CLM, Katongole-Mbidde E, Kaddu-Mukasa A, Atine I, Owor R, Lwanga S, Carswell W, Magrath IT. 1976. Treatment of Burkitt's lymphoma: randomized clinical trial of single agent versus combination chemotherapy. Int J Cancer 17:436–440.

Purtilo DT. 1980. Epstein-Barr virus-induced oncogenesis in immune-deficient individuals. Lancet 1:300–303.

Skipper HE, Schabel FM, Lloyd HH. 1978. Experimental therapeutics and kinetics: selection and overgrowth of specifically and permanently drug-resistant tumor cells. Semin Hematol 15:207–219.

Young RC, Canellos GP, Chabner BA, Schein PS, DeVita VT. 1973. Maintenance chemotherapy for advanced Hodgkin's disease in remission. Lancet 1:1339–1343.

Ziegler JL. 1972. Chemotherapy of Burkitt's lymphoma. Cancer 30:1534–1540.

Ziegler JL. 1977. Treatment results of 54 American patients with Burkitt's lymphoma are similar to the African experience. N Engl J Med 297:75–80.

Ziegler JL, Andersson M, Klein G, Henle W. 1976. Detection of Epstein-Barr virus DNA in American Burkitt's lymphoma. Int J Cancer 17:701–706.

Ziegler JL, Bluming AZ. 1971. Intrathecal chemotherapy in Burkitt's lymphoma. Br Med J 3:508–512.

Ziegler JL, Bluming AZ, Fass L., Morrow RH Jr. 1972. Relapse patterns in Burkitt's lymphoma. Cancer Res 32:1267–1272.

Ziegler JL, Magrath IT, Gerber P, Levine PH. 1977. Epstein-Barr virus and human malignancy. Ann Intern Med 86:323–336.

The Jeffrey A. Gottlieb Memorial Lecture

The Jeffrey A. Gottlieb Memorial Award

Edmund A. Gehan, Ph.D., the 1983 Jeffrey A. Gottlieb Memorial Award recipient, has had an important influence on cancer research through his expertise in design, analysis, and interpretation of clinical trials.

Dr. Gehan has served as chief of the Section of Biometrics in the Department of Biomathematics at UT M. D. Anderson Hospital and Tumor Institute since 1967. During his tenure, he has collaborated with clinicians on the statistical aspects of clinical trials and has been an important consultant on the controversial aspects of historical control studies. Determining prognostic factors is an important aspect of clinical trials, especially when historical controls are used. Dr. Gehan has made major contributions in this area of research and has developed techniques for adjusting for prognostic factors.

Before coming to UT M. D. Anderson Hospital, Edmund Gehan served as head of the Biometrics Section at the Cancer Chemotherapy National Service Center at the National Cancer Institute. He developed a statistical design for Phase II drug trials to determine how many patients must receive a drug before testing is continued or discontinued.

Dr. Gehan's international reputation was established early in the 1960s while he was a special fellow of the NCI at Birkbeck College of the University of London. At that time, he developed a test that allowed statistical comparisons between two treatment regimens when the end point for analysis was a measure of time. This method of analysis is commonly called the Gehan modification of the generalized Wilcoxon test.

Dr. Gehan received his doctorate in experimental statistics and public health from North Carolina State University in 1957. Even before completing this degree, he was awarded a fellowship in biostatistics from the United States Public Health Service and taught biostatistics at the University of North Carolina. He received his undergraduate degree in mathematics from Manhattan College.

The Jeffrey A. Gottlieb Memorial Award is given each year to recognize significant contributions to cancer therapy research. It was established by the friends and colleagues of Dr. Gottlieb who wanted to honor scientists who exemplified his spirit and dedication. Jeffrey Gottlieb was a respected leader in chemotherapy research with a special devotion to his patients.

Clearly, Dr. Gehan shared the dedication to solving the mystery of cancer with his close colleague, Dr. Gottlieb. Together, they designed and executed clinical trials that benefited and will continue to benefit patients with the disease.

UT M.D. Anderson Clinical Conference on Cancer,
Vol. 27, edited by R.J. Ford, L.M. Fuller, and
F.B. Hagemeister. Raven Press, New York © 1984.

Prognostic Factors in Clinical Studies: Examples from Acute Leukemia and Non-Hodgkin's Lymphoma

Edmund A. Gehan

*The University of Texas M.D. Anderson Hospital and Tumor Institute at Houston,
Department of Biomathematics, Houston, Texas 77030*

The objective of this chapter is to discuss the importance of knowing prognostic factors in clinical trials and to give some examples from studies in acute leukemia and non-Hodgkin's lymphoma. Statistical methodology for identifying and utilizing prognostic factors has been reviewed by Armitage and Gehan (1974).

First, the rationale will be reviewed for determining prognostic factors in clinical studies. Secondly, it will be demonstrated how prognostic factors can be used in the planning and analysis of clinical studies. Thirdly, the statistical methodology for determining and utilizing prognostic factors will be outlined briefly, and fourthly, some examples will be given from cancer clinical trials.

The word prognosis is derived from two Greek words that when combined mean "to know before." In a medical context, the word means the prediction of the duration, course, and outcome of disease for individual patients or groups of patients.

In making predictions, a doctor may rely on his accumulated experience or on the summaries of existing knowledge provided in recent scientific papers or textbooks. Observations on individual patients, however thorough, can give very little guidance about the prognosis for a future population of patients. Only by observing how the course of disease varies among groups of patients with different initial characteristics can one assess the merits of any potential prognostic variable.

REASONS FOR DETERMINING PROGNOSTIC FACTORS

From a general viewpoint, all clinicians who have treated patients with cancer, or any other disease, are aware that patients are quite heterogeneous. The identification and quantification of prognostic factors is an attempt to explain as much of this variability among patients as possible.

First, knowledge of prognostic features may provide insight into the mechanism of disease by revealing which of a number of variables influence the course and outcome of the disease. These variables may be used in constructing mathematical models that give predictions of probability of response, length of response, or survival.

Secondly, knowledge of prognostic characteristics may be used in the planning of clinical studies. For example, in non-Hodgkin's lymphoma, histology and stage are important patient characteristics related to chance of response. In a study designed to compare two treatments, patients could be stratified by these characteristics prior to allocation of treatment. Randomizing patients to treatments within each stratum would assure that patients on the two treatment regimens were comparable in prognosis and number. Also, treatments have been allocated to individual patients based upon mathematical models giving a prediction of the probability of response. An example of this will be given in acute leukemia.

Thirdly, knowledge of prognostic factors facilitates comparisons of treatments in randomized and nonrandomized clinical trials. There are three main reasons for allowing for prognostic factors in the analysis. When patients are randomized, there may still be certain differences among treatment groups in the distribution of prognostic variables. It is relevant to adjust treatment comparisons for important imbalances in prognostic factors, even when the imbalance itself may not be statistically significant. If the prognostic variables have a high correlation with the outcome, much of the random variation in response can be explained by prognostic features. Using a statistical adjustment procedure, the residual random variation can thereby be reduced and comparisons between treatments made correspondingly more precise. Interactions between treatments and prognostic variables may be detected, that is any tendency for the relative merits of the treatments to differ according to the prognostic variables. This is especially helpful when we desire to find the best treatment for each prognostic subgroup of patients.

Adjustment for prognostic factors is of particular importance in nonrandomized studies when two treatment regimens are being compared. The outstanding criticism of such studies is that patients may not be comparable between those in the current study and those in the historical group. The validity of such a study depends in an important way upon having knowledge of the prognostic factors and utilizing this knowledge in adjusting treatment comparisons.

Finally, knowledge of prognostic features may suggest remedial action. For example, if low serum calcium levels are related to poor prognosis, steps may be taken to raise the serum calcium levels prior to the start of treatment.

Prognostic variables may be determined from controlled clinical trials, observational studies, or retrospective studies. One should be aware that prognostic variables may change from one study to another and that a variable that has a high prognostic value in one study may have little value in a subsequent study. We know that selecting prognostic variables from within a study tends to exaggerate their importance, resulting in overoptimistic estimates of the precision of treatment comparisons. Consequently, it is important to confirm the relative importance of prognostic factors in several different studies.

A final, general point is that prognostic variables should not themselves be influenced by treatment. Otherwise, in correcting for differences in prognostic variables, one may remove some of the treatment effects.

STATISTICAL METHODS FOR PROGNOSTIC FACTORS STUDIES

The steps that can be identified in developing statistical regression models utilizing prognostic features are: univariate analyses, multivariate analyses, tests of regression models, tests for additional variables in models, and evolution of regression models.

Univariate Analyses

Usually, in a clinical trial, the number of possible variables is very large, too large for presentation of a compact summary of the data that reveals the important relationships. Consequently, the first step should be univariate analyses in which response rates, lengths of response, and survival rate are compared within groupings of patients that constitute possible subgroups. For example, if platelet count is considered as a possible prognostic feature, patients can be grouped by increasing levels of platelet count and prognoses compared among subgroups. This is an exploratory phase of the analysis in which the emphasis should not be so much on statistical significance tests as on assessments of the magnitude of the possible relationship to prognosis. A variable whose effect is not statistically significant might be retained on the grounds that evidence from other studies indicated that it was useful. Conversely, a variable might be rejected that has a statistically significant effect, if this effect is likely to be small.

Multivariate Analyses

The second stage of analysis should use regression models to relate the probability of complete remission or survival time to patient characteristics. A logistic regression model should be used to relate the probability of response to prognostic factors, and the form of the model is as follows:

$$\log\left\{\frac{p_i}{1 - p_i}\right\} = a_o + a_1 (x_{1i} - \bar{x}_1) + \ldots + a_k (x_{ki} - \bar{x}_k)$$

where p_i is the probability of response for the ith patient, the a's are regression coefficients to be estimated, the x's are patient characteristics possibly related to response, and the $\bar{x}$'s are the mean values of each patient characteristic. The model can be fit in step-wise fashion so that the first variable included is the one that gives the best prediction of probability of response; the second is the variable that, when added to the first, gives the best pair of variables for predicting response, and so on. The theory for fitting this model to experimental data was outlined in Cox (1970). A computer program for fitting the model in step-wise fashion was given by Lee (1974).

For finding patient characteristics related to disease-free intervals or survival time, Cox's regression model (1972) has been used. The form of the model is as follows:

$$\log\left\{\frac{\lambda_i(t)}{\lambda_o(t)}\right\} = b_1 (x_{1i} - \bar{x}_1) + \ldots + b_k (x_{ki} - \bar{x}_k)$$

where $\lambda_i(t)$ is the hazard function (or roughly the risk of failure per unit time) at time t for the ith individual, the b's are regression coefficients fitted in the model, the x's are patient characteristics, and the $\bar{x}$'s are mean values. The model can be fit in step-wise fashion so that the only x variables included in the analysis are those related to disease-free interval or survival. The theory for this model is outlined in Cox (1972).

Tests of Regression Models

Once a regression model has been fitted, it should be tested, both by application to the same data from which it was derived and to some data obtained prospectively. If a large enough set of data is available, it should be possible to utilize a jackknife-type procedure, i.e., to use the first half of the data for determining the appropriate model and the second half for testing it. Emphasis should be on finding prognostic factors that are consistently important in their relationship to endpoint.

Tests for Additional Variables in Models

Suppose we desire to test whether a new feature, say an immunological test or a lymphocyte surface marker, relates to probability of complete remission. If a logistic model is available with k variables, then it is possible to fit a logistic regression model for $k + 1$ variables and use a chi-square test to determine whether the additional variation explained is statistically significant. In this situation, the form of the model is as follows:

$$\log \left\{ \frac{p_i}{1 - p_i} \right\} = a_o + a_1(x_{1i} - \bar{x}_1) + \ldots + a_k(x_{ki} - \bar{x}_k) + a_{k+1}(x_{k+1,i} - \bar{x}_{k+1})$$

where x_{k+1} represents the new patient characteristic with the possible code $x_{k+1} = 0$ for patients with no lymphocyte surface marker and $x_{k+1} = 1$ for patients having the marker. A test of significance of treatment effect is simply whether the regression coefficient for type of treatment (a_{k+1}) is zero or not. This tests whether knowledge of the new patient characteristic adds to the predictability of response in addition to the other prognostic factors.

Further considerations in deciding whether to add a variable are: extent to which a confidence interval for predicted probability would become more narrow with the addition of the variable, the ease of determining the prognostic factor, the cost, and the possibility of transferring results of this model to other cancer centers. Regression models can evolve in this manner through addition or subtraction of variables related to prognosis.

EXAMPLE OF CLINICAL TRIAL IN ACUTE LEUKEMIA

An example of a clinical trial in acute leukemia conducted at the UT M. D. Anderson Hospital (protocol DT7995) is given to illustrate the use of prognostic factors in the planning and conducting of the study. The overall objective of the study is to evaluate new strategies of treatment for previously untreated patients so that benefit/risk ratios are maximized at defined time points during the patient's course of disease. Both at the beginning of remission induction and maintenance stages, statistical regression models were utilized to separate patients into prognostically favorable and unfavorable subgroups. The strategy was to administer innovative treatments to patients with unfavorable prognoses (either for induction of remission or length of remission), while administering more conventional treatments to patients with favorable prognoses. The ethical argument was that a patient expected to have an unfavorable prognosis after the administration of standard therapies would not be compromised by the administration of innovative treatments. As promising treatments are identified in patients with unfavorable prognoses, they will be administered to patients with favorable prognoses.

A logistic regression model was derived from a study of 325 previously untreated patients with acute leukemia, all of whom received a combination of doxorubicin and OAP (vincristine, arabinosyl cytosine, and prednisone) treatment between 1973 and 1977. More than 20 possible prognostic factors were considered for their relationship to probability of complete remission, length of complete remission, and survival. The final form of the regression model was as follows:

$$\log \left\{ \frac{p_i}{1 - p_i} \right\} = .495 - .744 \,(\text{Age} - 2.54) - 1.680 \,(\text{AHD} - .19)$$
$$- 1.109 \,(\text{Temp} - 1.34) - 1.031 \,(\text{BUN} - 1.12)$$
$$+ 1.039 \,(\text{Hgb} - 1.11) - 1.297 \,(\text{liver size} - .05)$$

where p_i = probability of complete remission for the ith patient. Age: 1 = less than 20 yrs, 2 = 20-49, 3 = 50-64, 4 = ⩾65. Antecedent hematological disorder: 0 = no, 1 = yes. Temperature: 1 = less than 101°F, 2 = greater than or equal to 101°F. BUN: 1 = less than 12 g/dl, 2 = greater than or equal to 12 g/dl. Liver: 0 = not enlarged, 1 = enlarged > 5 cm.

This logistic regression model was tested in two ways, firstly by fitting it to the data from which it was derived, and secondly, by fitting it to data from 107 patients studied prospectively (Keating et al. 1982, Smith et al. 1982). Observed complete remission rates were in close accord with the predicted probabilities of complete remission as obtained from the model.

In the clinical trial in acute leukemia (DT7995), patients were allocated to remission-induction treatment based upon the predicted probabilities of complete remission. When the predicted probability of complete remission was < .6, that is, when patients had a relatively low chance of responding to the standard remission induction treatment, patients received AMSA-OAP (amsacrine plus OAP) treatment in a protected environment, if one was available. When the predicted probability of complete remission was ⩾ .6, patients received Ad-OAP (doxorubicin plus OAP) as remission-induction treatment. The treatment of patients in the remission maintenance phase was also based upon logistic regression models; however details will not be given here. This clinical trial was closed to patient entry during 1983, and a final analysis of the data is underway. Preliminary analyses suggest that unfavorable-prognosis patients who received AMSA-OAP had a complete remission rate that was 10%–15% higher and a longer survival time than comparable patients who received Ad-OAP in 1973–1977.

EXAMPLE IN NON-HODGKIN'S LYMPHOMA

Since this conference has considered various aspects of the treatment of lymphoma patients, it seemed relevant to include an example of a prognostic factors study in non-Hodgkin's lymphoma. The objective is to determine patient characteristics related to survival of non-Hodgkin's lymphoma patients.

Table 1 gives a list of patient characteristics related to survival that was derived from a review of recent papers by Cabanillas et al. (1978,1983, Cabanillas 1983), Bartolucci et al. (1977), Bloomfield et al. (1977), and McKelvey et al. (1976). The prognostic features have been divided into three groups: tumor characteristics, host characteristics, and factors related to the effect of the tumor on the host.

Perhaps the prognostic feature receiving the most emphasis in the literature is the pathological characteristics of the tumor. Patients with nodular poorly differentiated lymphocytic tumors have more favorable prognoses than patients with tumors of other cell types. Patients with diffuse well-differentiated lymphocytic disease have more favorable prognoses than patients with other diffuse subtypes. Recently, a new pathological classification (Cabanillas 1983) has been used to

Table 1. *Prognostic Characteristics for Survival*
of Non-Hodgkin's Lymphoma Patients

Tumor characteristics
    Cell architecture (nodular vs diffuse)
    Cell type
        Nodular (PDL vs others)
        Diffuse (WDL vs others)
    Lymphocyte surface markers (B-cell vs others)
Host characteristics
    Age (young vs older)
    Sex (female vs male)
Effect of Tumor on Host
    Stage (III vs IV)
    Symptoms (none vs some)
    Performance status (active vs less active)
    Hemoglobin (high vs lower)
    Tumor bulkiness (nonbulky vs bulky)
    LDH (low vs higher)
    Prior treatment (none vs some)

PDL–poorly differentiated lymphocytic; WDL–well differentiated lymphocytic
The first word in the parentheses following each prognostic feature gives that value indicating a more favorable prognosis. For example, patients with nodular disease have more favorable prognoses for surviving than patients having diffuse disease.

divide patients into three major groupings according to the clinical grade: low, intermediate, or high. This classification has a significant relationship to survival rate; patients with low grade tumors have the best prognoses.

Table 2 gives some relevant data concerning two large non-Hodgkin's lymphoma studies conducted recently by the Southwest Oncology Group. In both studies, the patient populations consisted of all patients eligible for the study who had stages III or IV disease and no prior treatment. The CHOP (cyclophosphamide, doxorubicin, vincristine, and prednisone) vs HOP (CHOP minus cyclophosphamide) study was conducted from 1972–1974, and the results were reported by McKelvey et al. (1976). The second study, reported by Jones et al. (1983), utilized variations of the CHOP and COP (cyclophosphamide, vincristine, and prednisone) regimens of treatment. The objectives of the prognostic factors analysis were twofold, to identify prognostic features of the patients that were consistently related to survival time from the start of treatment and to perform a multivariate analysis to determine the combination of patient features that was best related to survival.

Table 3 summarizes the univariate analyses that were carried out relating each individual prognostic feature to survival time in the two studies. Surface marker data were not available for the two studies and have not been investigated. The relationship of patient characteristics to survival was reasonably consistent; all the tumor and host characteristics were significantly related to survival in both studies.

Table 4 gives the combination of patient variables that were related to survival after carrying out multivariate Cox regression analyses of the two studies. In the CHOP versus HOP study, cell architecture (nodular vs diffuse) and performance status were the only two patient characteristics entering the model at a highly statistically significant level $(P<.01)$. When the CHOP + BCG (CHOP plus *Bacillus Calmete Guérin*) study reported by Jones et al. (1983) was analyzed, cell architecture and performance status were the first two variables entering the model. However, sex, age, cell grade, mediastinal involvement, and stage were also highly statistically significantly related to survival.

The number of patients was over 450 in the Jones et al. (1983) study, whereas there were less than 300 patients in the study reported by McKelvey et al. (1976).

Table 2. *Non-Hodgkin's Lymphoma Studies**

	CHOP vs. HOP McKelvey et al. (1976)	CHOP + BCG vs. CHOP + BLEO vs. COP + BLEO Jones, et al. (1983)
Period of study	1972–1974	1974–1977
Total patients	506	652
Study population	323	520
Median follow-up time	444 wks	322 wks

*Study population: All eligible patients with stage III or IV disease and no prior treatment.

Table 3. *Patient Characteristics Related to Survival Based on Univariate Analyses of Survival in Two Non-Hodgkin's Lymphoma Studies*

	Studies	
Patient characteristics	CHOP vs. HOP (McKelvey 1976)	CHOP + BCG (Jones et al. 1983)
Cell architecture	**	**
Cell type		
Nodular	**	**
Diffuse	**	**
Age	*	**
Sex	*	**
Stage	**	**
Symptoms	**	**
Performance status	**	**
Liver biopsy	*	
Marrow biopsy		
Splenectomy	*	
Mediastinal involvement		
Nodal sites		
Hemoglobin		
Absolute lymphocyte count	**	**
Platelet count		

Two asterisks indicate a patient feature that was highly statistically significant ($P = .01$), one asterisk means that the variable was moderately strongly related to survival ($P = .05$), and no asterisk indicated that the patient feature was unrelated to survival. (See text for components of chemotherapeutic regimens.)

Table 4. *Values of Statistically Significant Regression Coefficients From Cox Regression Analyses of Two Non-Hodgkin's Lymphoma Studies*

	Studies		
Patient characteristics	CHOP vs. HOP (McKelvey 1976)	CHOP + BCG (Jones et al. 1983)	Favorable features
Cell architecture	−.9706	−.4168	Nodular
Performance status	+.4306	+.2702	Active
Sex		−.6446	Female
Age		+.3513	Young
Cell grade		+.6658	Low
Mediastinal involvement		−.5468	None
Stage		+.4042	III

(See text for components of chemotherapeutic regimens.)

It is possible that more variables were related to survival in the Jones et al. study because of the much larger number of patients.

It is well known that there is a high correlation between nodular versus diffuse tumors and low versus intermediate- to high-grade tumors. In the Jones et al. study

(1983), 89% of the nodular tumors were low grade, and 78% of the diffuse tumors were intermediate or high grade. This suggests that another multivariate analysis with low versus intermediate- to high-grade tumors as the first variable and performance status as the second would provide almost as good a fit to the data as cell architecture and performance status. Though details are not given here, this suggestion was confirmed by actually carrying out the analyses.

No new prognostic features related to survival time have been discovered by these analyses. Rather, patient characteristics identified in previous studies as prognostic have been confirmed, and it is strongly suggested that pathological characteristics and performance status are the two major patient characteristics related to survival.

ACKNOWLEDGMENT

I wish to thank the following individuals for their assistance in the preparation of this manuscript: Eugene McKelvey, Terry Smith, Dennis Dixon, Emil Freireich, Fernando Cabanillas, and Michael Keating.

This investigation was supported by grants CA-12014, CA-30138, and CA-28153 awarded by the National Cancer Institute, United States Department of Health and Human Services.

REFERENCES

Armitage P, Gehan EA. 1974. Statistical methods for the identification and use of prognostic factors. Int J Cancer 13:16–36.

Bartolucci A, Durant JR, Gams RA. 1977. Prognostic factors in non-Hodgkin's lymphoma. (Abstract) Proceedings of the American Society of Clinical Oncology 18:152.

Bloomfield CD, Kersey JH, Brunning RD, Gajl-Peczalska KJ. 1977. Prognostic significance of lymphocytic surface markers and histology in adult non-Hodgkin's lymphoma. Cancer Treat Rep 61:963–970.

Cabanillas F, Burke JS, Smith TL, Moon TE, Butler JJ, Rodriguez V. 1978. Factors predicting for response and survival in adults with advanced non-Hodgkin's lymphoma. Arch Intern Med 138:413–418.

Cabanillas F. 1983. Evolution of new combination chemotherapeutic regimens for malignant lymphomas. The U. T. M. D. Anderson Hospital Experience. The Cancer Bulletin 35:7–10.

Cabanillas F, Smith TL, Bodey GP, Gutterman JU, Freireich EJ. 1983. Nodular malignant lymphomas. Factors affecting complete response rate and survival. Cancer 44:1983–1989.

Cox DR. 1970. Analysis of Binary Data. Methuen and Co. London, pp. 87–91.

Cox DR. 1972. Regression models and life tables. Journal of the Royal Statistical Society 34:187–202.

Jones SE, Grozea PN, Metz EN, Haut A, Stephens R, Morrison FS, Talley R, Butler J, Byrne G, Hartsock R, Dixon D, Salmon S. 1983. Improved complete remission rates and survival for patients with large cell lymphoma treated with chemoimmunotherapy, Cancer 51:1083–1090.

Keating M, Smith TL, Gehan EA, McCredie KB, Bodey GP, Freireich EJ. 1982. A prognostic factor analysis for use in development of predictive models for response in adult acute leukemia, Cancer 50:457–465.

Lee ET. 1974. A computer program for linear logistic regression analysis. Computer Programs in Biomedicine 4:80–82.

McKelvey M, Gottlieb JA, Wilson HE, Haut A, Talley R, Stephens R, Lane M, Gamble J, Jones SE, Grozea P, Gutterman J, Coltman C, Moon TE. 1976. Hydroxyldaunomycin (Adriamycin) combination chemotherapy in malignant lymphoma, Cancer 38:1484–1493.

Smith TL, Gehan EA, Keating MJ, Freireich EJ. 1982. Prediction of remission in adult acute leukemia. Development and testing of predictive models. Cancer 50:466–474.

Author Index

Subject Index